Multidisciplinary Management of Gastric Neoplasms

Editors

KELLY L. OLINO
DOUGLAS S. TYLER

SURGICAL CLINICS
OF NORTH AMERICA

www.surgical.theclinics.com

Consulting Editor
RONALD F. MARTIN

April 2017 • Volume 97 • Number 2

ELSEVIER

1600 John F. Kennedy Boulevard • Suite 1800 • Philadelphia, Pennsylvania, 19103-2899

http://www.surgical.theclinics.com

SURGICAL CLINICS OF NORTH AMERICA Volume 97, Number 2
April 2017 ISSN 0039–6109, ISBN-13: 978-0-323-52433-9

Editor: John Vassallo, j.vassallo@elsevier.com
Developmental Editor: Colleen Dietzler

Surgical Clinics of North America (ISSN 0039–6109) is published bimonthly by Elsevier Inc., 360 Park Avenue South, New York, NY 10010-1710. Months of publication are February, April, June, August, October, and December. Business and Editorial Offices: 1600 John F. Kennedy Blvd., Suite 1800, Philadelphia, PA 19103-2899. Periodicals postage paid at New York, NY and additional mailing offices. Subscription prices are $386.00 per year for US individuals, $756.00 per year for US institutions, $100.00 per year for US students and residents, $469.00 per year for Canadian individuals, $958.00 per year for Canadian institutions, $525.00 for international individuals, $958.00 per year for international institutions and $250.00 per year for Canadian and foreign students/residents. To receive student/resident rate, orders must be accompanied by name of affiliated institution, date of term, and the signature of program/residency coordinator on institution letterhead. Orders will be billed at individual rate until proof of status is received. Foreign air speed delivery is included in all Clinics subscription prices. All prices are subject to change without notice. POSTMASTER: Send address changes to Surgical Clinics, Elsevier Health Sciences Division, Subscription Customer Service, 3251 Riverport Lane, Maryland Heights, MO 63043. **Customer Service (orders, claims, online, change of address): Telephone: 1-800-654-2452 (U.S. and Canada); 314-447-8871 (outside U.S. and Canada). Fax: 314-447-8029. E-mail: journalscustomerservice-usa@elsevier.com (for print support); journalsonline support-usa@elsevier.com (for online support).**

Reprints. For copies of 100 or more, of articles in this publication, please contact the Commercial Reprints Department, Elsevier Inc., 360 Park Avenue South, New York, New York 10010-1710. Tel. 212-633-3874, Fax: 212-633-3820, E-mail: reprints@elsevier.com.

The Surgical Clinics of North America is also published in Spanish by McGraw-Hill Interamericana Editores S.A., P.O. Box 5-237 06500 Mexico D.F. Mexico; and in Portuguese by Interlivros Edicoes Ltda., Rua Comandante Coelho 1085, CEP 21250, Rio de Janeiro, Brazil; and in Greek by Paschalidis Medical Publications, Athens Greece.

The Surgical Clinics of North America is covered in MEDLINE/PubMed (Index Medicus), EMBASE/Excerpta Medica, Current Contents/Clinical Medicine, Current Contents/Life Sciences, Science Citation Index, and ISI/BIOMED.

Contributors

CONSULTING EDITOR

RONALD F. MARTIN, MD, FACS
Colonel (ret.), United States Army Reserve, York Hospital, York, Maine

EDITORS

KELLY L. OLINO, MD
Assistant Professor of Surgery, University of Texas Medical Branch, Galveston, Texas

DOUGLAS S. TYLER, MD
John Woods Harris Distinguished Chair in Surgery, Professor and Chairman, Department of Surgery, University of Texas Medical Branch, Galveston, Texas

AUTHORS

SEIICHIRO ABE, MD
Endoscopy Division, National Cancer Center Hospital, Tokyo, Japan

BRIAN D. BADGWELL, MD, MS
Department of Surgical Oncology, The University of Texas MD Anderson Cancer Center, Houston, Texas

MICHAEL R. CASSIDY, MD
Department of Surgery, Memorial Sloan Kettering Cancer Center, New York, New York

HERBERT CHEN, MD, FACS
Chairman and Professor, Department of Surgery; Surgeon-in-Chief, UAB Hospital and Health System; Senior Advisor, UAB Comprehensive Cancer Center, Fay Fletcher Kerner Endowed Chair, University of Alabama at Birmingham, Birmingham, Alabama

BRITNEY COREY, MD
Assistant Professor, Department of Surgery, University of Alabama at Birmingham and Birmingham Veteran's Affairs Medical Center, Birmingham, Alabama

JEREMY L. DAVIS, MD
Center for Cancer Research, National Cancer Institute, NIH, Bethesda, Maryland

RYAN C. FIELDS, MD
Assistant Professor of Hepatobiliary, Pancreatic, Gastrointestinal, and Oncologic Surgery, Department of Surgery, Barnes-Jewish Hospital and Washington University School of Medicine, St Louis, Missouri

SEPIDEH GHOLAMI, MD
Department of Surgery, Memorial Sloan Kettering Cancer Center, New York, New York

GUILLERMO GOMEZ, MD
Granville T. Hall Chair and Professor of Surgery, General Surgery, The University of Texas Medical Branch, Galveston, Texas

MASAHARU HIGASHIDA, MD, PhD
Associate Professor, Department of Digestive Surgery, Kawasaki Medical School, Kurashiki, Okayama, Japan

MICHIHISA IIDA, MD, PhD
Assistant Professor, Department of Gastroentelogical, Breast and Endocrine Surgery, Yamaguchi University Graduate School of Medicine, Ube, Yamaguchi, Japan

NARUHIKO IKOMA, MD
Department of Surgical Oncology, The University of Texas MD Anderson Cancer Center, Houston, Texas

EMILY Z. KEUNG, MD
Clinical Fellow in Complex General Surgical Oncology, The University of Texas MD Anderson Cancer Center, Houston, Texas

HONG JIN KIM, MD, FACS
Division Chief, Professor of Surgery, Division of Surgical Oncology, University of North Carolina, Chapel Hill, North Carolina

HISAKO KUBOTA, MD, PhD
Associate Professor, Department of Digestive Surgery, Kawasaki Medical School, Kurashiki, Okayama, Japan

SHACHAR LAKS, MD, FACS
Fellow Surgical Oncology, Division of Surgical Oncology, University of North Carolina, Chapel Hill, North Carolina

ANNE O. LIDOR, MD, MPH
Professor of Surgery, Department of Surgery, University of Wisconsin, Madison, Wisconsin

ALBERT CRAIG LOCKHART, MD, MHS
Professor, Department of Medicine, Division of Oncology, Barnes-Jewish Hospital and Washington University School of Medicine, St Louis, Missouri

ELEFTHERIOS A. MAKRIS, MD, PhD
Department of Surgery, Stanford University School of Medicine, Stanford, California

PAUL F. MANSFIELD, MD
Vice President, Acute Care Services, The University of Texas MD Anderson Cancer Center, Houston, Texas

HIDEO MATSUMOTO, MD, PhD
Associate Professor, Department of Digestive Surgery, Kawasaki Medical School, Kurashiki, Okayama, Japan

MICHAEL O. MEYERS, MD, FACS
Professor of Surgery, Division of Surgical Oncology, University of North Carolina, Chapel Hill, North Carolina

HIROAKI NAGANO, MD, PhD
Professor and Chairman, Department of Gastroentelogical, Breast and Endocrine Surgery, Yamaguchi University Graduate School of Medicine, Ube, Yamaguchi, Japan

SAOWANEE NGAMRUENGPHONG, MD
Assistant Professor of Medicine, Division of Gastroenterology and Hepatology, Johns Hopkins Medicine, Johns Hopkins Medical Institutions, Baltimore, Maryland

ICHIRO ODA, MD
Endoscopy Division, National Cancer Center Hospital, Tokyo, Japan

YASUO OKA, MD, PhD
Associate professor, Department of Digestive Surgery, Kawasaki Medical School, Kurashiki, Okayama, Japan

IKENNA C. OKEREKE, MD
Associate Professor of Surgery; Chief, Thoracic Surgery, Division of Cardiothoracic Surgery, University of Texas Medical Branch, Galveston, Texas

MANISHA PALTA, MD
Assistant Professor, Department of Radiation Oncology, Duke University, Durham, North Carolina

GEORGE A. POULTSIDES, MD, MS, FACS
Associate Professor of Surgery, Department of Surgery, Stanford University School of Medicine, Stanford, California

CHANDRAJIT P. RAUT, MD, MSc
Associate Professor, Department of Surgery, Brigham and Women's Hospital; Center for Sarcoma and Bone Oncology, Dana-Farber Cancer Institute, Boston, Massachusetts

R. TAYLOR RIPLEY, MD
Center for Cancer Research, National Cancer Institute, NIH, Bethesda, Maryland

RYAN K. SCHMOCKER, MD, MS
Resident Physician, Department of Surgery, University of Wisconsin, Madison, Wisconsin

DAPHNA SPIEGEL, MD
Department of Radiation Oncology, Duke University, Durham, North Carolina

MATTHEW S. STRAND, MD
Resident Physician, Department of Surgery, Barnes-Jewish Hospital and Washington University School of Medicine, St Louis, Missouri

VIVIAN E. STRONG, MD
Gastric and Mixed Tumor Service, Department of Surgery, Memorial Sloan Kettering Cancer Center, New York, New York

SHIGERU TAKEDA, MD, PhD
Associate Professor, Department of Gastroentelogical, Breast and Endocrine Surgery, Yamaguchi University Graduate School of Medicine, Ube, Yamaguchi, Japan

ATUSHI TSURUTA, MD, PhD
Associate Professor, Department of Digestive Surgery, Kawasaki Medical School, Kurashiki, Okayama, Japan

TOMIO UENO, MD, PhD
Professor and Chairman, Department of Digestive Surgery, Kawasaki Medical School, Kurashiki, Okayama, Japan

HOPE URONIS, MD, MHS
Associate Professor, Division of Medical Oncology, Duke University, Durham, North Carolina

SHIGEFUMI YOSHINO, MD, PhD
Associate Professor, Department of Gastroentelogical, Breast and Endocrine Surgery, Yamaguchi University Graduate School of Medicine, Ube, Yamaguchi, Japan

Contents

Minimally invasive gastric resections carry several advantages, including less intraoperative blood loss, faster recovery time, reduced pain, and decreased hospital length of stay and quicker return to work. Numerous trials have proved that laparoscopic and robotic-assisted gastrectomy provides equivalent surgical and oncologic outcomes to open approaches. As with any minimally invasive approach, advanced minimally invasive training and good judgment by a surgeon are paramount in selecting patients in whom a minimally invasive approach is feasible. With increasing research in patient populations with more advanced disease, the indications are likely to continue to expand.

Gastroesophageal junction tumors have been increasing in incidence over time, with most tumors presenting at a locally advanced stage. The treatment plan depends on the stage at diagnosis. PET-CT and endoscopic ultrasound are used to determine clinical stage. Depending on the location of the tumor in the esophagus and stomach, treatment can include chemotherapy with or without radiation, followed by surgery if there is no disease progression. Prognosis is related to stage at diagnosis and response to preoperative treatment. Most surgery for gastroesophageal junction tumors can be performed minimally invasively, which helps decrease postoperative length of stay and morbidity from surgery.

Postgastrectomy syndromes result from altered form and function of the stomach. Gastrectomy disrupts reservoir capacity, mechanical digestion and gastric emptying. Early recognition of symptoms with prompt evaluation and treatment is essential. Many syndromes resolve with minimal intervention or dietary modifications. Re-operation is not common but often warranted for afferent and efferent loop syndromes and bile reflux gastritis. Preoperative nutritional assessment and treatment of common vitamin and mineral deficiencies after gastrectomy can reduce the incidence of chronic complications. An integrated team approach to risk assessment, patient education, and postoperative management is critical to optimal care of patients with gastric cancer.

Since Theodor Billroth and César Roux perfected the methods of postgastrectomy reconstruction in as early as the late nineteenth century, surgical management of gastric cancer has made incremental progress. The longstanding and contentious debate on the optimal extent of lymph node dissection for gastric cancer seems to have settled in favor of D2 dissection. Pylorus-preserving distal (central) gastrectomy has emerged as a less invasive, function-preserving option for T1N0 middle-third gastric cancers. Frozen section analysis of margins seems partially helpful in this direction. Last, the role of palliative gastrectomy in patients with metastatic seems less important than initially thought.

This article discusses the current National Comprehensive Cancer Network guidelines and other available Western and Eastern guidelines for the surveillance of gastric cancer following surgical resection. It reviews the literature assessing the utility of intensive surveillance strategies for gastric cancer, which fails to show an improvement in survival. The unique issues relating to follow-up of early gastric cancer and after endoscopic resection of early gastric cancer are discussed. This article also reviews the available modalities for follow-up. In addition, it briefly discusses the advancements in treatment of recurrent and metastatic disease and the implications for gastric cancer survival and surveillance strategies.

Gastric neuroendocrine tumors (NETs) are classified into three types. Type I gastric NETs are associated with chronic atrophic gastritis. They have a good prognosis and endoscopic resection is the mainstay of treatment. Type II gastric NETs are caused by hypergastrinemia. They have a poorer prognosis, and resection is required to control the disease. Endoscopic versus surgical resection is recommended for the gastric lesion. Type III gastric NETs are sporadic and not associated with any specific condition. They have the worst prognosis with the highest rate of metastatic disease, and oncologic resection is recommended. Medical therapies have some role.

Gastric cancer represents a major cause of cancer mortality worldwide despite a declining incidence. New molecular classification schemes developed from genomic and molecular analyses of gastric cancer have provided a framework for understanding this heterogenous disease, and early findings suggest these classifications will be relevant for designing and implementing new targeted therapies. The success of targeted therapy and immunotherapy in breast cancer and melanoma, respectively, has not been duplicated in gastric cancer, but trastuzumab and ramucirumab have demonstrated efficacy in select populations. New markers that predict therapeutic response are needed to improve patient selection for both targeted and immunotherapies.

Early gastric cancer (ECG) can be difficult to diagnose endoscopically. Endoscopists should be familiar with subtle changes and endoscopic features of EGC. Chromoendoscopy and image-enhanced endoscopy improve diagnostic accuracy and facilitate endoscopic resection. Endoscopic submucosal dissection is a preferred endoscopic technique for resection of EGC and offers a comparable overall survival to surgical resection. Endoscopic management of benign gastric epithelial polyps (fundic gland polyps, hyperplastic polyps, and gastric adenoma) depends on patient symptomatology, patient's comorbidities (eg, familial syndromes), lesions' characteristics, and risk of malignant transformation. This article provides an overview of endoscopic management of EGC and common premalignant gastric lesions.

Benign gastric lesions represent various pathologic entities and management considerations. Upper endoscopy serves as the primary diagnostic modality for gastric lesions. Persistent or giant gastric ulcers represent unique subtypes of ulcers, requiring investigation of the underlying cause. Medical management remains the mainstay of treatment; however, indications for surgical intervention remain. Gastric polyps also represent diverse etiologies, and accurate diagnosis requires pertinent information and tissue samples. Neoplastic lesions often present as polypoid lesions; a high index of suspicion is required when discovered endoscopically. Malignant transformation potential varies widely between the various lesions; therefore an accurate diagnosis is imperative to determine management.

Gastric lymphoma is rare, accounting for 3% of gastric neoplasms and 10% of lymphomas. Treatment should be stratified based on histologic type, stage, Helicobacter pylori infection, and t(11;18) translocation status. Surgery is no longer a mainstay for treatment and should be reserved for rare situations such as perforation, fistula formation, and severe bleeding. Multimodal treatment, including H pylori eradication, radiation therapy, chemotherapy, and immunotherapy, should be provided as appropriate and can result in excellent outcomes.

Gastric adenocarcinoma is the fifth most common cancer worldwide and
is often diagnosed at a late stage with nearly 50% of patients having locally
advanced, unresectable, or metastatic disease at the time of presentation.
Efforts to improve outcomes in patients with resected and unresectable
gastric cancer with various chemotherapy and radiation regimens are
ongoing. Appropriate evaluation and management is often not straightforward and requires the input of a multidisciplinary team. There is no
consensus as to the best approach for treatment of gastric cancer; however, the available data and our institutional approach to the management
of gastric cancer are discussed.

Gastrointestinal stromal tumors (GISTs) are the most common mesenchymal neoplasm of the gastrointestinal tract. The stomach is the most
common site of origin. Management of GISTs changed after the introduction of molecularly targeted therapies. Although the only potentially curative treatment of resectable primary GISTs is surgery, recurrence is
common. Patients with primary GISTs at intermediate or high risk of recurrence should receive imatinib postoperatively. Imatinib is also first-line
therapy for advanced disease. Cytoreductive surgery might be considered
in advanced GIST for patients with stable/responding disease or limited
focal progression on tyrosine kinase inhibitor therapy. GIST requires multidisciplinary management.

In recent decades, there has been considerable worldwide progress in the
treatment of gastric cancer. Gastrectomy with a modified D2 lymphadenectomy (sparing the distal pancreas and spleen) has increasingly gained
acceptance as a preferable standard surgical approach among surgeons
in the East and the West. Despite growing consensus significant differences still exist in surgical techniques in clinical trials and clinical practices
secondary to variations in epidemiology, clinicopathologic features, and
surgical outcomes among geographic regions. In addition, Western physicians tend to prefer adjuvant chemotherapy and radiotherapy after surgery
instead of using S-1 chemotherapy, as is the preference in the East.

Obesity has reached epidemic proportions worldwide and is associated
with a higher mortality from several diseases, including adenocarcinoma

of the esophagus and of the gastric cardia. Increased body mass index is associated with an increased incidence of gastroesophageal reflux disease (GERD), Barrett metaplasia, and adenocarcinoma of the cardia. Bariatric surgery remains the most effective therapy for morbid obesity and has the potential to improve weight-related GERD. A high index of suspicion is paramount for early detection of foregut neoplasia after bariatric surgery.

SURGICAL CLINICS
OF NORTH AMERICA

THE CLINICS ARE AVAILABLE ONLINE!
Access your subscription at:
www.theclinics.com

Foreword

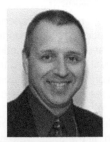

Ronald F. Martin, MD, FACS
Consulting Editor

As readers of our series know, we at the *Surgical Clinics of North America* try to cover the spectrum of issues that relate to general surgery on a somewhat cyclical basis. Every five or six years we make some attempt to come full circle on matters of interest. We make every effort to look at our topics from different vantage points or different subsets of the bigger topics in the hope that we continually keep our information fresh and of use. As our readers may also know, we constantly strive to strike a balance between in-depth detail and broad knowledge base on our topics. This latter aspiration provides one of the more interesting challenges in creating this series: how to balance what the generalist needs to know versus what the specialist can relay for a group of people with widely varying information needs and clinical responsibilities. Of course, as with most things in life, there is no absolute right answer as to how to accomplish this.

To achieve a balance in our series, we follow the educational requirements that are put on trainees by the educational oversight organizations. We also take into account the feedback that is available to us from our national organizations about how recent trainees perceive their training, as well as how those who hire them to the surgical workforce perceive the knowledge requirements of those who have recently trained. With that frame of reference, we also add focus on what is changing for everybody regardless of when we trained. It is undoubtedly imperfect and somewhat subjective, but probably serves as a reasonable starting point to help us know what to cover.

When one follows these trends for a while, one thing that becomes clear is the wide variety of forces that influence what we deem important. Sometimes new technology seems to overshadow fundamental principles. Other times, basic science eclipses matters of clinical expertise. Occasionally political forces, not wholly contained within medicine or surgery, creep in. Mostly, though, it is the inexorable march of collective re-evaluation that changes the way we perceive priority.

Gastric surgery is a fantastic example of how things change in surgery on many levels. Gastric operations were among the most common procedures done by surgical trainees in the 1950s and 1960s—the heyday of ulcer operations. Nonoperative means of treating the complications of acid-peptic disorders as well as treating hypersecretory states and bacterial infections to prevent those problems have significantly

Surg Clin N Am 97 (2017) xiii–xiv
http://dx.doi.org/10.1016/j.suc.2017.02.002
0039-6109/17/© 2017 Published by Elsevier Inc.

surgical.theclinics.com

reduced that kind of operative experience. The recent graduate from a residency program is highly likely to have performed very few, if any, major gastric operations.

The history and evolution of gastric surgery may be the finest example of excellence in surgical science. The logical progression of operative and nonoperative management based on the systematic development and a thorough and accurate understanding of the relation of anatomic structures and physiologic processes to overall function is unparalleled, in my opinion, elsewhere in surgery—especially if one considers the research tools that were available when most of the sentinel work was done. I don't believe it is a coincidence that many of the most notable names in surgical history are associated with their contributions to our understanding of gastric surgery.

Still, with all that we know about the stomach, with all the collective operative experience we have acquired about operating on the stomach, with all the tools we have available to us for managing the disorders of the stomach, gastric operations have largely left the sphere of the generalist and headed to the domain of the specialist or even subspecialist. I'll leave you to decide whether that is the path we should have chosen.

Independent of whether one specializes in gastric work or remains a generalist (or does both), a solid understanding of what we know and why we make clinical choices in gastric surgery is extremely useful knowledge to have. We owe a debt of gratitude to Dr Olino, Dr Tyler, and their colleagues for amassing this excellent collection of articles on gastric neoplasms. It will serve anybody well to review it.

As always, we desire feedback from our readership on whether or not we are meeting our goals of balancing the information we relay to you. We also are always interested in knowing whether there are topics we should consider covering that we are not already. Please let us know your thoughts.

Ronald F. Martin, MD, FACS
Colonel (ret.), United States Army Reserve
York Hospital
16 Hospital Drive, Suite A
York, ME 03909, USA

E-mail address:
rmartin@yorkhospital.com

Preface

Gastric Neoplasms

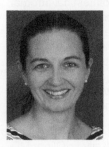 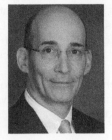

Kelly L. Olino, MD   Douglas S. Tyler, MD
Editors

Gastric neoplasms represent a heterogeneous group of lesions, all of which require multidisciplinary management in order to optimize patient outcomes. In this issue of the *Surgical Clinics of North America*, we have attempted to assemble a comprehensive compendium to guide the myriad of practitioners involved in the care of patients across all types of gastric neoplasms along the spectrum of premalignant to malignant disease.

The first section of this issue begins by providing an overview of findings typically seen during screening or incidentally discovered on upper endoscopy. Drs Schmocker and Lidor nicely summarize a variety of nonneoplastic lesions focusing on polyps, ulceration, and less commonly encountered benign growths. Drs Ngamruengphong, Abe, and Oda present a detailed overview of diagnostic and technical aspects of endoscopic interventions for premalignant and early stage gastric cancer. Finally, Dr Gomez lends his expertise as a bariatric surgeon with special considerations for the morbidly obese patient population, both prior to and following bariatric surgery.

We devoted a full section to gastric adenocarcinoma and gastroesophageal junction tumors given their worldwide prevalence. Drs Makris and Poultsides begin with a survey of the surgical considerations for management of gastric cancer, including different types of resection and lymphadenectomy options to palliative procedures. Drs Gholami, Cassidy, and Strong lend their expertise in minimally invasive surgery to detail technical considerations for the performance of these operations, while Dr Okereke provides an overview of gastroesophageal junction tumors. As gastric cancer is very common in Asia, we asked Dr Ueno and colleagues to offer their insight on how this disease is approached in the East as compared to Western countries.

The next section of this issue focuses on considerations following surgery, including nutrition and postgastrectomy syndromes reviewed by Dr Davis. The controversial question on how to best perform postresection surveillance is addressed by Drs Laks, Meyers, and Kim. Drs Spiegel, Palta, and Uronis provide a comprehensive comparison of the various neoadjuvant and adjuvant chemotherapy and radiation

Surg Clin N Am 97 (2017) xv–xvi
http://dx.doi.org/10.1016/j.suc.2017.02.001
0039-6109/17/© 2017 Published by Elsevier Inc.

surgical.theclinics.com

treatment regimens as well as current status of new clinical trials. Finally, Drs Strand, Lockhart, and Fields detail the advances in genetics, molecular biology, targeted therapies, and the potential role of immunotherapy.

The final section of this issue focuses on other common cancers found in the stomach and their multidisciplinary management. Management of gastrointestinal stromal tumors, including both the role and timing of surgery in combination with tyrosine kinase inhibitor treatment, is described by Drs Keung and Raut. Drs Corey and Chen discuss the subtypes of gastric neuroendocrine tumors and their management. Finally, Drs Ikoma, Badgwell, and Mansfield review the evidence-based multimodal treatment of gastric lymphoma.

We hope this issue will serve as a comprehensive reference for trainees and practitioners. We have focused on highlighting many of the recent advances as well as the future challenges oncologists face in the field.

Kelly L. Olino, MD
University of Texas Medical Branch
John Sealy Annex 6.100
301 University Boulevard
Galveston, TX 77555-0541, USA

Douglas S. Tyler, MD
Department of Surgery
University of Texas Medical Branch
John Sealy Annex 6.100
301 University Boulevard
Galveston, TX 77555-0541, USA

E-mail addresses:
keolino@utmb.edu (K.L. Olino)
dstyler@utmb.edu (D.S. Tyler)

Minimally Invasive Surgical Approaches to Gastric Resection

Sepideh Gholami, MD[a],*, Michael R. Cassidy, MD[a],
Vivian E. Strong, MD[b]

KEYWORDS

- Gastric cancer • Laparoscopic gastrectomy • Robotic gastrectomy
- Minimally invasive gastrectomy • Techniques in gastric resection

KEY POINTS

- Minimally invasive gastric resections carry several advantages, including less intraoperative blood loss, faster recovery time, reduced pain, and decreased hospital length of stay and quicker return to work.
- Numerous trials have proved that laparoscopic and robotic-assisted gastrectomy provides equivalent surgical and oncologic outcomes to open approaches.
- As with any minimally invasive approach, advanced minimally invasive training and good judgment by a surgeon are paramount in selecting patients in whom a minimally invasive approach is feasible.
- With increasing research in patient populations with more advanced disease, the indications are likely to continue to expand.

INTRODUCTION

Gastric cancer is an important contributor of cancer deaths and is associated with worse survival in the West compared with countries in Asia.[1] An estimated 951,600 new diagnoses of gastric cancer and 723,100 deaths were reported worldwide in 2012.[2] Recent reports have also shown that the incidence of gastroesophageal junction and gastric cardia tumors is increasing in the United States. Perhaps even more alarming is the 70% increase in the incidence of noncardia distal gastric cancer among 25 to 39 year olds in the United States over the past few years.[3] Because gastric cancer may manifest in a variety of histologic, anatomic, and genetic patterns, a customized and multimodality treatment plan for each patient leads to the best outcomes. Gastrectomy with curative intent remains the only strategy offering hope for

[a] Department of Surgery, Memorial Sloan Kettering Cancer Center, 1275 York Avenue, C-1272, New York, NY 10065, USA; [b] Gastric and Mixed Tumor Service, Department of Surgery, Memorial Sloan Kettering Cancer Center, 1275 York Avenue, H-1217, New York, NY 10065, USA
* Corresponding author.
E-mail address: gholamis@mskcc.org

Surg Clin N Am 97 (2017) 249–264
http://dx.doi.org/10.1016/j.suc.2016.11.003
surgical.theclinics.com
0039-6109/17/© 2016 Elsevier Inc. All rights reserved.

long-term survival and cure in gastric cancer patients. Recent advances in minimally invasive techniques have enhanced the surgical armamentarium for accomplishing both complete gastric cancer staging and curative resection. More importantly, randomized trials comparing laparoscopic with open gastrectomy have not only proved oncologic equivalency of the 2 approaches but also demonstrated favorable outcomes in postoperative recovery with minimally invasive approaches.[4-8] As a result, minimally invasive surgery is emerging as a preferred option in the treatment of gastric cancer. This article discusses the technical aspects of both laparoscopic and robot-assisted approaches to gastric cancer management.

LEARNING CURVE FOR LAPAROSCOPIC AND ROBOTIC GASTRECTOMY

Several factors influence the learning curve for laparoscopic and robotic gastrectomy. Part of the technical complexity arises from the different types of gastric resection and the range of technical skills required (as an example, an esophagojejunostomy after total gastrectomy is more challenging to perform than a stapled gastrojejunostomy after distal gastrectomy). Although technical factors of the operations influence the acquisition of skill, the training of the surgeon, experience with both open gastrectomy and minimally invasive techniques in general, and case volume also play a role.

There is a dearth of literature to address the question of learning curve in a systematic way for laparoscopic and robotic gastrectomy. Additionally, much of the knowledge about the learning curve has been generated in Eastern countries, where gastric cancer is far more common than in the United States. For laparoscopic gastrectomy, 1 study reports the outcomes of a series of laparoscopic distal gastrectomies performed during the learning curve of a single surgeon in South Korea.[9] The surgeon had prior extensive experience with open gastrectomy; 102 laparoscopic gastrectomies, divided into early (n = 50) and late (n = 51) groups, were compared with a series of 71 open gastrectomies. All the operations were for early gastric cancer. In the late laparoscopic group, the mean lymph node retrieval was greater and operative time was shorter compared with the early laparoscopic group. The open group, however, had the fastest operative times and greatest lymph node retrieval.

In another study, a series of 100 laparoscopic gastrectomies were divided into 5 groups based on the level of the surgeon's experience.[10] If the surgeon had performed more than 60 laparoscopic gastrectomies, there were no conversions to open and the operative time for the laparoscopic approach was similar to that of the open gastrectomy comparison group. Blood loss decreased after 20 laparoscopic gastrectomies, and hospital length of stay was shorter after 60 laparoscopic gastrectomies.

Other small studies of learning curve in laparoscopic gastrectomy similarly suggest a case volume of approximately 50 to 60 cases to achieve proficiency.[11] Most series, however, report only on the experience with early gastric cancer in highly selected patients. The learning curve for more advanced disease may be more difficult to overcome, particularly where extended lymphadenectomy is required[12] (**Fig. 1**).

There is some evidence that the learning curve for robotic gastrectomy may require fewer cases to achieve proficiency. For example, 1 study reported the experience of a single surgeon, dividing cases into early-experience laparoscopic, late-experience laparoscopic, and early-experience robotic gastrectomy.[13] Early-experience robotic gastrectomies showed nearly equivalent outcomes to late-experience laparoscopic gastrectomies. Robotic gastrectomies had less blood loss, shorter hospital length of stay, faster diet initiation, and better lymph node retrieval than early-experience laparoscopic gastrectomies. Most experience with robotic gastrectomy is reported for surgeons already proficient in laparoscopic gastrectomy, which enhances the

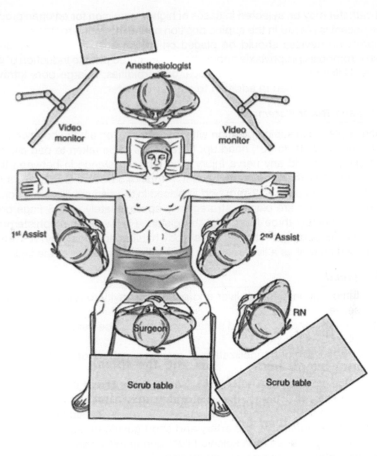

Fig. 1. Position for a patient undergoing laparoscopic gastrectomy. (© 2017, Memorial Sloan Kettering Cancer Center.)

learning curve. In these reports, the learning curve to proficiency in robotic gastrectomy has been described as 20 to 25 cases.[14,15]

SURGICAL TECHNIQUE
Preoperative Planning

Prior to any surgical intervention for gastric cancer, the patient has to undergo a complete staging work-up, including an upper endoscopy with biopsy; endoscopic ultrasound to assess for T stage and potential nodal involvement; CT of the chest, abdomen, and pelvis; and, for locally invasive tumors, a positron tomography scan. Patients with T3 or higher disease or positive lymph nodes require additional staging laparoscopy with washings for cytology. If no intra-abdominal deposits are noted and washings are negative for malignant cells, upfront surgical resection is recommended. Otherwise, patients should undergo neoadjuvant chemotherapy with possible additional radiation as indicated.[16,17]

Preparation and Patient Positioning

Like any other abdominal operation, the patient should be on clear fluids the day before and nothing by mouth after midnight the night prior to the operation. An epidural catheter may be selected in cases of higher suspicion for an open procedure. Once the patient is placed in the supine position on the operating room table, sequential compression devices should be placed on the lower extremities and chemical deep vein thrombosis prophylaxis should be administered prior to induction of general anesthesia. Unless the patient has medical comorbidities, 2 large bore intravenous catheters should be placed in addition to a Foley catheter.

Positioning and Trocar Placement

The patient is placed in supine position with the legs split on a bean bag, with the bed tilted approximately 30° to 40°, head up. Care needs to be taken to pad all pressure points properly to avoid any nerve injury. The surgeon stands in-between the legs with an assistant to either side of the patient. A total of 5 trocars are usually sufficient to complete the operation. A 12-mm port is placed in the periumbilical position, and 4 additional 5-mm ports are placed strategically approximately 4 to 5 fingerbreadths apart at approximately three-fourths of the distance between the xiphisternum and the umbilicus, depending on the patient's body habitus and anatomy. A 10-mm 30° camera is used as well as a liver retractor to elevate the left lobe of the liver.

Surgical Approach

1. Identify tumor and inspect the liver and peritoneal cavity to rule out grossly metastatic disease.
   a. Intraoperative endoscopy and a marking stitch can be used for tumors that are difficult to identify externally.
2. Entry into lesser sac and mobilization of greater curvature of the stomach toward the spleen
   a. Lift up the stomach and enter lesser sac over the top of the transverse colon, avoiding damage to the colonic mesentery. Stay close to the posterior wall of the stomach and open the greater curve toward the left side of the patient.
   b. Divide the left gastroepiploic artery and short gastric vessels.
   c. Remove lymph nodes from splenic hilum during this dissection.
3. Mobilization of greater curvature and pylorus
   a. Continue with omentectomy along the transverse colon in the direction toward gallbladder.
   b. Divide the right gastroepiploic vessels with a stapling device of clips and avoid injury to the pancreas.
   c. The dissection finishes approximately 2 cm distal to the pylorus, freeing up periduodenal and peripancreatic tissue.
   d. Transect the duodenum with an endo-GIA stapler verifying that the nasogastric tube and temperature probe (if present) have been removed prior to transection. The authors typically use a stapler with reinforcement (Seamguard), which is an option at the discretion of the surgeon.
4. Mobilization of the lesser curvature of the stomach
   a. Mobilize the lesser curvature toward the esophagus, including the gastrohepatic ligament, avoiding injury to an accessory left hepatic artery.
   b. The right gastric vessels are then divided.
   c. Divide the left gastric artery along the posterior wall of stomach with its associated lymph node bundle.
   d. Station 12 lymph nodes (hepatoduodenal) are gradually divided and taken en bloc with the stomach.
   e. Transect the stomach at an oncologically appropriate location based on judgment of adequate margin.

   f. Place the gastrectomy specimen with en bloc lymph nodes in an Endo Catch bag and send specimen for a frozen to check on the entire proximal margin.
5. Reconstruction with Roux-en-Y
   a. Position the patient in Trendelenburg position.
   b. Find the ligament of Treitz and transect the jejunum 30 cm to 50 cm distal to it, creating the Roux limb proximally and biliopancreatic limb distally.
   c. Prepare the Roux limb, taking care to avoid injury to the vascular arch.
   d. Measure 60 cm to 70 cm of length along the Roux limb and choose a point for the jejunojejunostomy.
   e. Align the 2 antimesenteric limbs of the biliopancreatic limb and Roux limb to make an enterotomy in both limbs of jejunum and fire the linear GIA load.
   f. Close the resultant enterostomy with a running 2-0 silk suture.
   g. Reapproximate the mesenteric defect with an absorbable suture to prevent internal hernias when technically feasible.[18]
   h. The Roux limb is then brought up to the esophagus/proximal stomach in an antecolic fashion.
   i. The nasogastric tube is pulled back.
   j. Using a circular EEA stapler, an end-to-end esophagojejunostomy/gastrojejunostomy anastomosis is created, or
   k. Create a gastrostomy 1 cm away from the transection point and bring the Roux limb parallel to it; then create an enterotomy in the Roux limb.
   l. Ensure hemostasis and that there is no kinking or tension on the future anastomosis.
   m. Fire an endo-GIA stapler to create a large anastomotic opening and close the defect with a running 2-0 silk suture.
   n. A gastrostomy tube is placed back through the Roux limb.
   o. A water-bubble test can be performed to rule out a leak.

Immediate Postoperative Care

In general, no nasogastric tube or surgical drains are routinely indicated. Patient-controlled anesthesia is used for postoperative analgesia unless an epidural has been placed. Transfer to the surgical floor is safe, if the patient has been in recovery and stable for 4 hours to 6 hours.

From day 1, the patient should be up out of bed, ambulating, and using an incentive spirometer to help with mobilization.

In general, the patient can be started on ice chips and sips of clear fluids on postoperative day 1. Assuming the patient tolerates clear fluids well, full liquids can be started on postoperative day 2. Diet can be advanced to a postgastrectomy diet when the patient has return of bowel function, usually by postoperative day 3 or 4. Nutritional consultation prior to discharge is crucial to educate the patient about expectations and anticipated changes in eating habits after undergoing a gastrectomy.

Rehabilitation and Recovery

After discharge, patients are usually seen within 2 weeks for routine postoperative check. Surveillance for gastric cancer involves routinely a CT scan in 3-month intervals for a year and 6-month intervals the year after, followed by yearly follow-up for a total of at least 5 years, depending on stage of tumor. It is crucial to keep track of patient weights at each visit to ensure proper nutrition.

Clinical Results in the Literature

Multiple studies have shown the effectiveness and oncologic results of the laparoscopic technique. In a recent review by Son and colleagues,[19] cumulative results from multiple trials did not show significant differences in terms of survival rate or recurrence after surgery based on long-term follow-up evaluation, although multiple trials and review articles have shown that the number of lymph node retrieved were equivalent in the 2 groups.[19] A summary of results is demonstrated in **Tables 1** and **2**.

ROBOTIC GASTRECTOMY
Robotic Setup and Patient Positioning

Patient positioning for robotic gastrectomy is similar to that of laparoscopic gastrectomy, as discussed previously. The patient's arms may be tucked at the side or may be extended on arm boards. Proper padding of the pressure points should be assured. Because of the steep positioning required for robotic gastrectomy, at least 45° of reverse Trendelenburg position, the patient should be well secured to the table by straps at the shoulders, hips, and knees. Foot boards may also be used for additional security. In contrast to the laparoscopic setup, the patient must be fully positioned prior to robot docking, and, once the robotic arms are in place, the patient's position cannot be changed unless the robot is fully undocked (**Fig. 2**).

Port placement for robotic gastrectomy is demonstrated in **Fig. 3**. The camera port should be placed 15 cm to 20 cm from the xiphoid of the patient, with additional ports placed at least 8 cm from each other. The positioning of the camera port is critical and may not always be placed at the umbilicus in heavier patients. All other ports are positioned based on the camera port and this must accommodate good visualization of the stomach but enough distance to see and protect the transverse colon and to perform the jejununojejunostomy or other anastomosis with enough room for adequate visualization.

Procedural Details

Conversion to open

The entire operative team should be familiar with robotic instrumentation and the detailed plan for conversion to an open operation in the event of an emergency that cannot be resolved robotically. Roles of each team member should be discussed during the preoperative timeout. There should be a low threshold for conversion based on the clinical experience and judgment of the surgeon.

Procedural Setup

Pneumoperitoneum may be established in routine fashion, either using a Veress needle in the left upper quadrant or via one of the ports after a direct cutdown technique. Once adequate pneumoperitoneum is achieved, the remaining ports are placed. These include a 10-mm to 12-mm midline port and two 8-mm ports at the left midclavicular line and left anterior axillary line, respectively. On the right, a 10-mm to 12-mm port is placed in the midclavicular line and a 5-mm port is placed in the anterior axillary line. A liver retractor can be helpful to expose the stomach, in particular the esophageal hiatus, and can be placed through a small subxiphoid stab incision.

After port placement but before docking the robot, the abdomen should be explored laparoscopically for radiographically occult peritoneal disease and for identification of the primary tumor. If the tumor is not visualized, especially in cases of tumors at the gastroesophageal junction, endoscopy should be used to locate it. A judgment must be made regarding surgical resectability with a 2-cm to 4-cm margin. If

Table 1
Recent randomized clinical trials of laparoscopic versus open gastrectomy for the treatment of gastric cancer

Study, Year	Eligibility	Procedure	LND Extent	Number of Patients	Operative Time Less	Blood Loss Less	Number of Lymph Nodes Retrieved	Hospital Stay	Morbidity	Mortality
Kitano et al,[8] 2002	cT1	LADG/ODG	NR	14/14	ODG	LADG	Equivalent	Equivalent	Equivalent	Equivalent
Fujii et al,[25] 2003	cT1	LADG/ODG	NR	10/10	ODG	Equivalent	NR	NR	Equivalent	Equivalent
Hayashi et al,[26] 2005	cT1	LADG/ODG	NR	14/14	ODG	Equivalent	Equivalent	LADG	NR	Equivalent
Huscher et al,[6] 2005	cT1-4 N0-2	TLGD/ODG	D1, D2	30/29	Equivalent	TLGD	Equivalent	TLGD	Equivalent	Equivalent
Lee et al,[7] 2005	cT1	LADG/ODG	D2	24/23	ODG	Equivalent	Equivalent	Equivalent	LADG	NR
Kim et al,[5] 2008	cT1 N0-1	LADG/ODG	D1, D2	82/82	ODG	LADG	ODG	LADG	NR	NR
Kim et al,[4] 2010	cT1-2N0-1	LADG/ODG	D1, D2	179/163	ODG	LADG	NR	NR	Equivalent	Equivalent
Cai et al,[27] 2011	cT2-3	LAD/OG	D2	49/47	OG	Equivalent	Equivalent	Equivalent	Equivalent	NR
Sakuramoto et al,[28] 2013	cT1	LADG/ODG	D1	31/32	ODG	LADG	Equivalent	Equivalent	Equivalent	NR
Takiguchi et al,[29] 2013	cTNMI	LADG/ODG	D1, D2	20/20	ODG	LADG	Equivalent	LADG	NR	NR
Aoyama et al,[30] 2014	cTNMI	LADG/ODG	D1, D2	13/13	ODG	LADG	Equivalent	NR	Equivalent	Equivalent

Abbreviations: DG, Distal gastrectomy; LADG, Laparoscopic distal gastrectomy; LAG, Laparoscopy-assisted gastrectomy; LN, Lymph node; LND, Lymph node dissection; ODG, Open distal gastrectomy; OG, Open gastrectomy; PG, Proximal gastrectomy; TG, Total gastrectomy; TLDG, Totally laparoscopic distal gastrectomy.
From Son T, Hyung WJ. Laparoscopic gastric cancer surgery: current evidence and future perspectives. World J Gastroenterol 2016;22(2):731; with permission.

Table 2
Summary of nonrandomized clinical trials comparing robotic, laparoscopic, and open gastrectomy

Reference, Year	Study Design	Type of Approach	Type of Surgery (TG/STG)	Op Time (minutes)	Estimated Blood Loss	Retrieval No. of Lymph Nodes	Conversion (%)	Morbidity (%)	Mortality (%)
Pugliese et al,[31] 2010	Nonrandomized Retrospective	R 18	0/18	344	90	25	2	6	6.2
		L 52	0/52	235	148	31	3	12.5	2
Kim et al,[32] 2009	Nonrandomized Retrospective	R 16	0/16	259.2	30.3	41.1	0	0	0
		L 11	0/11	203.9	44.7	37.4	0	9	0
		O 12	0/12	126.7	78.8	43.3	—	16	—
Caruso et al,[33] 2011	Nonrandomized Retrospective	R 29	12/17	290	197.6	28.0	—	41.4	0
		O 120	37/83	222	386.1	31.7	—	42.5	3.3
Woo et al,[34] 2011	Nonrandomized Retrospective	R 236	62/172	219.5	91.6	39.0	0	11	0.3
		L 591	108/481	170.7	147.9	37.4	0	13.7	0.4
Eom et al,[35] 2012	Nonrandomized Retrospective	R 30	0/30	229.1	152.8	30.2	0	13	0
		L 62	0/62	189.4	88.3	33.4	0	6	0
Kang et al,[36] 2012	Nonrandomized Retrospective	R 100	16/84	202	93.2	—	—	14.0	0
		L 282	37/245	173	173.4	—	—	10.3	0
Yoon et al,[37] 2012	Nonrandomized Retrospective	R 36	36/0	305.8	214.2	42.8	0	16.7	0
		L 65	65/0	210.2	150.3	39.4	0	15.4	0
Huang et al,[14] 2012	Nonrandomized Retrospective	R 39	7/32	430	50	32	—	15.4	—
		L 64	7/57	350	100	26	—	15.6	—
		O 586	179/407	320	400	34	—	14.7	—

Kim et al,[38] 2012	Nonrandomized	R 436	109/327	226	85	40.2	—	10.1	0.5
	Retrospective	L 861	158/703	176	112	37.6	—	9.4	0.3
		O 4542	1232/3309	158	192	40.5	—	10.7	0.5
Park et al,[39] 2012	Nonrandomized	R 30	0/30	218	75	34	0	5	0
	Prospective	L 120	0/120	140	60	35	0	9	0
Uyama et al,[40] 2012	Nonrandomized	R 25	0/25	361	51.8	44.3	0	11.2	0
	Retrospective	L 225	0/225	345	81.0	43.2	0	16.9	0
Hyun et al,[41] 2013	Nonrandomized	R 38	9/29	234.4	131.3	32.8	0	47.3	0
	Retrospective	L 83	18/65	220.0	130.5	32.6	0	38.5	0
Suda et al,[42] 2014	Nonrandomized	R 88	30/58	381	46	40	0	2.3	1.1
	Retrospective	L 438	136/302	361	34	38	0	11.4	0.2
Son et al,[43] 2014	Nonrandomized	R 51	51/0	264.1	163.4	47.2	0	15.7	2.0
	Retrospective	L 58	58/0	210.3	210.7	42.8	—	22.4	0
Noshiro et al,[44] 2014	Nonrandomized	R 21	0/21	439	96	44	0	9.5	0
	Retrospective	L 161	0/160	315	115	40	0	10.0	0
Junfeng et al,[45] 2014	Nonrandomized	R 120	26/92 (PG:2)	234.8	118.3	34.6	0	5.8	—
	Retrospective	L 394	118/261 (PG:15)	221.3	137.6	32.7	0	4.3	—
Huang et al,[46] 2014	Nonrandomized	R 72	8/64	357.9	79.6	30.6	—	12.5	1.4
	Retrospective	L 73	10/63	319.8	116.0	28.1	—	—	—

Abbreviations: L, laparoscopic; LN, lymph nodes; O, open; PG, proximal gastrectomy; R, robotic; STG, subtotal gastrectomy; TG, total gastrectomy.

From Obama K, Sakai Y. Current status of robotic gastrectomy for gastric cancer. Surg Today 2016;46(5):529; with permission.

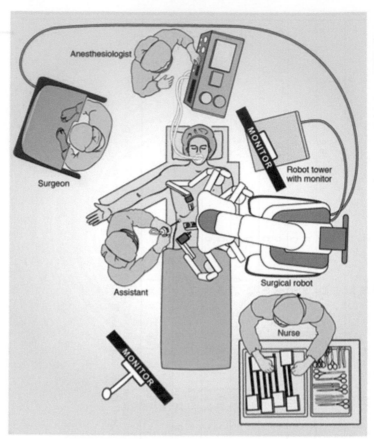

Fig. 2. Position for a patient undergoing robotic total gastrectomy. The operation is generally performed in steep reverse Trendelenburg position and the patient must be positioned prior to docking the robot. (© 2017, Memorial Sloan Kettering Cancer Center.)

technically possible to proceed, the patient is placed in steep reverse Trendelenburg position and the robot is docked. Arms 1 and 3 are placed in the left ports and arm 2 is placed in the 12-mm port. Helpful instruments include the fenestrated bipolar grasper (typically in arm 2), monopolar scissors or an energy sealant device (in arm 1), and grasping forceps (in arm 3).

1. Omentectomy
   a. To start, the greater omentum is retracted cephalad and the omentum is divided from the colon from by entering the avascular plane between the 2. Entrance to the lesser sac is confirmed by visualization of the posterior wall of the stomach.
   b. The bedside assistant should retract the stomach anteriorly and to the right.
   c. The omentectomy proceeds by progressing toward the splenic flexure, dividing and ligating the short gastric vessels with the energy sealant device.
   d. Then, the omentectomy can be completed by dividing the colonic attachments to the omentum toward the hepatic flexure.
   e. Once entirely separated, the omentum can be placed in the right upper quadrant until removed later.
2. Dissection of the greater curvature

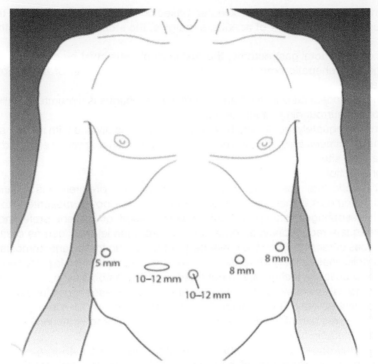

Fig. 3. Port placement for robotic total gastrectomy. (© 2017, Memorial Sloan Kettering Cancer Center.)

    a. The stomach is now freed from its posterior attachments to the pancreas, using either the energy sealant device or sharp dissection.

    b. The right gastroepiploic vessels are dissected at their origin from the gastroduodenal vessels and divided with a linear stapler, either by robotic attachment or by removing arm 2 of the robot from the 12-mm port in the right midclavicular line and allowing the bedside assistant to introduce a stapler.

3. Division of the proximal duodenum

    a. A window must now be created at the level of the pylorus.

    b. The gastrohepatic attachments are divided and the right gastric artery is ligated.

    c. Lymphatic tissues following the common and proper hepatic arteries are mobilized toward the specimen.

    d. A linear stapler is used to divide the proximal duodenum.

4. Lymphadenectomy

    a. After division of the duodenum, the stomach may now be reflected toward the left upper quadrant and lymphadenectomy may commence.

    b. The lymphadenectomy, which was begun along the proper hepatic artery, is carried along the common hepatic artery toward the celiac axis and splenic artery.

    c. The lymphatic tissue following the left gastric artery and vein is dissected toward the specimen.

    d. The vessels are divided with a linear vascular stapler.

5. Division of the stomach or distal esophagus

    a. The tumor location and extent of involvement are assessed by endoscopy influence the proximal division point on the stomach.

    b. Once the location has been selected based on oncologic principles and the surgeon's best judgment of adequate margins, the stomach is divided with linear staplers.

    c. In cases of total gastrectomy, the distal esophagus must be divided.

    d. The gastrohepatic omentum must be divided to the level of the esophageal hiatus.

    e. The peritoneal fat is incised and the distal esophagus is circumferentially freed from its surrounding attachments.

    f. Once adequately mobilized, the distal esophagus is divided with a linear stapler.

    g. The specimens are generally removed in a specimen bag via an enlarged umbilical port site.

6. Reconstruction

    For robotic total gastrectomy, typically the authors' preference is an antecolic anastomosis if there is redundancy in the small bowel mesentery to reach the esophageal stump without tension. Based on patient preference and adequate redundancy, an omega pouch from the jejunum can be created. In cases of tension when the mesentery is brought up for the anastomosis, a retrocolic anastomosis with a direct Roux-en-Y reconstruction is preferred. There are 3 possible techniques to consider for the anastomosis:

    a. A transoral anvil device (25 French) is one option for esophagojejunostomy after total gastrectomy. This technique is preferable especially for a total gastrectomy that requires part of the distal esophagus where the reconstruction is positioned in the thoracic cavity

    b. A second option is a linear stapled anastomosis where a 45-mm stapler is inserted into the Roux limb of the jejunum and positioned anterior to the esophageal stump and the other part of the stapler is positioned posteriorly in the esophagus via a small entry point for the stapler in the anterior wall of the esophagus. The remaining enterotomy is closed with a running 3-0 PDS suture.

    c. A third option is a hand-sewn end-to-end esophagojejunostomy, which is done in 1 or 2 layers, interrupted with 3-0 PDS suture. This anastomosis may be preferable for a smaller patient with a narrow esophagus.

Postoperative Care

After robotic gastrectomy, as with laparoscopic gastrectomy, nasoenteric drainage is not necessary.[20] In addition, the authors do not advocate routine use of jejunostomy tubes after total gastrectomy. Patients may begin sips of clear liquids on the first postoperative day and their diets may be advanced as tolerated in the subsequent days. Early enteric feeding is advantageous in patients who are clinically well.[21] Patients should be encouraged to ambulate and their pain should be controlled with multimodality therapy. Limiting narcotic use may speed recovery and prevent postoperative ileus. A benefit of the robotic approach is decreased pain compared with open approach.

Potential Complications

An anastomotic leak is the most feared complication of gastrectomy.[22] Patients with anastomotic leak may manifest fever, tachycardia, or leukocytosis. Any such signs or symptoms should prompt radiographic evaluation with an upper gastrointestional series using oral water-soluble contrast or a contrast-enhanced CT. Other complications can include intraluminal bleeding, intraabdominal bleeding, ileus, bowel obstruction, and infectious complications.[22]

Postoperative Outcomes in the Literature

Knowledge of the outcomes of robotic gastrectomy comes from retrospective series and nonrandomized prospective studies. In a meta-analysis of short-term outcomes comparing robotic, laparoscopic, and open gastrectomy, robotic gastrectomy was associated with shorter length of stay compared with open gastrectomy but longer operative times.[23] Compared with laparoscopic gastrectomy, there was less intraoperative blood loss in the robotic group. Overall morbidity was equivalent between the approaches. Few data are available on long-term oncologic outcomes after robotic gastrectomy, but current evidence suggests that oncologic outcomes are similar with robotic gastrectomy as with other approaches, albeit in well-selected patients.[24]

SUMMARY

Minimally invasive techniques are the preferred approach in the treatment of gastric cancer in well-selected patients today. Minimally invasive gastric resections carry several advantages, including less intraoperative blood loss, faster recovery time, reduced pain, and decreased hospital length of stay and quicker return to work. Comparing minimally invasive to open techniques, complications rates have been reported to occur with equal and/or lesser frequency, in addition to the numerous other advantages known to minimally invasive approaches (discussed previously), including fewer long-term effects, such as incisional hernias and adhesions/bowel obstructions. Numerous trials have proved that laparoscopic and robotic-assisted gastrectomy provide equivalent surgical and oncologic outcomes to open approaches. As with any minimally invasive approach, good judgment by the surgeon is paramount in selecting patients in which a minimally invasive approach is feasible. Patients with large tumors, widely diffuse cancers (ie, linitis plastica), very elderly patients, or patients with significant comorbidities may not be good candidates for this approach. There is a clear place, however, for minimally invasive approaches in the treatment of gastric cancer for well-selected patients and when performed by surgeons with advanced minimally invasive training. With increasing research in patient populations with more advanced disease, the indications are likely to continue to expand.

REFERENCES

1. Strong VE, Song KY, Park CH, et al. Comparison of gastric cancer survival following R0 resection in the United States and Korea using an internationally validated nomogram. Ann Surg 2010;251(4):640–6.
2. Torre LA, Bray F, Siegel RL, et al. Global cancer statistics, 2012. CA Cancer J Clin 2015;65(2):87–108.
3. Anderson WF, Camargo MC, Fraumeni JF, et al. Age-specific trends in incidence of noncardia gastric cancer in US adults. JAMA 2010;303(17):1723–8.
4. Kim H-H, Hyung WJ, Cho GS, et al. Morbidity and Mortality of Laparoscopic Gastrectomy Versus Open Gastrectomy for Gastric Cancer An Interim Report—A Phase III Multicenter, Prospective, Randomized Trial (KLASS Trial). Ann Surg 2010;251(3):417–20.
5. Kim Y-W, Baik YH, Yun YH, et al. Improved quality of life outcomes after laparoscopy-assisted distal gastrectomy for early gastric cancer: results of a prospective randomized clinical trial. Ann Surg 2008;248(5):721–7.
6. Huscher CG, Mingoli A, Sgarzini G, et al. Laparoscopic versus open subtotal gastrectomy for distal gastric cancer: five-year results of a randomized prospective trial. Ann Surg 2005;241(2):232–7.

7. Lee JH, Han HS. A prospective randomized study comparing open vs laparoscopy-assisted distal gastrectomy in early gastric cancer: early results. Surg Endosc 2005;19(2):168–73.

8. Kitano S, Shiraishi N, Fujii K, et al. A randomized controlled trial comparing open vs laparoscopy-assisted distal gastrectomy for the treatment of early gastric cancer: an interim report. Surgery 2002;131(Suppl 1):S306–11.

9. Yoo CH, Kim HO, Hwang SI, et al. Short-term outcomes of laparoscopic-assisted distal gastrectomy for gastric cancer during a surgeon's learning curve period. Surg Endosc 2009;23(10):2250–7.

10. Kunisaki C, Makino H, Yamamoto N, et al. Learning curve for laparoscopy-assisted distal gastrectomy with regional lymph node dissection for early gastric cancer. Surg Laparosc Endosc Percutan Tech 2008;18(3):236–41.

11. Zhang X, Tanigawa N. Learning curve of laparoscopic surgery for gastric cancer, a laparoscopic distal gastrectomy-based analysis. Surg Endosc 2009;23(6):1259–64.

12. Jin SH, Kim DY, Kim H, et al. Multidimensional learning curve in laparoscopy-assisted gastrectomy for early gastric cancer. Surg Endosc 2007;21(1):28–33.

13. Song J, Kang WH, Oh SJ, et al. Role of robotic gastrectomy using da Vinci system compared with laparoscopic gastrectomy: initial experience of 20 consecutive cases. Surg Endosc 2009;23(6):1204–11.

14. Huang K-H, Lan Y-T, Fang W-L, et al. Initial experience of robotic gastrectomy and comparison with open and laparoscopic gastrectomy for gastric cancer. J Gastrointest Surg 2012;16(7):1303–10.

15. Park SS, Kim MC, Park MS, et al. Rapid adaptation of robotic gastrectomy for gastric cancer by experienced laparoscopic surgeons. Surg Endosc 2012;26(1):60–7.

16. Macdonald JS, Smalley SR, Benedetti J, et al. Chemoradiotherapy after surgery compared with surgery alone for adenocarcinoma of the stomach or gastroesophageal junction. N Engl J Med 2001;345(10):725–30.

17. Cunningham D, Allum WH, Stenning SP, et al. Perioperative chemotherapy versus surgery alone for resectable gastroesophageal cancer. N Engl J Med 2006;355(1):11–20.

18. Kelly KJ, Allen PJ, Brennan MF, et al. Internal hernia after gastrectomy for cancer with Roux-Y reconstruction. Surgery 2013;154(2):305–11.

19. Son T, Hyung WJ. Laparoscopic gastric cancer surgery: current evidence and future perspectives. World J Gastroenterol 2016;22(2):727–35.

20. Davis JL, Selby LV, Chou JF, et al. Patterns and Predictors of Weight Loss After Gastrectomy for Cancer. Ann Surg Oncol 2016;23(5):1639–45.

21. Lassen K, Fetveit T, Horn A, et al. Allowing normal food at will after major upper gastrointestinal surgery. Ann Surg 2008;247(5):721–9.

22. Selby LV, Vertosick EA, Sjoberg DD, et al. Morbidity after total gastrectomy: Analysis of 238 patients. J Am Coll Surg 2015;220(5):863–71.e2.

23. Marano A, Young Choi Y, Hyung WJ, et al. Robotic versus laparoscopic versus open gastrectomy: a meta-analysis. J Gastric Cancer 2013;13(3):136–48.

24. Nakauchi M, Suda K, Susumu S, et al. Comparison of the long-term outcomes of robotic radical gastrectomy for gastric cancer and conventional laparoscopic approach: a single institutional retrospective cohort study. Surg Endosc 2016;30(12):5444–52.

25. Fujii K, Sonoda K, Izumi K, et al. T lymphocyte subsets and Th1/Th2 balance after laparoscopy-assisted distal gastrectomy. Surg Endosc 2003;17(9):1440–4.

26. Hayashi H, Ochiai T, Shimada H, et al. Prospective randomized study of open versus laparoscopy-assisted distal gastrectomy with extraperigastric lymph node dissection for early gastric cancer. Surg Endosc 2005;19(9):1172–6.

27. Cai J, Wei D, Gao CF, et al. A prospective randomized study comparing open versus laparoscopy-assisted D2 radical gastrectomy in advanced gastric cancer. Dig Surg 2011;28(5–6):331–7.

28. Sakuramoto S, Yamashita K, Kikuchi S, et al. Laparoscopy versus open distal gastrectomy by expert surgeons for early gastric cancer in Japanese patients: short-term clinical outcomes of a randomized clinical trial. Surg Endosc 2013; 27(5):1695–705.

29. Takiguchi S, Fujiwara Y, Yamasaki M, et al. Laparoscopy-assisted distal gastrectomy versus open distal gastrectomy. A prospective randomized single-blind study. World J Surg 2013;37(10):2379–86.

30. Aoyama T, Yoshikawa T, Hayashi T, et al. Randomized comparison of surgical stress and the nutritional status between laparoscopy-assisted and open distal gastrectomy for gastric cancer. Ann Surg Oncol 2014;21(6):1983–90.

31. Pugliese R, Maggioni D, Sansonna F, et al. Subtotal gastrectomy with D2 dissection by minimally invasive surgery for distal adenocarcinoma of the stomach: results and 5-year survival. Surg Endosc 2010;24(10):2594–602.

32. Kim M-C, Heo G-U, Jung G-J. Robotic gastrectomy for gastric cancer: surgical techniques and clinical merits. Surg Endosc 2009;24(3):610–5.

33. Caruso S, Patriti A, Marrelli D, et al. Open vs robot-assisted laparoscopic gastric resection with D2 lymph node dissection for adenocarcinoma: a case-control study. Int J Med Robot 2011;7(4):452–8.

34. Woo Y, Hyung WJ, Pak K-H, et al. Robotic gastrectomy as an oncologically sound alternative to laparoscopic resections for the treatment of early-stage gastric cancers. Arch Surg 2011;146(9):1086–92.

35. Eom BW, Yoon HM, Ryu KW, et al. Comparison of surgical performance and short-term clinical outcomes between laparoscopic and robotic surgery in distal gastric cancer. Eur J Surg Oncol 2012;38(1):57–63.

36. Kang BH, Xuan Y, Hur H, et al. Comparison of surgical outcomes between robotic and laparoscopic gastrectomy for gastric cancer: the learning curve of robotic surgery. J Gastric Cancer 2012;12(3):156–63.

37. Yoon HM, Kim Y-W, Lee JH, et al. Robot-assisted total gastrectomy is comparable with laparoscopically assisted total gastrectomy for early gastric cancer. Surg Endosc 2012;26(5):1377–81.

38. Kim KM, An JY, Kim HI, et al. Major early complications following open, laparoscopic and robotic gastrectomy. Br J Surg 2012;99(12):1681–7.

39. Park JY, Jo MJ, Nam B-H, et al. Surgical stress after robot-assisted distal gastrectomy and its economic implications. Br J Surg 2012;99(11):1554–61.

40. Uyama I, Kanaya S, Ishida Y, et al. Novel integrated robotic approach for suprapancreatic D2 nodal dissection for treating gastric cancer: technique and initial experience. World J Surg 2012;36(2):331–7.

41. Hyun M-H, Lee C-H, Kwon Y-J, et al. Robot Versus Laparoscopic Gastrectomy for Cancer by an Experienced Surgeon: Comparisons of Surgery, Complications, and Surgical Stress. Ann Surg Oncol 2013;20(4):1258–65.

42. Suda K, Man-i M, Ishida Y, et al. Potential advantages of robotic radical gastrectomy for gastric adenocarcinoma in comparison with conventional laparoscopic approach: a single institutional retrospective comparative cohort study. Surg Endosc 2014;29(3):673–85.

43. Son T, Lee JH, Kim YM, et al. Robotic spleen-preserving total gastrectomy for gastric cancer: comparison with conventional laparoscopic procedure. Surg Endosc 2014;28(9):2606–15.
44. Noshiro H, Ikeda O, Urata M. Robotically-enhanced surgical anatomy enables surgeons to perform distal gastrectomy for gastric cancer using electric cautery devices alone. Surg Endosc 2014;28(4):1180–7.
45. Junfeng Z, Yan S, Bo T, et al. Robotic gastrectomy versus laparoscopic gastrectomy for gastric cancer: comparison of surgical performance and short-term outcomes. Surg Endosc 2014;28(6):1779–87.
46. Huang K-H, Lan Y-T, Fang W-L, et al. Comparison of the operative outcomes and learning curves between laparoscopic and robotic gastrectomy for gastric cancer. PLoS One 2014;9(10):e111499.

Management of Gastroesophageal Junction Tumors

Ikenna C. Okereke, MD

KEYWORDS

- Barrett • Adenocarcinoma • Neoadjuvant • Minimally invasive

KEY POINTS

- Gastroesophageal junction tumors have increased in overall incidence.
- Multimodality treatment is the standard of care for gastroesophageal junction tumors.
- Most surgery for gastroesophageal junction tumors can be performed through a minimally invasive approach.

INTRODUCTION

Cancers of the esophagus and stomach are among the most prevalent malignancies globally and are a major cause of cancer-related mortality. Overall approximately 1.4 million new cases of cancers of the esophagus and stomach arise worldwide each year.[1] Gastroesophageal junction tumors refer to tumors that arise close to the gastroesophageal junction. This subset of tumors has increased in prevalence in the past decade, increasing by approximately 10% over the past 40 years.[2] Overwhelmingly the most common histology is adenocarcinoma, accounting for more than 90% of all gastroesophageal tumors.[3]

Traditionally, the management of esophageal cancers has differed slightly from the management of gastric cancers. As such, there has been some controversy about the exact definition of a gastroesophageal tumor and the appropriate treatment plan to undertake once a diagnosis of gastroesophageal tumor is made.

The most commonly used classification system to define a gastroesophageal tumor was created by Jörg Rüdiger Siewert, a German surgeon who created a classification system for gastroesophageal junction tumors based on the location of the epicenter of the given tumor (**Table 1**).[4] Siewert type I tumors have their epicenter located between 1 cm and 5 cm above the gastroesophageal junction. Siewert type II tumors are

Disclosures: None.
Thoracic Surgery, Division of Cardiothoracic Surgery, University of Texas Medical Branch, 301 University Boulevard, Galveston, TX 77555, USA
E-mail address: ikokerek@utmb.edu

Table 1 Siewert classification system	
	Description
Type I	Adenocarcinoma of the distal esophagus with the center located within 1 cm above and 5 cm above the anatomic esophagogastric junction.
Type II	Adenocarcinoma of the cardia with the tumor center within 1 cm above and 2 cm below the anatomic esophagogastric junction
Type III	Subcardial adenocarcinoma with the tumor center between 2 cm and 5 cm below the anatomic esophagogastric junction

From Xiao J, Liu Z, Ye P, et al. Clinical comparison of antrum-preserving double tract reconstruction vs roux-en-Y reconstruction after gastrectomy for Siewert types II and III adenocarcinoma of the esophagogastric junction. World J Gastroenterol 2015;21:9999; with permission.

centered from 1 cm above to 2 cm below the gastroesophageal junction. Siewert type III tumors have their epicenter in the cardia of the stomach, from 2 cm to 5 cm below the gastroesophageal junction, with infiltration proximal to the gastroesophageal junction. The American Joint Committee on Cancer changed the system for gastroesophageal junction tumors thereafter, including all tumors in the Siewert system as esophageal cancers. The National Comprehensive Cancer Network, alternatively, recommends that Siewert type III tumors should be treated as gastric cancers, noting that their nodal drainage differs slightly and that overall prognosis for Siewert type III tumors is worse than for Siewert type I and type II tumors.[5]

RISK FACTORS

Multiple risk factors have been identified for development of gastroesophageal junction tumors. Gastroesophageal reflux disease has been shown associated with gastroesophageal junction tumors.[6] The risk of disease seems to increase with the severity of gastroesophageal reflux disease, as measured by frequency and/or duration of symptoms.[7]

Barrett esophagus, which can be a sequela of chronic inflammation from gastroesophageal reflux disease, is also a risk factor for gastroesophageal junction tumors.[8] Long-segment Barrett esophagus, defined as a length of Barrett esophagus greater than or equal to 3 cm, has a higher risk of development of gastroesophageal junction tumors than short-segment Barrett esophagus.

Obesity has been shown an independent risk factor for gastroesophageal junction tumors. Possibly the increase in obesity rates worldwide has contributed to the increased incidence of gastroesophageal junction tumors that have been diagnosed. As body mass index increases, the risk of gastroesophageal junction cancer seems to increase as well.[9]

Dietary composition seems to have an association with gastroesophageal tumors. In particular, diets high in fats and red meats have been associated with an increased incidence of gastroesophageal cancer. In contrast, diets high in fruits, fish, and vegetables have been associated with a decreased incidence of gastroesophageal tumors.[10]

Smoking seems to lead to an increased incidence of gastroesophageal junction tumors. When compared with never-smokers, ex-smokers have a relative risk of 1.62 and current smokers having a relative risk of 2.32 of developing gastroesophageal cancer. Furthermore, the risk of gastroesophageal junction tumors increases with an increasing amount of smoking, as measured by pack-years.[11]

PRESENTATION

Most patients present with vague symptoms of dysphagia and weight loss, with an occasional patient presenting with a gastrointestinal bleed manifesting as hematemesis or dark blood per rectum. Given the ability of the esophagus and stomach to distend, most patients remain asymptomatic until presenting later with locally advanced disease. Approximately 80% of patients with gastroesophageal junction tumors present with locally advanced or diffuse metastatic disease.[12]

Many patients with gastroesophageal junction tumors also have positive lymph nodes at the time of presentation. This high incidence of lymphadenopathy occurs as a result of the anatomic configuration of the esophagus. As opposed to other organs, the esophagus has a rich submucosal plexus of lymphatic vessels and lacks a serosal layer. This rich plexus allows for spread to lymph nodes, even for superficial lesions.

DIAGNOSIS AND STAGING

Patients who present with dysphagia should have an upper gastrointestinal barium swallow as their initial diagnostic test. An example of a typical barium swallow is shown in **Fig. 1**. A result such as this should prompt an esophagogastroduodenoscopy and biopsy of the mass (**Fig. 2**).

Once a diagnosis of malignancy has been made, PET-CT scan and endoscopic ultrasound should be performed to define the full extent of disease. PET-CT scan is useful to determine whether any distant disease is present, such as in the liver or retroperitoneum. Although PET-CT is helpful for evaluation of distant metastases, it is less helpful in defining the depth of tumor invasion or presence of locoregional lymph node metastases. Endoscopic ultrasound, however, does clearly define depth of invasion and can show enlarged lymph nodes, which can be biopsied during endoscopic ultrasound if needed.

The depth of tumor invasion is an important determinant of prognosis and treatment plan. The relationship of the tumor to the muscularis propria is a useful guide to

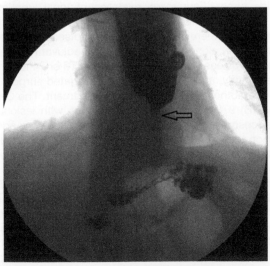

Fig. 1. Upper gastrointestinal series demonstrating narrowing of distal esophagus and gastroesophageal junction; arrow shows the area of tapering.

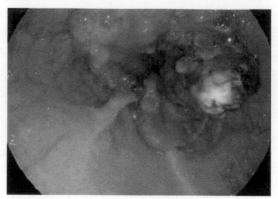

Fig. 2. Endoscopy showing gastroesophageal adenocarcinoma.

understanding T staging. Tumors that are superficial to the muscularis propria are T1 lesions. Tumors that are within the muscularis propria are T2 lesions. Tumors that extend past the muscularis propria are T3 lesions. Tumors that invade adjacent structures are classified as T4 lesions. T4 lesions are further broken down into T4a or T4b. T4a lesions involve the pleura, pericardium, or diaphragm but are still resectable. T4b lesions involve structures, such as the aorta or trachea, and are, as such, unresectable. Although histologic grade does affect prognosis in several studies, it is generally not used to determine the initial treatment plan.

PREOPERATIVE TREATMENT

Once a diagnosis is made, a treatment plan can be determined. All patients with gastroesophageal junction tumors should have a complete multimodality treatment plan determined in a multidisciplinary tumor conference. The need for preoperative chemotherapy or radiation treatment depends on the stage and location of the gastroesophageal junction tumor. Early-stage gastroesophageal junction tumors, which have not invaded the muscularis propria and have no apparent lymphadenopathy, are treated with surgery. If there is no up-staging of disease after pathologic results are reviewed, then surgery alone is sufficient and no adjuvant treatment is required.

For locally advanced disease, which is defined as a T3 or T4 lesion, or a lesion with regional lymphadenopathy, multiple trials have investigated surgery alone compared with preoperative chemotherapy and/or radiation treatment. The Cancer and Leukemia Group B (CALGB) 9781 study examined patients with lesions of the thoracic esophagus or gastroesophageal junction and showed that the addition of chemotherapy and radiation treatment prior to surgery increased the median survival from 1.79 years to 4.48 years. The overall 5-year survival rate in the same study increased from 16% to 39%.[13]

Another study, the ChemoRadiotherapy for Oesophageal cancer Followed by Surgery Study (CROSS) trial, enrolled 366 patients and evaluated preoperative chemoradiation therapy followed by surgery compared with surgery alone for esophageal and gastroesophageal junction cancers[14]; 25% of these patients had gastroesophageal junction tumors. Complete R0 resection was performed in 92% of patients who underwent preoperative treatment, compared with 69% of patients who had surgery alone. And 5-year survival was 47% in the chemoradiation treatment group compared with 24% in the group who had surgery alone.

The Medical Research Council Adjuvant Gastric Cancer Infusional Chemotherapy (MAGIC) trial investigated 503 patients with resectable cancer of the stomach, gastroesophageal junction or lower esophagus[15]; 253 patients underwent surgery alone, whereas 250 patients were given 3 cycles of preoperative chemotherapy, using epirubicin, cisplatin and 5-fluorouracil, surgery, and then an additional 3 cycles of chemotherapy after surgery; 90% of patients completed the preoperative chemotherapy, whereas only 50% of patients completed their postoperative chemotherapy. The overall 5-year survival was 36% in the perioperative chemotherapy group and 23% in the surgery alone group. It was also observed that down-staging occurred on pathologic examination due to treatment response in both the primary tumor and nodal basins. Perioperative complication rate and mortality were similar between the groups.

Recently, the role of the HER2 receptor has been investigated in patients with gastroesophageal junction tumors. HER2, a part of the human epithelial growth factor receptor group, has been studied extensively in breast cancer. Recently, however, its role in esophageal cancer has been examined. HER2 is overexpressed in approximately one-quarter of all gastroesophageal junction tumors.[16] Overexpression is associated with a more aggressive clinical course and an overall worse outcome. Trastuzumab is a recombinant humanized monoclonal antibody, which is directed against the HER2 receptor, and its role in the clinical management of patients with gastroesophageal junction tumors is being investigated in a multi-institutional phase III trial. In this trial, patients with locally advanced esophageal cancers that overexpress HER2 are randomized to receive preoperative chemoradiation with or without trastuzumab. A previous study evaluating patients with unresectable esophageal cancers showed that the addition of trastuzumab to a standard chemotherapy regimen increased survival.[17]

SURGERY

Patients who undergo preoperative treatment are restaged after completion of treatment. Regardless of the Siewert classification, the surgical management of gastroesophageal junction tumors involves resection of the esophagus and stomach with wide margins around the tumor. In general, it is best to achieve at least 5 cm margins both proximal and distal to the gastroesophageal junction tumor. This margin distance is based on numerous studies that have shown that microscopic disease can be present centimeters away from the mass.[18] One study showed that patients with gastroesophageal junction tumors who had fewer than 7 positive lymph nodes experienced increased survival when surgical margin was greater than 3.8 cm. Patients with 7 or more positive lymph nodes did not experience the same survival benefit with this surgical margin.[19]

There are several open approaches that can be used to perform an esophagectomy. For a transhiatal esophagectomy, a midline laparotomy and a left cervical incision are made. The stomach is mobilized and the thoracic esophagus is bluntly dissected. This approach avoids a thoracotomy and the potential resultant pulmonary morbidity but is less desirable for midesophageal lesions, which would be less amenable to blunt dissection away from surrounding mediastinal structures. Also, subcarinal and upper paraesophageal lymph nodes are not accessible when performing a transhiatal esophagectomy.

A left thoracoabdominal incision allows excellent access to the distal esophagus and stomach. This technique is less frequently used, however, because the wound is large and it is a painful incision.

Although a majority of esophagectomies worldwide are performed as open procedures, minimally invasive approaches are increasing in prevalence with time. The author's center performs almost all of the gastroesophageal junction tumor resections minimally invasively, and the Ivor Lewis esophagectomy is the preferred technique. The approach is described.

General endotracheal anesthesia should be administered using a double-lumen endotracheal tube. It is appropriate and more efficient to intubate the patient just once with a double-lumen tube as opposed to intubating initially with a single-lumen tube and then exchanging endotracheal tubes prior to entering the chest. An arterial line should be placed for blood pressure monitoring. Two large-bore intravenous lines are adequate for resuscitation, and a central line should rarely be needed. Most procedures can be completed minimally invasively and an epidural catheter is usually not needed for postoperative analgesic relief. An orogastric tube should be placed for gastric decompression.

The configuration of the port sites for the abdomen and chest is shown in **Fig. 3**. After the abdomen is prepped and draped, a 12-mm port is placed in the left epigastric area for the camera. Another 12-mm port is placed in the right epigastric area, approximately 1 handbreadth away from the camera port. Two 5-mm ports are placed in the right upper quadrant, with the port furthest to the patient's right side acting as the liver retractor. One 5-mm port is placed in the left upper quadrant.

Dissection should begin with division of the gastrohepatic ligament. This division should be performed with an energy device, such as an ultrasonic scalpel instrument. Rarely, an accessory left hepatic vessel may course through this ligament. This dissection should proceed to the level of the right crus of the diaphragm. At this point the left gastric pedicle can be dissected as well.

Next, the greater curvature is mobilized by dividing the gastrocolic and gastrosplenic ligaments, and the short gastric vessels that course along this area. At least

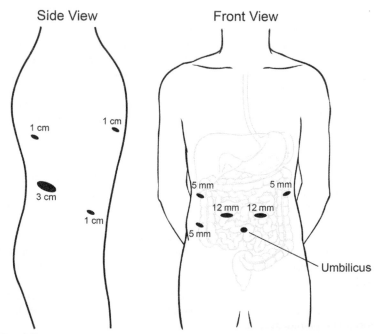

Fig 3. Minimally invasive port placement sites in the chest and abdomen for minimally invasive Ivor Lewis esophagectomy.

40% to 50% of the greater curvature should be mobilized to ensure adequate length of the gastric conduit. When retracting along the greater curvature, excessive force can lead to splenic injury and significant bleeding and possibly the need for a splenectomy. The principal blood supply of the gastric conduit is the right gastroepiploic artery, and care must be taken to preserve this artery and prevent damage to it during the dissection of the greater curvature. During the dissection, the energy device should be no closer than several millimeters away from the gastroepiploic artery, to prevent inadvertent thermal damage to the artery. Injury to the right gastroepiploic artery may lead to gastric conduit necrosis, a condition associated with high morbidity and mortality.

Once the lesser and greater curvatures have been mobilized, the esophagus and gastroesophageal junction are encircled. With this maneuver, the left gastric pedicle should be fully isolated. The left gastric pedicle can then be divided with a vascular stapling device. The stapler should be placed as close to the retroperitoneum as possible, to allow for as wide a lymph node retrieval as possible in this area.

The gastric conduit should then be divided after the orogastric tube has been removed. The author's practice is to make the conduit approximately 4 cm to 5 cm in width. The specimen is then temporarily sutured to the distal esophagus, to allow delivery of the stomach into the chest during the thoracic portion of the operation. A Kocher maneuver is then performed to ensure adequate length of the conduit. There are different strategies used to address gastric emptying across different centers. At the author's institution, a pyloromyotomy is performed. Many centers alternatively perform a pyloroplasty, injection of botulinum toxin into the pylorus, or no procedure at all for gastric emptying. The author performs a pyloromyotomy in Heineke-Mikulicz fashion. The first step is to divide the muscle layer of the pylorus longitudinally for approximately 4 cm, centered across the pylorus. The muscle layer is then closed transversely, thereby avoiding excessive narrowing of the pylorus.

A jejunal feeding catheter should be considered to be placed in all cases, because the patient may require supplemental nutrition for several weeks before oral intake can meet metabolic demands. The port furthest to the patient's left side is used as the insertion site for the catheter, to avoid an additional puncture through the abdomen, and a 14-French soft red rubber catheter is used as the tube. Each of the 12-mm ports has its fascia closed prior to skin closure.

Four small incisions are made in the chest. The camera is inserted in the midaxillary line through a 1-cm incision at the seventh or eighth intercostal space, depending on the patient's body habitus. A posterior 1-cm incision in the eighth intercostal space is created for retraction. A 1-cm incision is created anteriorly in the sixth intercostal space at the anterior axillary line. Finally, a 1-cm incision is created anteriorly in the fourth intercostal space at the anterior axillary line. The inferior pulmonary ligament is divided and the lung is retracted anteriorly. With the patient rotated slightly anteriorly, the lung should retract without the need of an additional lung retractor of any kind.

The pleura overlying the esophagus is divided and the esophagus is encircled. A pliable Penrose drain can be placed around the esophagus and used for retraction, or the esophagus can be grabbed directly if care is taken not to tear it. The dissection of the esophagus should proceed to the level of the azygous vein. Direct feeding vessels from the aorta should be divided using an energy device. Mediastinal lymph nodes in the inferior pulmonary ligament, paraesophageal area, and subcarinal regions should be dissected and sent for pathologic review. The azygous vein should be encircled and divided using a vascular stapler.

The esophagus is then divided at approximately the level of the azygous vein. The gastric conduit should be pulled completely into the chest to make sure there is adequate length before deciding on the proximal division point. The specimen is placed into an impermeable plastic or mesh bag, to prevent port site implantation of tumor. The incision with the camera is then lengthened to allow for removal of the specimen.

To perform the anastomosis a small gastrotomy is made, close to the tip of the gastric conduit and just large enough to allow a circular 25-mm stapler to fit. The accepting anvil can be placed transorally by the anesthesia team and passed down to the staple line on the esophagus. A small hole, just large enough to accept the anvil, is then created on the esophagus. The hole should be created within 2 mm to 3 mm of the staple line but not on the staple line directly. The anastomosis is then performed in end-to-side fashion. The gastrotomy and excess stomach are divided using a linear stapler. The author's practice is to perform an esophagogastroscopy after the stapling to assess the anastomosis and to place a nasogastric tube in the appropriate position. Almost all patients can be extubated at the end of the case. Most patients should not need to go to the intensive care unit postoperatively.

If the tumor involves a large amount of the stomach or the stomach cannot be used for any particular reason, the colon is an excellent alternative as a conduit. The author's preferred approach is to use the ascending colon in an isoperistaltic fashion. The colon is routed substernally and the proximal anastomosis performed between the esophagus and the colon. The distal anastomosis is between the colon and the remaining stomach, or a Roux-en-Y jejunal limb can be used if the entire stomach has to be resected.

POSTOPERATIVE CARE

Tube feeds can be begun early in the postoperative course as the patient recovers and the esophagogastric anastomosis heals. A gastrograffin swallow should be performed on postoperative days 5 to 7, although many centers do not routinely perform this test. Most patients can be discharged to home with a soft oral diet and maintenance tube feeds.

An anastomotic leak after an Ivor Lewis esophagectomy can be a fatal complication if not recognized early but in most cases can be treated with minimal morbidity to the patient. Tachycardia is often the first presenting sign of an anastomotic leak. Fever and rising white blood cell count can accompany an anastomotic leak as well. Diagnosis should be made with a gastrograffin swallow and confirmed with esophagoscopy. Once recognized, placement of an esophageal stent across the anastomosis often resolves most cases. Any pleural effusion that has accumulated should be drained by tube thoracostomy. Overall the incidence of anastomotic leak has decreased significantly over the past 2 decades, and the average incidence of anastomotic leak after Ivor Lewis esophagectomy is approximately 3%.[20]

Although rare, chylothorax can be a persistent and burdensome complication of esophagectomy. An increased amount of drainage from the chest tube, especially after initiation of jejunal feeds or an oral diet, can be the first sign of chylothorax. Classically the character of the chest tube drainage is thin, milky fluid, but the chest tube drainage can also be serous. Measurement of the triglyceride level is diagnostic, with levels usually greater than 500 mg/dL. Initial treatment should be cessation of diet and total parenteral nutrition. A low-fat diet can be maintained if chest tube drainage does not remain excessive. If these initial measures do not work, then surgery to ligate the thoracic duct may be necessary. At many centers, the interventional radiology team may be able to perform a thoracic duct embolization percutaneously using lymphoscintigraphy.

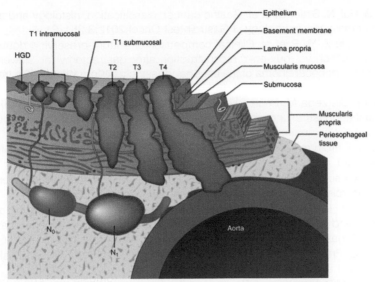

Fig. 4. Staging system for gastroesophageal junction tumors and survival by stage. HGD, high grade dysplasia. (*From* Spicer JD, Dhupar R, Kim JY, et al. Esophagus. In: Townsend CM, editor. Sabiston textbook of surgery. 20th edition. Philadelphia: Elsevier, 2017. p. 1031; with permission.)

Overall 30-day mortality rates range from 1% to 10%.[21] Centers that perform a high volume of esophagectomies, defined as greater than 20 esophagectomies each year, tend to experience lower mortality rates than low-volume centers.[22]

PROGNOSIS

Fig. 4 shows the 5-year survival for each stage. Among patients who undergo preoperative chemoradiation treatment, those who achieve a complete pathologic response have a 55% 5-year survival compared with 27% 5-year survival in patients who have persistent disease.[23]

SUMMARY

Gastroesophageal junction tumors have increased in incidence over the past 40 years. Management of patients with these tumors should be conducted using a multidisciplinary approach, because the majority of these patients present with locally advanced disease. Among patients with locally advanced disease, perioperative chemoradiation or treatment with chemotherapy seems to confer a survival advantage compared with surgery alone. Most surgeries can be performed minimally invasively with excellent outcomes. Prognosis varies by stage and patients who experience a complete pathologic response to preoperative chemoradiation treatment have the best long-term outcomes.

REFERENCES

1. Zhang Y. Epidemiology of esophageal cancer. World J Gastroenterol 2013;19: 5598–606.
2. Buas M, Vaughan T. Epidemiology and risk factors for gastroesophageal junction tumors: understanding the rising incidence of this disease. Semin Radiat Oncol 2013;23:3–9.

3. Hu B, Hajj N, Sittler S, et al. Gastric cancer: classification, histology and application of molecular pathology. J Gastrointest Oncol 2012;3:251–61.
4. Xiao J, Liu Z, Ye P, et al. Clinical comparison of antrum-preserving double tract reconstruction vs roux-en-Y reconstruction after gastrectomy for Siewert types II and III adenocarcinoma of the esophagogastric junction. World J Gastroenterol 2015;21:9999–10007.
5. Kulig P, Sierzega M, Pach R, et al. Differences in prognosis of Siewert II and III oesophagogastric junction cancers are determined by the baseline tumour staging but not its anatomical location. Eur J Surg Oncol 2016;42:1215–21.
6. Souza R. From reflux esophagitis to esophageal adenocarcinoma. Dig Dis 2016; 34:483–90.
7. Chak A, Faulx A, Eng C, et al. Gastroesophageal reflux symptoms in patients with adenocarcinoma of the esophagus or cardia. Cancer 2006;107:2160–6.
8. Weston A, Krmpotich P, Makdisi W, et al. Short segment Barrett's esophagus: clinical and histological features, associated endoscopic findings, and association with gastric intestinal metaplasia. Am J Gastroenterol 1996;91:981–6.
9. Abnet C, Freedman N, Hollenbeck A. A prospective study of BMI and risk of oesophageal and gastric adenocarcinoma. Eur J Cancer 2008;44:465–7.
10. Jiang G, Li B, Liao X, et al. Poultry and fish intake and risk of esophageal cancer: a meta-analysis of observational studies. Asia Pac J Clin Oncol 2016;12:82–91.
11. Kabat G, Ng S, Wynder E. Tobacco, alcohol intake, and diet in relation to adenocarcinoma of the esophagus and gastric cardia. Cancer Causes Control 1993;4: 123–32.
12. Markar S, Karthikesalingam A, Low DE. Outcomes assessment of the surgical management of esophageal cancer in younger and older patients. Ann Thorac Surg 2012;94:1652–8.
13. Tepper J, Krasna M, Niedzwiecki D, et al. Phase III trial of trimodality therapy with cisplatin, fluorouracil, radiotherapy, and surgery compared with surgery alone for esophageal cancer: CALGB 9781. J Clin Oncol 2008;26:1086–92.
14. Van Hagen P, Hulshof J, Van Lanschot E, et al. Preoperative chemoradiotherapy for esophageal or junctional cancer. N Engl J Med 2012;366:2074–84.
15. Cunningham D, Allum W, Stenning S, et al. Perioperative chemotherapy versus surgery alone for resectable gastroesophageal cancer. N Engl J Med 2006; 355:11–20.
16. Niu J, Weber J, Gelbspan D. Change of HER2 status in metastatic esophageal adenocarcinoma: heterogeneity of the disease? Case report and review of literature. J Gastrointest Oncol 2012;3:358–61.
17. Safran H, DiPetrillo T, Akerman P, et al. Phase I/II study of trastuzumab, paclitaxel, cisplatin and radiation for locally advanced, HER2 overexpressing, esophageal adenocarcinoma. Int J Rad Oncol 2007;67:405–9.
18. Casson A, Darnton S, Subramanian S. What is the optimal distal resection margin for esophageal carcinoma? Ann Thorac Surg 2000;69:205–9.
19. Barbour A, Rizk N, Gonen M, et al. Adenocarcinoma of the gastroesophageal junction: influence of esophageal resection margin and operative approach on outcome. Ann Surg 2007;246:1–8.
20. Van Daele E, Van de Putte D, Ceelen W. Risk factors and consequences of anastomotic leakage after Ivor Lewis oesphagectomy. Interact Cardiovasc Thorac Surg 2016;22:32–7.
21. Stavrou E, Ward R, Pearson S. Oesophagectomy rates and post-resection outcomes in patients with cancer of the oesophagus and gastro-oesophageal

junction: a population-based study using linked health administrative linked data. BMC Health Serv Res 2012;12:384.

22. Metzger R, Bollschweiler E, Vallbohmer D, et al. High volume centers for esophagectomy: what is the number needed to achieve low postoperative mortality? Dis Esophagus 2004;17:310–4.

23. Donahue J, Nichols F, Li Z, et al. Complete pathologic response after neoadjuvant chemoradiotherapy for esophageal cancer is associated with enhanced survival. Ann Thorac Surg 2009;87:392–8.

Postgastrectomy Syndromes and Nutritional Considerations Following Gastric Surgery

CrossMark

Jeremy L. Davis, MD*, R. Taylor Ripley, MD

KEYWORDS

- Postgastrectomy syndromes • Nutritional deficiencies • Dumping • Bile reflux
- Roux-en-Y

KEY POINTS

- Postgastrectomy syndromes are common sequelae of surgery for gastric cancer.
- Dumping syndrome is a common postgastrectomy complication diagnosed in the presence of classic symptoms and appropriate clinical history.
- Afferent and efferent loop syndromes most often require operative intervention for syndrome resolution.
- Nutritional deficiencies and perioperative nutritional supplementation are common, especially after total gastrectomy.

INTRODUCTION

Late postoperative complications of gastrectomy may present as a constellation of symptoms and signs referred to as postgastrectomy syndromes. These syndromes result from alterations in anatomy and function of the stomach and proximal small intestine. Although some syndromes occur in isolation, patients may present with various symptoms that warrant a thorough understanding of both cause and treatment. Historically, elective operations for both benign and malignant disorders of the stomach provided surgeons with experience in recognition and treatment of these syndromes. Elective operation for peptic ulcer disease has declined dramatically and is associated with both decreased prevalence and familiarity with postgastrectomy syndromes.[1–3] Meanwhile, bariatric surgery volume has grown substantially, making it the most likely cause of postgastrectomy syndromes and nutritional deficiencies.[4–6] The low incidence of gastric cancer in the western hemisphere also suggests that variations in the resection and reconstruction that are reported to prevent or treat

Surgical Oncology Section, Thoracic & Gastrointestinal Oncology Branch, National Cancer Institute, 10 Center Drive, MSC1201, Room 4-3940, Bethesda, MD 20892, USA
* Corresponding author.
E-mail address: Jeremy.Davis@nih.gov

Surg Clin N Am 97 (2017) 277–293
http://dx.doi.org/10.1016/j.suc.2016.11.005
0039-6109/17/Published by Elsevier Inc.

surgical.theclinics.com

postgastrectomy syndromes are doubtful routine for surgeons performing gastrectomy for malignancy in the United States.[7] This article focuses on the cause, diagnosis, and treatment of classic postgastrectomy syndromes (**Table 1**) and nutritional considerations in patients with gastric cancer.

ANATOMY AND PATHOPHYSIOLOGY

The proximal and distal stomach, including the pylorus, has separate and distinct functions, including storage, mechanical breakdown, preliminary digestion, and emptying of food. Extrinsic and intrinsic innervation of the stomach, endocrine and paracrine signaling, and duodenogastric feedback each provide coordinated control of normal gastric function. The proximal stomach undergoes vagal-mediated receptive relaxation and accommodation during ingestion of a meal and generates tonic contractions to aid in transport of contents to the distal stomach. The distal stomach produces slow-wave, circumferential contractions (3 per minute) that result in the transport and mechanical trituration of large food particles.[8] Control of gastric emptying varies based on the pressure gradient between the stomach and duodenum and resistance to flow across the pylorus, signaling via various gastrointestinal hormones, and coordinated duodenal contractions. Even though parasympathetic vagal innervation speeds gastric emptying, the effect of vagotomy on emptying is variable depending on the level of transection of the vagi and associated gastric resection, specifically related to the elimination of the antrum and pylorus.[9] Emptying of liquids occurs before solids and is aided by tonic contraction of the proximal stomach.[10] Thus, vagotomy can eliminate the receptive relaxation and accommodation of the proximal stomach and may result in more rapid emptying of liquids. Digestible solid food is retained until the mechanical process reduces particles to 1 mm followed by the coordinated transport of chyme into the duodenum. Loss of truncal vagal tone releases normal suppression of antral pacemakers and can therefore disrupt normal emptying; in contrast, highly selective vagotomy (parietal cell vagotomy) induces

Table 1 Postgastrectomy syndromes		
Syndrome	**First-line Therapy**	**Second-line Therapy**
Dumping	Dietary modifications	Roux-en-Y gastrojejunostomy
Small gastric remnant	Dietary modifications	Jejunal pouch[a]
Postvagotomy diarrhea	Dietary modification	Antiperistaltic jejunal segment
Delayed gastric emptying/gastric atony	Prokinetic medication	Completion gastrectomy, conversion to Roux-en-Y
Afferent loop syndrome	Address obstruction based on cause	Roux-en-Y gastrojejunostomy
Efferent loop syndrome	Assess obstruction based on cause	None
Roux stasis	Completion gastrectomy, Roux-en-Y gastrojejunostomy	Feeding jejunostomy
Bile reflux gastritis	Attempt medical therapy (eg, cholestyramine)	Roux-en-Y gastrojejunostomy; Braun enteroenterostomy; jejunal interposition

[a] Not advocated routinely.

faster transit of liquids but normal solid emptying.[11] In addition to altered gastric anatomy and innervation, the normal function of gastric mucosa to secrete acid and enzymes, and produce mucus, hormones, and intrinsic factor, is also disrupted by gastrectomy and contributes to the increased incidence of postgastrectomy syndromes (**Fig. 1**).[9]

DUMPING SYNDROME

The syndrome of rapid emptying of gastric contents was first described more than a century ago and the term dumping was applied soon after.[12,13] Dumping is characterized based on timing of onset and constellation of symptoms. It is a frequent postgastrectomy syndrome for which diagnosis is based primarily on inciting factors and the presence of classic symptoms (**Box 1**). Vasomotor symptoms include diaphoresis, flushing, dizziness, and palpitations. Gastrointestinal symptoms may consist of abdominal fullness, crampy pain, nausea, and diarrhea. Early dumping begins within 30 minutes of food consumption and manifests with both gastrointestinal and vasomotor symptoms, whereas late dumping occurs 2 to 4 hours after a meal and consists primarily of vasomotor symptoms and associated hypoglycemia. Both forms of the syndrome occur in response to rapid gastric emptying of hyperosmolar contents into the proximal intestine.[14] Patients with this distressing syndrome may react by decreasing oral intake, often resulting in weight loss and malnutrition. Incidence is variable and ranges from 20% to more than 50% of patients showing some symptoms, depending on the type of operation.[15–18] In a survey of Japanese patients after gastrectomy, the incidence of at least 1 symptom of early dumping syndrome was greater than 60%, whereas the incidence of late dumping was nearly 50%.[19]

Emptying of the distal stomach is controlled primarily by cyclic contractions of the antrum and coordinated pyloric resistance. Under normal conditions the distal stomach functions to retain, grind, and control emptying of small food particles into the duodenum. The rapid transit of hyperosmolar carbohydrate into the small intestine results in fluid shift from the intravascular space into the bowel lumen and release of multiple enteric hormones, including vasoactive inhibitory peptide, gastric inhibitory peptide, neurotensin, and serotonin.[20–22] Gastrointestinal hormone release is thought to affect gastrointestinal secretion, motility, and splanchnic blood flow. The relative intravascular hypovolemia induces release of epinephrine, resulting in the classic

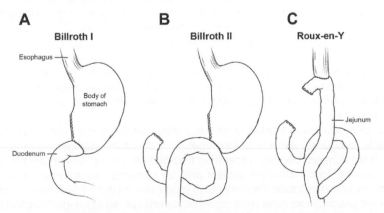

Fig. 1. Common postgastrectomy reconstruction; Billroth I gastroduodenostomy (*A*), Billroth II gastrojejunostomy (*B*), and Roux-en-Y esophagojejunostomy (*C*).

> **Box 1**
> **Dumping syndromes**
>
> *Early dumping (10–30 minutes after meal)*
> - Gastrointestinal symptoms: abdominal pain, diarrhea, bloating, nausea, borborygmus
> - Vasomotor symptoms: flushing, palpitations, diaphoresis, tachycardia, syncope, hypotension
>
> *Late dumping (2–4 hours after meal)*
> - Hypoglycemia
> - Vasomotor symptoms: flushing, palpitations, diaphoresis, syncope, tremulousness, hunger

vasomotor symptoms of the syndrome.[23] Luminal carbohydrate also stimulates release of enteroglucagon, resulting in hyperinsulinism and hypoglycemia, which also contribute to vasomotor symptoms and adrenaline response in late dumping.[24]

Rapid gastric emptying associated with dumping is the potential consequence of multiple surgical alterations. Operations resulting in loss of receptive relaxation and accommodation of the proximal stomach (as with vagotomy), loss of gastric capacity or control of emptying, and loss of duodenal feedback inhibition of emptying may all lead to dumping.[25–27] Extensive gastrectomy that impairs accommodation and reservoir function of the proximal stomach results in additional rapid emptying of liquids. Operations that not only eliminate the distal stomach but also bypass duodenal feedback on the stomach, such as Billroth II, may result in higher incidence of dumping compared with other gastric procedures. Thus, it is expected that total and subtotal (≥80%) gastrectomy are associated with a greater incidence of dumping than antrectomy.[16] Although the mode of reconstruction after distal gastrectomy may contribute to symptom development, it probably has less of an impact than extent of resection.[28,29] A study by Nunobe and colleagues[30] showed no difference in symptoms of dumping between distal gastrectomy patients undergoing Roux-en-Y and Billroth I reconstruction. Even so, operative techniques designed to maintain pyloric function via preservation, reconstruction, and normal gastrointestinal transit have been proposed.[7,31,32]

Empiric treatment based on symptoms alone often substantiates the diagnosis, but diagnostic tests can be used. Assessment of gastric emptying using a technetium-labeled meal can be a helpful adjunct; if gastric emptying is normal, dumping can be excluded.[33,34] A clinical scoring system developed by Sigstad[35] may aid in diagnosis, as can provocative oral glucose challenge, which was found to be highly sensitive and specific for dumping.[35,36] Quality-of-life questionnaires commonly used to assess gastrointestinal symptoms also can be useful in identifying patients with this and other syndromes.[37,38] Endoscopy and contrast-enhanced fluoroscopic imaging of the upper gastrointestinal tract serves to define anatomy and aid in diagnosis of other syndromes.

Dumping syndrome is treated most frequently through dietary modifications. Our practice is to counsel patients before operation about the postgastrectomy diet of at least 6 small meals per day, separating liquids from solids, limiting simple sugars, and consuming foods with high protein and fat contents. Attempts to slow gastric emptying by increasing food viscosity using guar gum or pectin are generally not tolerated. Some practitioners have recommended acarbose, an alpha-glycosidase hydrolase inhibitor, to interfere with carbohydrate absorption, thereby limiting symptoms associated with late dumping.[39,40] If symptoms become refractory to dietary modifications, medical treatment with somatostatin analogues is recommended.[41–43] Short-acting and long-acting formulations of octreotide slow gastric emptying, impede intestinal transit, and inhibit gastrointestinal hormone release.[44] The largest study evaluating symptom control with short-acting and long-acting octreotide showed improvement in both early and late dumping symptoms with favorable quality of life in patients receiving long-acting octreotide.[41] Despite disadvantages of long-term somatostatin analogue use, improvements in quality of life may be worthwhile for patients in whom this treatment is necessary.

Surgical treatment of dumping syndrome refractory to dietary and medical therapy is uncommon and depends on the preceding type of gastrectomy. Operations to restore duodenal transit by converting Billroth type II to Billroth type I or to delay emptying by narrowing the gastroenterostomy have been proposed.[27,45] Conversion to Roux-en-Y is considered the most desirable procedure, whereas reconstruction of a previously ablated pylorus and interposition of an antiperistaltic jejunal segment have been described.[31,34] Numerous methods of pouch construction are designed to increase receptive capacity after total gastrectomy. A meta-analysis suggests lower incidence of dumping syndrome and improved quality of life in patients with a pouch.[46]

SMALL GASTRIC REMNANT

Loss of reservoir function of the stomach may result in small gastric remnant syndrome, also referred to as early satiety syndrome. Symptoms include early satiety, epigastric pain soon after eating, and vomiting. Symptoms occur most often when greater than 80% of the stomach is removed. Weight loss is common and vitamin and mineral deficiencies are present as in other postgastrectomy syndromes. The cause is loss of gastric capacity through resection or vagotomy resulting in loss of receptive relaxation and accommodation. Similar symptoms may be seen in patients with delayed gastric emptying, or gastric atony. The primary mode of treatment is dietary modification.

DELAYED GASTRIC EMPTYING

Although delayed gastric emptying is observed in settings besides gastrectomy, its clinical presentation warrants mention. Retention of food within the gastric remnant has been observed on endoscopy in patients after distal gastrectomy; however, most studies have found no association between retention and symptoms.[47,48] Delayed emptying is seen more frequently after Billroth I than Billroth II or Roux-en-Y. Medical treatment with prokinetic agents may help symptoms and complete resection of the gastric remnant for chronic gastric atony is rare.[49]

POSTVAGOTOMY DIARRHEA

Although any type of gastrectomy can result in postoperative diarrhea, it is most frequently associated with vagotomy. Incidence is highest with truncal vagotomy, and lowest among selective vagotomy procedures. The diarrhea is usually episodic, explosive, and unrelated to oral intake, and therefore distinguishable from diarrhea associated with dumping. The mechanisms are multifactorial and attributed to alterations in the rate of flow of enteric contents, including gastric emptying of liquids, consequences of small bowel and biliary vagal denervation, and relative malabsorption related to altered anatomy and transit. Diagnosis can be challenging and common causes of diarrhea must be considered. Although symptoms may resolve over the course of several months, dietary modification to avoid instigating foods and fiber supplementation may be effective. Medical therapy with antidiarrheal agents, such as loperamide, and the bile acid sequestrant cholestyramine can be useful.[50] Surgical therapy is not routine, although antiperistaltic jejunal segments have been described to slow intestinal transit.[51]

ROUX STASIS SYNDROME

Roux stasis syndrome manifests in patients as postprandial fullness, pain or gas bloating, and nausea, followed by vomiting that relieves the pain.[52–55] When the syndrome becomes chronic with severe symptoms, weight loss and malnutrition may develop. Patients often adapt by consuming a diet of only liquids. The pathophysiology is likely secondary to vagotomy and transection of the proximal small bowel during Roux creation. Vagotomy results in delayed gastric emptying, whereas small bowel transection disrupts action potentials that coordinate small bowel contractions.[56] As expected, patients with Roux-en-Y gastroenterostomy are at higher risk than patients with esophagojejunostomy.[55,57] A retrospective review performed at the Mayo Clinic revealed that 30% of 202 patients had symptoms consistent with Roux stasis syndrome after gastrojejunostomy.[58] However, they reported that only 6% (2 out of 32) had symptoms consistent with Roux stasis syndrome after esophagojejunostomy. These findings suggest that the atonic gastric remnant is often responsible for the disorder. Characteristics of the Roux are also causal factors, as noted by scintigraphic measurements of Roux limb transit time that are noted to be decreased in both animal and human studies.[57,59,60]

Diagnosis depends on timing and is defined as early (<90 days postoperatively) or late. In the early syndrome, small bowel obstruction must be ruled out with a computed tomography (CT) scan. In the late setting, CT scan helps rule out internal hernia, adhesive bowel obstruction, malignant recurrence, and possible anastomotic stricture. Endoscopy and fluoroscopic upper gastrointestinal studies should be performed to look for other disorder because this syndrome is a diagnosis of exclusion. Scintigraphic imaging can measure gastric emptying and Roux limb transit and is the most useful test for this syndrome; regardless of results, treatment depends on severity of symptoms and not radiographic findings.[61]

Dietary management is preferred because both medical and surgical treatment often have unsatisfactory results. Small, frequent meals are recommended and liquids often are tolerated better than a solid diet. If small meals do not provide enough calories, nutritional supplements can augment caloric intake. Medical management consists of metoclopramide and erythromycin; however, these drugs are better at acute management rather than long-term symptom relief. Surgical treatment consists of resection of the remnant stomach with Roux-en-Y esophagojejunostomy. If the patient has already had a total gastrectomy or the Roux limb is the cause of this syndrome, this approach will not work. Often, the only surgical management consists of placing a jejunostomy tube to maintain adequate nutrition.

BILE (ALKALINE) REFLUX GASTRITIS

Symptoms of bile reflux gastritis are burning epigastric pain, nausea with vomiting that does not relieve the pain, and pain that is only partially associated with meals.[62,63] The vomitus contains bile mixed with food. Over time, patients can experience weight loss and anemia. Symptoms usually occur 1 to 3 years after gastrectomy.[64] Bile reflux gastritis is attributed to chronic exposure of the gastric remnant to biliopancreatic secretions caused by loss of the pylorus. It is most frequently found after Billroth II, with decreased incidence after Billroth I and pyloroplasty. This syndrome is less common given both the reduction in gastrectomy for peptic ulcer disease and preference for Roux-en-Y reconstruction. A prospective randomized trial reported fewer symptoms and reduced histologic evidence of inflammation for patients undergoing Roux-en-Y versus Billroth II reconstruction.[65,66]

For accurate diagnosis, the most important findings are pain, nausea, and bilious vomiting associated with endoscopic findings of bile and inflammation in the distal stomach. However, diagnosis can be difficult because almost all patients have some bile reflux and inflammation without symptoms. No correlation between the degree of inflammation and symptoms has been established. Ruling out other causes before establishing a diagnosis is critical. The differential diagnosis includes peptic ulcer disease, afferent loop syndrome, efferent loop syndrome, adhesive or malignant bowel obstruction, and marginal ulceration. The bilious reflux mixed with food without relief of pain distinguishes this syndrome from afferent loop syndrome. A CT scan should be obtained to rule out small bowel obstruction. A hepatobiliary iminodiacetic acid (HIDA) scan may reveal pooling of bile in the stomach and scintigraphy may reveal lack of gastric emptying. Endoscopy is critical to assess the anastomosis and the gastric remnant. Findings that indicate bile reflux include erythema, bile in the stomach, thickened gastric folds, atrophy, and petechiae.[67] Biopsy is required and may reveal chronic inflammation, foveolar hyperplasia, intestinal metaplasia, and acute inflammation.[67]

Medical treatment is usually ineffective, although it should be attempted before considering surgical options. Theoretically, cholestyramine should bind bile acids and reduce inflammation and reflux. However, a study randomizing patients to cholestyramine versus placebo found no symptom relief or differences in histologic findings.[68] Studies of ursodeoxycholic acid and sucralfate have shown minimal effect.[69,70] Other options include antacids, promotility agents, histamine receptor blockers, proton pump inhibitors, and anticholinergic agents. However, no medical treatment seems to lead to consistent symptom relief.

Surgical therapy is the mainstay of treatment, which consists of Roux-en-Y gastrojejunostomy to divert biliopancreatic contents away from the gastric remnant.[64,71–75] Regardless of whether patients have undergone Billroth II or Billroth I, reconstruction with a Roux-en-Y is recommended with at least a 60-cm Roux limb. The remnant stomach may need revision to a smaller volume depending on preoperative assessment of gastroparesis in order to decrease the incidence of Roux-en-Y syndrome, which develops in 10% to 15% of patients. Despite Roux-en-Y reconstruction, up to 40% of patients still experience reflux. Other operations include Braun enteroenterostomy, the Henley jejunal interposition, and the duodenal switch.[76–78] Braun enteroenterostomy is the simplest operation to correct reflux gastritis. It consists of an anastomosis between the afferent and efferent limbs after a Billroth II gastrojejunostomy. The anastomosis should be 45 to 60 cm distal to the gastrojejunostomy. Occlusion of the afferent limb between the enteroenterostomy and the gastrojejunostomy may further decrease reflux. The Henley jejunal interposition consists of an isoperistaltic 40-cm segment of proximal jejunum placed between the gastric remnant and duodenum.[76] This reconstruction can be used after either Billroth I or II. The duodenal switch procedure is used for patients with reflux through an intact pylorus. The duodenum is transected 2 to 4 cm distal to the pylorus, the distal duodenal end is closed, and the proximal end is connected to a Roux-en-Y jejunal limb.[79] The enteroenterostomy should be 60 cm distal to the duodenojejunostomy. One study compared Roux-en-Y with a long Roux limb with Henley loop and with the duodenal switch operation.[77] This comparison showed that all of these operations are reasonable in appropriately selected patients with the emphasis on creating longer Henley loops and Roux limbs.

AFFERENT LOOP SYNDROME

Patients with afferent loop syndrome have classic symptoms of immediate postprandial pain and cramping, followed by vomiting that completely relieves the pain without food debris in the vomitus. This syndrome is extremely uncommon, occurring in less than 1% of patients, particularly given the infrequency of gastrectomy with Billroth II gastrojejunostomy. Afferent loop obstruction has several causes, including hernias, volvulus, kinking at the anastomosis, marginal ulceration, adhesions, recurrent cancer, and intussusception. Some reports suggest that longer afferent limbs and anastomosis to the lesser curve may increase this risk.

Both acute and chronic afferent loop syndromes may develop.[80] Acute afferent loop syndrome usually occurs within 1 to 2 weeks postoperatively and may be attributed to gastroparesis or ileus, but the distinction is critical because acute afferent loop syndrome may lead to duodenal stump leak. Preventing duodenal stump leak during an acute obstruction is a surgical emergency. In the absence of a duodenal leak, biliopancreatic secretions result in increased pressure with a distended duodenum. The lack of routine decompression leads to a blind loop with bacterial overgrowth, vitamin B_{12} deficiency, bile salt deconjugation, steatorrhea, and iron deficiency. In the chronic, partially obstructive form, the closed loop is intermittently decompressed into the gastric remnant, which results in the characteristic bilious emesis without food.

CT is the primary imaging modality, in which a distended afferent limb is commonly seen and evaluation for malignant disease or sites of obstruction also can be appreciated. Endoscopy can aid in diagnosis but is more useful at evaluating for bile reflux. HIDA scan may reveal secretion into the duodenum without transit into the stomach, but is rarely necessary to confirm the diagnosis.

Primary treatment is surgical. In the acute setting, operation is emergent and, if delayed, necrosis of all or part of the duodenum is possible. With partial necrosis, the afferent limb can be preserved. Although rare, complete necrosis of the afferent limb requires pancreaticoduodenectomy. In the absence of limb necrosis, 2 surgical options are common. If the afferent limb is sufficient in length a Braun enteroenterostomy between the afferent and efferent limbs allows decompression of the afferent limb with minimal dissection and no bowel transection. Conversion to Roux-en-Y gastrojejunostomy is the most frequent reconstructive option.[53] The jejunojejunostomy should be at least 50 cm to 60 cm distal to the gastrojejunostomy. Percutaneous and endoscopic relief of the obstruction also have been reported. For patients with malignant recurrences and short survival, surgery may be avoided by endoscopic placement of a self-expanding stent within the obstructed afferent limb. Alternatively, for patients with obstructive jaundice and dilated biliary ducts, percutaneous transhepatic self-expanding nitinol stenting has been described.[81]

EFFERENT LOOP SYNDROME

Efferent loop syndrome is a mechanical obstruction at the Billroth II gastrojejunostomy site or beyond. The obstruction is similar to a small bowel obstruction and presents with distention, nausea, and emesis. The obstruction can be acute or chronic, partial or complete. Bilious emesis may be present, similar to bile reflux gastritis, afferent loop syndrome, or delayed gastric emptying. The underlying causes of the obstruction include anastomotic stricture, adhesions, retroanastomotic herniation in the mesocolon, jejunogastric intussusception, marginal ulceration, and recurrent cancer or carcinomatosis.

Evaluation and diagnosis consists of CT scan and endoscopy. Occasionally, a HIDA scan can help differentiate efferent loop syndrome from bile reflux gastritis for patients with chronic symptoms. Treatment is surgical, consisting of lysis of adhesions, reduction and repair of hernias, or revision of the anastomosis. For malignant obstruction or isolated strictures, self-expanding intraluminal stents may be used. In addition, self-limiting, functional disturbances of the efferent limb may occur and can be managed with nasogastric tube decompression and fluids.[82]

NUTRITIONAL CONSIDERATION
Deficiencies

Nutritional deficiencies are ubiquitous after gastrectomy.[83] Given that gastric cancer is asymptomatic or minimally symptomatic for an extended period before diagnosis, preoperative nutritional deficiencies and weight loss can develop insidiously.[84,85] As the stage of gastric cancer advances, the extent of nutritional deficiencies increases, affecting 80% of patients in advanced stages.[86] The extent of preoperative deficiencies has been directly linked to overall and disease-specific survival after gastrectomy.[87] Correlations between poor preoperative nutrition and increased postoperative morbidity, including infectious, wound healing, and pulmonary complications, and mortality have been reported in several studies.[88–91]

Nutritional deficiencies should be evaluated preoperatively. Several nutritional screening surveys have been developed and validated.[92–94] Preoperative Nutritional Risk Screening (NRS) 2002 scores correlate with postoperative complications.[92] Other tools, such as the Short Nutritional Assessment Questionnaire, may predict postoperative mortality.[95] Additional risk stratification methods have been used to create prognostic nutritional indices with routine laboratory tests such as albumin, lymphocytes, platelets, or neutrophils.[96–99] Regardless of the method used to assess and monitor nutrition, preoperative and postoperative assessment of nutrition is critical to improve outcomes after gastrectomy. Nutritional counseling in addition to routine assessment may also have benefit in maintaining weight.[100] Our group combines the NRS tool and evaluation by a registered dietitian for all patients at presentation and throughout treatment; the frequency of contact is determined by the degree of preoperative deficiency.

Postoperative nutritional deficiencies are broadly split between immediate perioperative and long-term sequelae of gastrectomy. This article focuses on long-term postgastrectomy nutritional considerations. Given that bariatric surgery is more common than gastrectomy for cancer or ulcer disease, recent literature on nutritional deficiencies largely focuses on this group of patients. Although intended for bariatric patients, the American Society of Metabolic and Bariatric Surgery guidelines are useful for monitoring and supplementing specific nutritional deficiencies.[101] This society recommends monitoring multiple nutritional components, including vitamins B_1, B_6, B_{12}, A, D, E, and K, and folate, iron, zinc, and protein. Among these nutrients, a few are commonly deficient after gastrectomy and warrant specific attention.

Iron deficiency leads to anemia in approximately 50% of patients. The primary cause for iron deficiency is lack of absorption from decreased gastric acid secretion, decreased intrinsic factor production, and bypass of the duodenum.[102–104] The degree of anemia is correlated with the operation performed. For example, patients have a higher degree of anemia after total gastrectomy versus partial gastrectomy, and after Roux-en-Y gastrojejunostomy versus Billroth I reconstruction.[105,106] Clearly, the duodenum is bypassed after Roux-en-Y reconstruction and less gastric acid and intrinsic factor are produced after a total gastrectomy. Although vitamin C deficiency is rare, iron deficiency is exacerbated by vitamin C deficiency, and supplemental vitamin C, regardless of its level, can increase iron absorption. Vitamin B_{12} deficiency is common after gastrectomy and often develops in less than 1 year.[107] If unrecognized, it may result in fatigue, paresthesias, emotional changes, and even dementia. Unlike iron deficiency, B_{12} does not depend on the type of reconstruction, rather on the loss of intrinsic factor.[108] Vitamin D loss results in calcium deficiency, which may lead to early-onset osteoporosis.[109] Osteoporosis and fracture risk also are related to calcium malabsorption caused by decreased gastric acid production, therefore total calcium, ionized calcium, and parathyroid hormone levels should be checked to evaluate calcium deficiencies.[110]

Fat malabsorption occurs to some degree in all patients after a gastrectomy. It is more common when the duodenum is bypassed; however, rapid transit even with the duodenum in continuity can still result in malabsorption of fat.[111–113] Bacterial overgrowth is another contributing factor to both fat malabsorption and mineral deficiencies. Fat malabsorption also leads to deficiencies in fat-soluble vitamins, including vitamin D. Protein deficiencies are common and are usually related to patient intolerance of high-protein food. Testing for albumin, prealbumin, and lymphocyte counts should reveal these deficiencies. Dietary factors are interrelated and individual deficiencies may exacerbate others. Specific symptoms and syndromes have been described for all of these deficiencies, but the best management is prevention by monitoring rather than recognition and treatment after symptoms develop.

Supplementation

Dietary supplementation following gastrectomy often centers on replacing essential vitamins and minerals lost through alterations in natural absorption mechanisms as well as maintaining body mass in patients who inevitably lose weight after, and often before, gastrectomy for cancer. Nutritional supplementation using enteral and parenteral forms of feeding have been debated for decades. All patients lose weight after gastric resection, which is the purpose of restrictive and malabsorptive operations for obesity. Analysis of 376 consecutive patients undergoing gastrectomy for gastric cancer revealed that extent of postoperative weight loss depended on preoperative body mass index and the extent of gastric resection, with greater resection associated with greater weight loss.[114] The degree of postoperative weight loss is important because it not only affects quality of life but is also linked to cancer-specific outcomes. Some investigators have suggested that postoperative weight loss is associated with lower likelihood of continuation of systemic chemotherapy and worse cancer outcomes.[115–117]

Optimizing postoperative nutrition begins with optimal preoperative assessment. Even so, intraoperative and postoperative nutritional support is the focus here. Options for perioperative nutritional support include oral dietary supplements, appetite stimulants, enteral feeding, and total parenteral nutrition (TPN). The merits of enteral nutrition compared with TPN have been argued elsewhere, and enteral nutrition is preferred because of its immediate effects on preserving mucosal integrity and normal flora, reducing length of hospital stay, and associated decreases in infectious and noninfectious complications.[118,119] Vitamin and mineral deficiencies should be monitored and replenished along with monitoring of peripheral blood levels to guide therapy. Our practice is to provide a multivitamin supplement that includes vitamin B_{12}, vitamin D, calcium, and iron. At 1, 3, 6, 9, and 12 months after surgery, patients are weighed, evaluated by a registered dietitian, and peripheral blood is tested for thiamine, red blood cell folate, iron panel, vitamin B_{12}, methylmalonic acid, zinc, 25-hydroxy vitamin D, prealbumin, c-reactive protein, complete blood count, and basic metabolic panel.

SUMMARY

Alterations in form and function of the stomach result in the postgastrectomy syndromes. Gastric resection disrupts normal reservoir capacity, mechanical digestion, and emptying into the intestine. Physiologic function is also impaired by operations that eliminate vagal innervation and bypass the duodenum or remove the pylorus. Patients and clinicians can benefit from an appreciation of these common sequelae of gastrectomy. Efficient recognition of symptoms and prompt evaluation with common modalities such as endoscopy and contrast-enhanced imaging are essential. Although many syndromes resolve with minimal intervention, dietary modifications and medical management are most commonly used for patients with dumping, small gastric remnant, gastric atony, and diarrhea. Surgical intervention is often warranted for afferent and efferent loop syndromes, and bile reflux gastritis. Preoperative nutritional deficiencies are common in patients with gastric cancer. Nutritional assessment and preoperative management with a focus on preventive treatment are likely to decrease the incidence of severe complications. Care of patients after gastrectomy is enhanced through an integrated team approach to preoperative assessment, patient education, and effective management of postoperative symptoms.

REFERENCES

1. Wang YR, Richter JE, Dempsey DT. Trends and outcomes of hospitalizations for peptic ulcer disease in the United States, 1993 to 2006. Ann Surg 2010;251(1): 51–8.
2. Paimela H, Tuompo PK, Perakyl T, et al. Peptic ulcer surgery during the H2-receptor antagonist era: a population-based epidemiological study of ulcer surgery in Helsinki from 1972 to 1987. Br J Surg 1991;78(1):28–31.
3. Gustavsson S, Kelly KA, Melton LJ 3rd, et al. Trends in peptic ulcer surgery. A population-based study in Rochester, Minnesota, 1956-1985. Gastroenterology 1988;94(3):688–94.
4. Shibata C, Shiiba KI, Funayama Y, et al. Outcomes after pylorus-preserving gastrectomy for early gastric cancer: a prospective multicenter trial. World J Surg 2004;28(9):857–61.
5. Tomita R, Tanjoh K, Fujisaki S. Novel operative technique for vagal nerve- and pyloric sphincter-preserving distal gastrectomy reconstructed by interposition of a 5 cm jejunal J pouch with a 3 cm jejunal conduit for early gastric cancer and postoperative quality of life 5 years after operation. World J Surg 2004; 28(8):766–74.
6. Livingston EH. The incidence of bariatric surgery has plateaued in the U.S. Am J Surg 2010;200(3):378–85.
7. Oh SY, Lee HJ, Yang HK. Pylorus-preserving gastrectomy for gastric cancer. J Gastric Cancer 2016;16(2):63–71.
8. Duthie HL, Kwong NK, Brown BH, et al. Pacesetter potential of the human gastroduodenal junction. Gut 1971;12(4):250–6.
9. Hocking MP, Vogel SB. Physiology of gastric secretion and motility in normal and postgastrectomy (postvagotomy) states. In: Hocking MP, Vogel SB, editors. Woodward's Postgastrectomy syndromes. 2nd edition. Philadelphia: WB Saunders; 1991. p. 29–46.
10. Bortoff A. Smooth muscles of the gastrointestinal tract. In: Christensen J, Wingate DL, editors. A guide to gastrointestinal motility. Boston: John Wright; 1983. p. 48–74.

11. Wilbur BG, Kelly KA. Effect of proximal gastric, complete gastric, and truncal vagotomy on canine gastric electric activity, motility, and emptying. Ann Surg 1973;178(3):295–303.
12. Hertz AF. IV. The cause and treatment of certain unfavorable after-effects of gastro-enterostomy. Ann Surg 1913;58(4):466–72.
13. Wyllys E, Andrews E, Mix CL. "Dumping stomach" and other results of gastro-jejunostomy: operative cure by disconnecting old stoma. Surg Clin Chicago 1920;(4):879–92.
14. Machella TE. The mechanism of the post-gastrectomy "dumping" syndrome. Ann Surg 1949;130(2):145–59.
15. Vecht J, Masclee AA, Lamers CB. The dumping syndrome. Current insights into pathophysiology, diagnosis and treatment. Scand J Gastroenterol Suppl 1997; 223:21–7.
16. Herrington JL Jr, Edwards LW, Classen KL, et al. Vagotomy and antral resection in the treatment of duodenal ulcer: results in 514 patients. Ann Surg 1959;150: 499–516.
17. Jordan GL Jr, Bolton BF, De Bakey ME. Experience with gastrectomy at a veterans hospital. J Am Med Assoc 1956;161(17):1605–8.
18. Sawyers JL, Herrington JL Jr, Burney DP. Proximal gastric vagotomy compared with vagotomy and antrectomy and selective gastric vagotomy and pyloroplasty. Ann Surg 1977;186(4):510–7.
19. Mine S, Sano T, Tsutsumi K, et al. Large-scale investigation into dumping syndrome after gastrectomy for gastric cancer. J Am Coll Surg 2010;211(5):628–36.
20. Drapanas T, McDonald JC, Stewart JD. Serotonin release following instillation of hypertonic glucose into the proximal intestine. Ann Surg 1962;156(4):528–36.
21. Sagor GR, Bryant MG, Ghatei MA, et al. Release of vasoactive intestinal peptide in the dumping syndrome. Br Med J (Clin Res Ed) 1981;282(6263):507–10.
22. Sirinek KR, O'Dorisio TM, Howe B, et al. Neurotensin, vasoactive intestinal peptide, and Roux-en-Y gastrojejunostomy. Their role in the dumping syndrome. Arch Surg 1985;120(5):605–9.
23. Roberts KE, Randall HT, Farr HW, et al. Cardiovascular and blood volume alterations resulting from intrajejunal administration of hypertonic solutions to gastrectomized patients: the relationship of these changes to the dumping syndrome. Ann Surg 1954;140(5):631–40.
24. Shultz KT, Neelon FA, Nilsen LB, et al. Mechanism of postgastrectomy hypoglycemia. Arch Intern Med 1971;128(2):240–6.
25. Winner RB, Clarke JS. The relation between plasma volume fall and movement of fluid into the jejunum during dumping. Am J Surg 1962;104:169–76.
26. Humphrey CS, Johnston D, Walker BE, et al. Incidence of dumping after truncal and selective vagotomy with pyloroplasty and highly selective vagotomy without drainage procedure. Br Med J 1972;3(5830):785–8.
27. Vogel SB, Hocking MP. Postgastrectomy dumping and diarrhea. In: Hocking MP, Vogel SB, editors. Woodward's postgastrectomy syndromes. 2nd edition. Philadelphia: WB Saunders; 1991. p. 89–111.
28. Wallensten S. Results of the surgical treatment of peptic ulcer by partial gastrectomy according to Billroth I and II methods; a clinical study based on 1256 operated cases. Acta Chir Scand Suppl 1954;191:1–161.
29. Moore HG Jr, Schlosser RJ, Stevenson JK, et al. Clinical analysis of Billroth I and Billroth II subtotal gastric resections. AMA Arch Surg 1953;67(1):4–22.
30. Nunobe S, Okaro A, Sasako M, et al. Billroth 1 versus Roux-en-Y reconstructions: a quality-of-life survey at 5 years. Int J Clin Oncol 2007;12(6):433–9.

31. Sawyers JL, Herrington JL Jr. Superiority of antiperistaltic jejunal segments in management of severe dumping syndrome. Ann Surg 1973;178(3):311–21.

32. Koruth NM, Krukowski ZH, Matheson NA. Pyloric reconstruction. Br J Surg 1985; 72(10):808–10.

33. Abell TL, Camilleri M, Donohoe K, et al. Consensus recommendations for gastric emptying scintigraphy: a joint report of the American Neurogastroenterology and Motility Society and the Society of Nuclear Medicine. Am J Gastroenterol 2008;103(3):753–63.

34. Vogel SB, Hocking MP, Woodward ER. Clinical and radionuclide evaluation of Roux-Y diversion for postgastrectomy dumping. Am J Surg 1988;155(1):57–62.

35. Sigstad H. A clinical diagnostic index in the diagnosis of the dumping syndrome. Changes in plasma volume and blood sugar after a test meal. Acta Med Scand 1970;188(6):479–86.

36. van der Kleij FG, Vecht J, Lamers CB, et al. Diagnostic value of dumping provocation in patients after gastric surgery. Scand J Gastroenterol 1996;31(12): 1162–6.

37. Tanizawa Y, Tanabe K, Kawahira H, et al. Specific features of dumping syndrome after various types of gastrectomy as assessed by a newly developed integrated questionnaire, the PGSAS-45. Dig Surg 2016;33(2):94–103.

38. Nakada K, Ikeda M, Takahashi M, et al. Characteristics and clinical relevance of Postgastrectomy Syndrome Assessment Scale (PGSAS)-45: newly developed integrated questionnaires for assessment of living status and quality of life in postgastrectomy patients. Gastric Cancer 2015;18(1):147–58.

39. Hasegawa T, Yoneda M, Nakamura K, et al. Long-term effect of alpha-glucosidase inhibitor on late dumping syndrome. J Gastroenterol Hepatol 1998;13(12):1201–6.

40. Lyons TJ, McLoughlin JC, Shaw C, et al. Effect of acarbose on biochemical responses and clinical symptoms in dumping syndrome. Digestion 1985;31(2–3): 89–96.

41. Arts J, Caenepeel P, Bisschops R, et al. Efficacy of the long-acting repeatable formulation of the somatostatin analogue octreotide in postoperative dumping. Clin Gastroenterol Hepatol 2009;7(4):432–7.

42. Deloose E, Bisschops R, Holvoet L, et al. A pilot study of the effects of the somatostatin analog pasireotide in postoperative dumping syndrome. Neurogastroenterol Motil 2014;26(6):803–9.

43. Vecht J, Lamers CB, Masclee AA. Long-term results of octreotide-therapy in severe dumping syndrome. Clin Endocrinol (Oxf) 1999;51(5):619–24.

44. Hasler WL, Soudah HC, Owyang C. Mechanisms by which octreotide ameliorates symptoms in the dumping syndrome. J Pharmacol Exp Ther 1996; 277(3):1359–65.

45. Yang YS, Chen LQ, Yan XX, et al. Preservation versus non-preservation of the duodenal passage following total gastrectomy: a systematic review. J Gastrointest Surg 2013;17(5):877–86.

46. Gertler R, Rosenberg R, Feith M, et al. Pouch vs. no pouch following total gastrectomy: meta-analysis and systematic review. Am J Gastroenterol 2009; 104(11):2838–51.

47. Jung HJ, Lee JH, Ryu KW, et al. The influence of reconstruction methods on food retention phenomenon in the remnant stomach after a subtotal gastrectomy. J Surg Oncol 2008;98(1):11–4.

48. Kubo M, Sasako M, Gotoda T, et al. Endoscopic evaluation of the remnant stomach after gastrectomy: proposal for a new classification. Gastric Cancer 2002; 5(2):83–9.

49. Speicher JE, Thirlby RC, Burggraaf J, et al. Results of completion gastrectomies in 44 patients with postsurgical gastric atony. J Gastrointest Surg 2009;13(5): 874–80.

50. Storer EH. Postvagotomy diarrhea. Surg Clin North Am 1976;56(6):1461–8.

51. Sawyers JL. Management of postgastrectomy syndromes. Am J Surg 1990; 159(1):8–14.

52. Jordan GL Jr. The afferent loop syndrome. Surgery 1955;38(6):1027–35.

53. Brooke-Cowden GL, Braasch JW, Gibb SP, et al. Postgastrectomy syndromes. Am J Surg 1976;131(4):464–70.

54. Miedema BW, Kelly KA. The Roux stasis syndrome. Treatment by pacing and prevention by use of an 'uncut' Roux limb. Arch Surg 1992;127(3):295–300.

55. Mathias JR, Fernandez A, Sninsky CA, et al. Nausea, vomiting, and abdominal pain after Roux-en-Y anastomosis: motility of the jejunal limb. Gastroenterology 1985;88(1 Pt 1):101–7.

56. Eckhauser FE, Knol JA, Raper SA, et al. Completion gastrectomy for postsurgical gastroparesis syndrome. Preliminary results with 15 patients. Ann Surg 1988;208(3):345–53.

57. Perino LE, Adcock KA, Goff JS. Gastrointestinal symptoms, motility, and transit after the Roux-en-Y operation. Am J Gastroenterol 1988;83(4):380–5.

58. Gustavsson S, Ilstrup DM, Morrison P, et al. Roux-Y stasis syndrome after gastrectomy. Am J Surg 1988;155(3):490–4.

59. Hocking MP, Vogel SB, Falasca CA, et al. Delayed gastric emptying of liquids and solids following Roux-en-Y biliary diversion. Ann Surg 1981;194(4):494–501.

60. Vogel SB, Vair DB, Woodward ER. Alterations in gastrointestinal emptying of 99m-technetium-labeled solids following sequential antrectomy, truncal vagotomy and Roux-Y gastroenterostomy. Ann Surg 1983;198(4):506–15.

61. van der Mijle HC, Kleibeuker JH, Limburg AJ, et al. Manometric and scintigraphic studies of the relation between motility disturbances in the Roux limb and the Roux-en-Y syndrome. Am J Surg 1993;166(1):11–7.

62. Kauer WK, Peters JH, DeMeester TR, et al. Mixed reflux of gastric and duodenal juices is more harmful to the esophagus than gastric juice alone. The need for surgical therapy re-emphasized. Ann Surg 1995;222(4):525–31 [discussion: 531–3].

63. Stoker DL, Williams JG. Alkaline reflux oesophagitis. Gut 1991;32(10):1090–2.

64. Zobolas B, Sakorafas GH, Kouroukli I, et al. Alkaline reflux gastritis: early and late results of surgery. World J Surg 2006;30(6):1043–9.

65. Csendes A, Burgos AM, Smok G, et al. Latest results (12-21 years) of a prospective randomized study comparing Billroth II and Roux-en-Y anastomosis after a partial gastrectomy plus vagotomy in patients with duodenal ulcers. Ann Surg 2009;249(2):189–94.

66. Fukuhara K, Osugi H, Takada N, et al. Correlation between duodenogastric reflux and remnant gastritis after distal gastrectomy. Hepatogastroenterology 2004;51(58):1241–4.

67. Vere CC, Cazacu S, Comanescu V, et al. Endoscopical and histological features in bile reflux gastritis. Rom J Morphol Embryol 2005;46(4):269–74.

68. Nicolai JJ, Speelman P, Tytgat GN, et al. Comparison of the combination of cholestyramine/alginates with placebo in the treatment of postgastrectomy biliary reflux gastritis. Eur J Clin Pharmacol 1981;21(3):189–94.

69. Stefaniwsky AB, Tint GS, Speck J, et al. Ursodeoxycholic acid treatment of bile reflux gastritis. Gastroenterology 1985;89(5):1000–4.

70. Buch KL, Weinstein WM, Hill TA, et al. Sucralfate therapy in patients with symptoms of alkaline reflux gastritis. A randomized, double-blind study. Am J Med 1985;79(2C):49–54.

71. Bondurant FJ, Maull KI, Nelson HS Jr, et al. Bile reflux gastritis. South Med J 1987;80(2):161–5.

72. Capussotti L, Marucci MM, Arico S, et al. Long-term results of surgical treatment for alkaline reflux gastritis in gastrectomized patients. Am J Gastroenterol 1984; 79(12):924–6.

73. Davidson ED, Hersh T. The surgical treatment of bile reflux gastritis: a study of 59 patients. Ann Surg 1980;192(2):175–8.

74. Tasse D, Ghosn PO, Gagnon M, et al. Alkaline reflux gastritis: Roux-en-Y diversion is effective. Can J Surg 1982;25(3):337–9.

75. Tireli M. The results of the surgical treatment of alkaline reflux gastritis. Hepatogastroenterology 2012;59(119):2352–6.

76. Aranow JS, Matthews JB, Garcia-Aguilar J, et al. Isoperistaltic jejunal interposition for intractable postgastrectomy alkaline reflux gastritis. J Am Coll Surg 1995;180(6):648–53.

77. Mabrut JY, Collard JM, Romagnoli R, et al. Oesophageal and gastric bile exposure after gastroduodenal surgery with Henley's interposition or a Roux-en-Y loop. Br J Surg 2004;91(5):580–5.

78. Klingler PJ, Perdikis G, Wilson P, et al. Indications, technical modalities and results of the duodenal switch operation for pathologic duodenogastric reflux. Hepatogastroenterology 1999;46(25):97–102.

79. Strignano P, Collard JM, Michel JM, et al. Duodenal switch operation for pathologic transpyloric duodenogastric reflux. Ann Surg 2007;245(2):247–53.

80. Mitty WF Jr, Grossi C, Nealon TF Jr. Chronic afferent loop syndrome. Ann Surg 1970;172(6):996–1001.

81. Gwon DI. Percutaneous transhepatic placement of covered, self-expandable nitinol stent for the relief of afferent loop syndrome: report of two cases. J Vasc Interv Radiol 2007;18(1 Pt 1):157–63.

82. Bodon GR, Ramanath HK. The gastrojejunostomy efferent loop syndrome. Surg Gynecol Obstet 1972;134(5):777–80.

83. Rosania R, Chiapponi C, Malfertheiner P, et al. Nutrition in patients with gastric cancer: an update. Gastrointest Tumors 2016;2(4):178–87.

84. Deans DA, Tan BH, Wigmore SJ, et al. The influence of systemic inflammation, dietary intake and stage of disease on rate of weight loss in patients with gastro-oesophageal cancer. Br J Cancer 2009;100(1):63–9.

85. Ravasco P, Monteiro-Grillo I, Vidal PM, et al. Cancer: disease and nutrition are key determinants of patients' quality of life. Support Care Cancer 2004;12(4):246–52.

86. Donohoe CL, Ryan AM, Reynolds JV. Cancer cachexia: mechanisms and clinical implications. Gastroenterol Res Pract 2011;2011:601434.

87. Wadhwa R, Taketa T, Sudo K, et al. Modern oncological approaches to gastric adenocarcinoma. Gastroenterol Clin North Am 2013;42(2):359–69.

88. Rey-Ferro M, Castano R, Orozco O, et al. Nutritional and immunologic evaluation of patients with gastric cancer before and after surgery. Nutrition 1997;13(10):878–81.

89. Sungurtekin H, Sungurtekin U, Balci C, et al. The influence of nutritional status on complications after major intraabdominal surgery. J Am Coll Nutr 2004; 23(3):227–32.

90. Wu GH, Liu ZH, Wu ZH, et al. Perioperative artificial nutrition in malnourished gastrointestinal cancer patients. World J Gastroenterol 2006;12(15):2441–4.

91. Kuzu MA, Terzioglu H, Genc V, et al. Preoperative nutritional risk assessment in predicting postoperative outcome in patients undergoing major surgery. World J Surg 2006;30(3):378–90.

92. Guo W, Ou G, Li X, et al. Screening of the nutritional risk of patients with gastric carcinoma before operation by NRS 2002 and its relationship with postoperative results. J Gastroenterol Hepatol 2010;25(4):800–3.

93. Kruizenga HM, Seidell JC, de Vet HC, et al. Development and validation of a hospital screening tool for malnutrition: the short nutritional assessment questionnaire (SNAQ). Clin Nutr 2005;24(1):75–82.

94. van Venrooij LM, van Leeuwen PA, Hopmans W, et al. Accuracy of quick and easy undernutrition screening tools–Short Nutritional Assessment Questionnaire, Malnutrition Universal Screening Tool, and modified Malnutrition Universal Screening Tool–in patients undergoing cardiac surgery. J Am Diet Assoc 2011; 111(12):1924–30.

95. Tegels JJ, de Maat MF, Hulsewe KW, et al. Value of geriatric frailty and nutritional status assessment in predicting postoperative mortality in gastric cancer surgery. J Gastrointest Surg 2014;18(3):439–45 [discussion: 445–6].

96. Asher V, Lee J, Innamaa A, et al. Preoperative platelet lymphocyte ratio as an independent prognostic marker in ovarian cancer. Clin Transl Oncol 2011; 13(7):499–503.

97. Chua W, Charles KA, Baracos VE, et al. Neutrophil/lymphocyte ratio predicts chemotherapy outcomes in patients with advanced colorectal cancer. Br J Cancer 2011;104(8):1288–95.

98. Ejaz A, Spolverato G, Kim Y, et al. Impact of body mass index on perioperative outcomes and survival after resection for gastric cancer. J Surg Res 2015; 195(1):74–82.

99. Sakurai K, Tamura T, Toyokawa T, et al. Low preoperative prognostic nutritional index predicts poor survival post-gastrectomy in elderly patients with gastric cancer. Ann Surg Oncol 2016;23(11):3669–76.

100. Poulsen GM, Pedersen LL, Osterlind K, et al. Randomized trial of the effects of individual nutritional counseling in cancer patients. Clin Nutr 2014;33(5):749–53.

101. Allied Health Sciences Section Ad Hoc Nutrition Committee, Aills L, Blankenship J, et al. ASMBS allied health nutritional guidelines for the surgical weight loss patient. Surg Obes Relat Dis 2008;4(Suppl 5):S73–108.

102. Tovey FI, Clark CG. Anaemia after partial gastrectomy: a neglected curable condition. Lancet 1980;1(8175):956–8.

103. Mimura EC, Bregano JW, Dichi JB, et al. Comparison of ferrous sulfate and ferrous glycinate chelate for the treatment of iron deficiency anemia in gastrectomized patients. Nutrition 2008;24(7–8):663–8.

104. Munoz M, Villar I, Garcia-Erce JA. An update on iron physiology. World J Gastroenterol 2009;15(37):4617–26.

105. Geokas MC, McKenna RD. Iron-deficiency anemia after partial gastrectomy. Can Med Assoc J 1967;96(7):411–7.

106. Imamura M, Kimura Y, Ito T, et al. Effects of antecolic versus retrocolic reconstruction for gastro/duodenojejunostomy on delayed gastric emptying after

pancreatoduodenectomy: a systematic review and meta-analysis. J Surg Res 2016;200(1):147–57.

107. Bae JM, Park JW, Yang HK, et al. Nutritional status of gastric cancer patients after total gastrectomy. World J Surg 1998;22(3):254–60 [discussion: 260–1].

108. Okuda K. Discovery of vitamin B12 in the liver and its absorption factor in the stomach: a historical review. J Gastroenterol Hepatol 1999;14(4):301–8.

109. Mellstrom D, Johansson C, Johnell O, et al. Osteoporosis, metabolic aberrations, and increased risk for vertebral fractures after partial gastrectomy. Calcif Tissue Int 1993;53(6):370–7.

110. Zittel TT, Zeeb B, Maier GW, et al. High prevalence of bone disorders after gastrectomy. Am J Surg 1997;174(4):431–8.

111. Leth RD, Abrahamsson H, Kilander A, et al. Malabsorption of fat after partial gastric resection. A study of pathophysiologic mechanisms. Eur J Surg 1991; 157(3):205–8.

112. Rieu PN, Jansen JB, Joosten HJ, et al. Effect of gastrectomy with either Roux-en-Y or Billroth II anastomosis on small-intestinal function. Scand J Gastroenterol 1990;25(2):185–92.

113. Stael von Holstein C, Walther B, Ibrahimbegovic E, et al. Nutritional status after total and partial gastrectomy with Roux-en-Y reconstruction. Br J Surg 1991; 78(9):1084–7.

114. Davis JL, Selby LV, Chou JF, et al. Patterns and predictors of weight loss after gastrectomy for cancer. Ann Surg Oncol 2016;23(5):1639–45.

115. Aoyama T, Yoshikawa T, Shirai J, et al. Body weight loss after surgery is an independent risk factor for continuation of S-1 adjuvant chemotherapy for gastric cancer. Ann Surg Oncol 2013;20(6):2000–6.

116. Lee SE, Lee JH, Ryu KW, et al. Changing pattern of postoperative body weight and its association with recurrence and survival after curative resection for gastric cancer. Hepatogastroenterology 2012;59(114):430–5.

117. Sierzega M, Choruz R, Pietruszka S, et al. Feasibility and outcomes of early oral feeding after total gastrectomy for cancer. J Gastrointest Surg 2015;19(3): 473–9.

118. Gabor S, Renner H, Matzi V, et al. Early enteral feeding compared with parenteral nutrition after oesophageal or oesophagogastric resection and reconstruction. Br J Nutr 2005;93(4):509–13.

119. Kamei H, Hachisuka T, Nakao M, et al. Quick recovery of serum diamine oxidase activity in patients undergoing total gastrectomy by oral enteral nutrition. Am J Surg 2005;189(1):38–43.

Surgical Considerations in the Management of Gastric Adenocarcinoma

Eleftherios A. Makris, MD, PhD, George A. Poultsides, MD, MS*

KEYWORDS

- Gastric cancer • Gastrectomy • Reconstruction • Lymphadenectomy • Margins

KEY POINTS

- Complete surgical resection of the tumor and regional lymph nodes remains the only potentially curative modality for gastric adenocarcinoma; this may require a total or distal gastrectomy depending on the type, location, and extent of the tumor.
- Roux-en-Y reconstruction has the theoretic advantage of avoiding alkaline (bile) reflux gastritis and/or esophagitis and may be preferred to Billroth II reconstruction.
- Routine use of feeding jejunostomy tubes and external drains is not supported by the existing literature but is encouraged in select situations where less than optimal anastomotic healing is expected.
- A pylorus-preserving Billroth I distal (central) gastrectomy has recently emerged as an option for early T1N0 middle-third gastric cancers as an effort to improve long-term postgastrectomy functional outcomes.
- Based on the recently published 15-year follow-up of the Dutch D1 versus D2 lymphadenectomy trial, a distal pancreas-preserving and spleen-preserving D2 lymphadenectomy should be considered standard practice during resection of gastric adenocarcinoma.
- Although surgeons should strive to achieve negative margins during gastric cancer resection, confirmed by intraoperative frozen section, conversion of an R1 frozen section margin to R0 by extending the resection intraoperatively does not seem to yield long-term outcomes comparable to an upfront R0 resection.
- REGATTA (a phase III, randomized controlled trial) demonstrated no added survival benefit from palliative D1 gastrectomy for gastric cancer patients with a single site of metastasis receiving systemic chemotherapy.

Disclosure Statement: The authors have nothing to disclose.
Department of Surgery, Stanford University School of Medicine, 300 Pasteur Drive, H3680, Stanford, CA 94305, USA
* Corresponding author. Stanford University School of Medicine, 300 Pasteur Drive, H3680, Stanford, CA 94305.
E-mail address: gpoultsides@stanford.edu

Surg Clin N Am 97 (2017) 295–316
http://dx.doi.org/10.1016/j.suc.2016.11.006
0039-6109/17/© 2016 Elsevier Inc. All rights reserved.

surgical.theclinics.com

TOTAL, DISTAL, AND CENTRAL GASTRECTOMY (OPEN APPROACH WITH RECONSTRUCTION)

Although chemotherapy has made significant progress over the past decade in the management of locally advanced or metastatic gastric adenocarcinoma, complete surgical resection of the primary tumor and regional lymph nodes remains the cornerstone of therapy for localized disease. This can be accomplished through a total or partial gastric resection, depending on the location, extent, and histology of the tumor.

Total Gastrectomy

Indications and contraindications

Total gastrectomy is commonly indicated for gastric adenocarcinoma involving the entire or proximal stomach.[1] Total gastrectomy might also be necessary for patients with signet ring cell gastric carcinoma due to the commonly encountered diffuse submucosal spread and difficulty in obtaining negative margins with a subtotal gastrectomy[2] or in patients with hereditary diffuse gastric cancer (CDH1 mutation carriers), who typically exhibit a multifocal pattern of involvement throughout the entire organ.[3] Total gastrectomy should not be recommended, however, in situations where wide (4–6 cm) negative margins can be achieved with a partial gastrectomy, because the partial gastrectomy has a significantly improved safety and long-term functional outcome profile, especially in patients with advanced age, malnutrition, and extensive comorbidities.

Resection

For the vast majority of patients where a total gastrectomy is contemplated, an upper midline laparotomy (from the xiphoid process to the umbilicus) with the patient in the supine position provides adequate exposure. If the operation is performed for a bulky cardia or fundus tumor with extension along the proximal esophagus, a left thoracoabdominal incision (starting as an anterolateral 7th intercostal space left thoracotomy and terminating as an upper midline laparotomy through the left costal cartilage) with the patient in the right semilateral decubitus position provides the best exposure for dissection of the distal thoracic esophagus above the diaphragm up to the level of the inferior pulmonary ligament. A double-lumen endotracheal tube is necessary in this situation.

A thorough exploration of the abdomen should be performed to exclude any sites of radiographically occult metastasis in the liver or peritoneum. This step should preferably be performed through a diagnostic laparoscopy, especially in the case of a locally advanced tumor. Particular attention should be paid toward any potential tumor infiltration into the hepatoduodenal ligament or the root of the mesentery, both of which preclude the likelihood of a curative resection. Otherwise, a total gastrectomy should be carried out through the following operative steps:

- The left triangular ligament of the liver should be divided, and the left lateral section of the liver should be retracted superiorly and to the right to expose the gastroesophageal junction.
- The greater omentum should be detached from the transverse colon and its epiploic appendages using electrocautery.
- If technically feasible, the anterior layer of the transverse mesocolon should be dissected from the mesocolic vessels (**Fig. 1**) all the way to the peritoneum overlying the anterior pancreas. These 2 structures comprise the omental bursa and should be resected with a radical gastrectomy, provided the integrity of the mesocolon and the pancreas can be preserved.

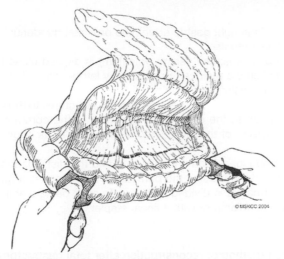

Fig. 1. The anterior layer of the mesocolon is sharply dissected from the mesocolonic vessels in an avascular plane. (*From* Fischer JE, editor. Fischer's mastery of surgery, 6th edition. Philadelphia: Lippincott Williams & Wilkins; with permission.)

- The right gastroepiploic artery and vein should be ligated at their origins from the gastroduodenal artery and the gastrocolic trunk of the superior mesenteric vein, respectively (**Fig. 2**).
- The short gastric vessels should be divided close to the spleen, facilitating ligation of the left gastroepiploic artery close to its origin from the distal splenic artery.

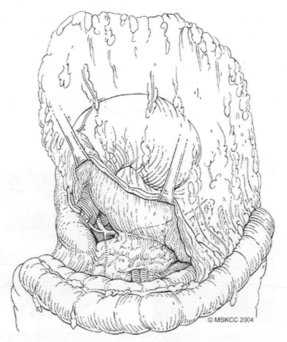

Fig. 2. The right gastroepiploic vessels should be ligated close to their origin. (*From* Fischer JE, editor. Fischer's mastery of surgery, 6th edition. Philadelphia: Lippincott Williams & Wilkins; with permission.)

- After ligation of the right gastric artery, the proximal duodenum is divided, typically with a linear stapler.
- The gastrohepatic ligament (lesser omentum) is divided close to the liver, with caution not to injure a replaced or accessory left hepatic artery.
- With the stomach reflected cephalad, dissection of porta, hepatic artery, and celiac axis nodes is completed, skeletonizing the structures to the left of the left hepatic artery, back to the celiac, and posterior to the common hepatic artery, followed by division of the left gastric artery close to its origin from the celiac axis (**Fig. 3**).
- The phrenoesophageal ligament is divided and the distal esophagus is circumferentially dissected, excising the paracardial lymph nodes (**Fig. 4**).
- The distal esophagus is divided with a knife after being stabilized with a noncrushing vascular clamp or with a linear stapler.

Reconstruction
The most common method of reconstruction after total gastrectomy is an end-to-side Roux-en-Y esophagojejunostomy (**Fig. 5**). The length of the Roux limb should be at least 40 cm from the downstream jejunojejunostomy to minimize alkaline reflux toward the esophagus. An additional advantage of this method of reconstruction is that the anastomosis is defunctionalized, that is, there is no passage of enteric contents (except saliva) if the patient is kept nothing by mouth. This way a small leak from this anastomosis can be managed conservatively with bowel rest, provided the resulting fistula is controlled with an external drain. The esophagojejunostomy can be performed in a hand-sewn fashion (typically in a single layer interrupted or running suture, **Fig. 6**) or with an EEA circular stapler. An anvil stapler can be inserted through the open end of the esophagus, which is subsequently closed with a purse-string suture over the anvil (**Fig. 7**). Alternatively, the distal end of the esophagus can be maintained stapled and the anvil is placed through an orogastric tube delivery system by an anesthesiologist.

The Hunt-Lawrence J pouch (**Fig. 8**) with a Roux-en-Y reconstruction is one of the most commonly selected techniques to augment the capacity of the functional reservoir. To create the pouch, the jejunum can be folded back onto itself and the 2 limbs can be held together using traction sutures. A caudal incision is made in

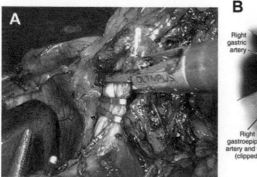
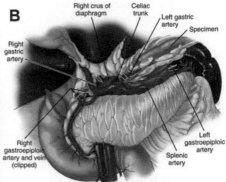

Fig. 3. Division of the left gastric artery (LN station 7). Laparoscopic view (*A*). Medical illustration view (*B*). (*From* Kitano S, Kono Y, Shiraishi N. Laparoscopy-assisted distal gastrectomy for cancer. In: Frantzides CT, editor. Video atlas of advanced minimally invasive surgery. Philadelphia: Elsevier Saunders. p. 105; with permission.)

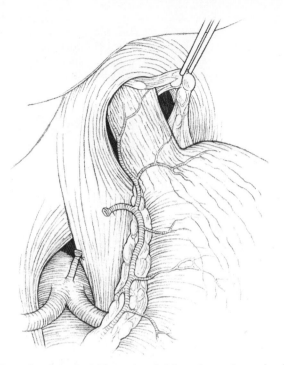

Fig. 4. Mobilization of esophageal hiatus by dividing the peritoneal reflection from the diaphragm and dissection of the paracardial lymph nodes.

each loop and a side-to-side anastomosis is created with a linear stapler-cutter. At this point, the anastomosis between the pouch and the esophagus can be created with an EEA circular stapling device, as previously described, and the caudal pouch opening is closed transversely using the stapler. Although the optimal pouch length has yet to be defined, the results of a small trial found a 9-cm pouch associated with a greater likelihood of regaining preoperative oral intake levels and body weight maintenance compared with a 12-cm pouch.[4] Traditionally the value of pouch formation has been a subject of debate; however, recent literature has shown that pouch creation can improve functional outcomes and quality of life.[5–7] These results have been confirmed in a recent meta-analysis of pooled outcomes data from 9 randomized trials with up to 15 months' postgastrectomy follow-up.[7] Compared with patients who did not undergo pouch reconstruction, those who did had significantly improved oral intake and complained less frequently of dumping and heartburn. Quality of life was significantly improved in patients with a pouch compared with patients without a pouch, and this incremental improvement was more profound over time from 6 months to 12 months to 24 months postoperatively. Although several different pouch reconstruction techniques were assessed in the meta-analysis, the type of pouch technique did not increase patient morbidity, mortality, length of the operation, or hospital stay. Similar to these results, an additional trial found the preoperative quality of life for patients who underwent pouch reconstruction was regained within 2 years of the procedure compared with 5 years in patients who did not undergo this reconstructive approach.[8] These results suggest that pouch reconstruction may play an important role in functional and quality-of-life outcomes

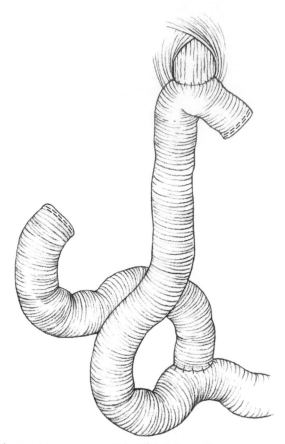

Fig. 5. Completed Roux-en-Y reconstruction after total gastrectomy.

after total gastrectomy, especially in patients with early gastric cancer, where a long life expectancy is anticipated.

Additional considerations should be given for patients with preoperative weight loss or risk factors for complicated or delayed postoperative recovery. In such cases, a jejunal feeding tube should be considered. This should be placed distal to the jejunojejunostomy in a Stamm or Witzel fashion. This tube serves several important purposes, such as allowing early enteral feeding, and the delivery of enterally administered postoperative medications. Additionally, it can be used to ensure a period of prolonged enteral access as a contingency against the development of anastomotic complications. Routine use of jejunal feeding tubes, however, is a subject of controversy due to conflicting data regarding the risk of infectious complications.[9,10]

Although studies evaluating the use of external drains after gastrectomy for gastric cancer are heterogeneous and few, individual prospective trials,[11–13] meta-analyses,[14,15] and multi-institutional retrospective studies[16] do not demonstrate any consistent benefit from the use of prophylactic external drains on several postoperative outcomes. Conversely, however, there seems to be a concerning increase in postoperative complications and length of hospital stay associated with the use of external drains among some studies. Based on existing data, routine use of external drains after total gastrectomy for gastric cancer is not recommended. An exception

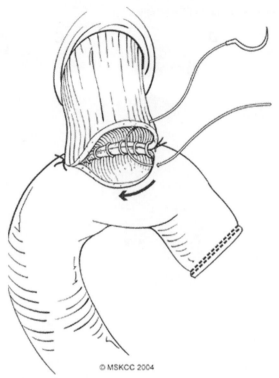

© MSKCC 2004

Fig. 6. Hand-sewn end-to-side esophagojejunostomy. (*From* Fischer JE, editor. Fischer's mastery of surgery, 6th edition. Philadelphia: Lippincott Williams & Wilkins; with permission.)

to this recommendation is the unusual situation when there is concern for the integrity of the pancreatic capsule during dissection.

A water-soluble upper gastrointestinal contrast study can be performed on postoperative day 5 or sooner to assure the integrity of the anastomosis before initiation of oral intake, although this does not necessarily represent routine practice and can be dictated by the individual patient factors and the trajectory of the postoperative recovery.

Parenteral vitamin B_{12} supplementation is required long term after a total gastrectomy due to lack of intrinsic factor production from the stomach. This can be accomplished through monthly intramuscular injections, weekly nasal sprays, or daily sublingual pills, based on patient preference.

Distal Gastrectomy

Indications and contraindications

For patients with tumors of the gastric body or antrum, in whom a 4-cm to 6-cm proximal margin can be obtained without a total gastrectomy, while maintaining a reasonably sized gastric remnant, a more conservative distal gastric resection should be performed, because this confers an equivalent survival outcome with less morbidity and better long-term quality of life than does a total gastrectomy. Nonetheless, a total gastrectomy should be performed if necessary to achieve an R0 resection (commonly in the case of signet ring cell histology), because positive resection margins lead to poor survival after gastric cancer resection. Similarly, patients with hereditary diffuse

End to side anastomosis with EEA stapler

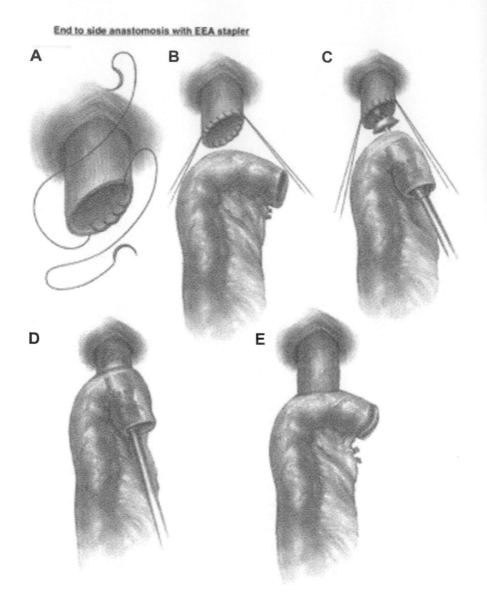

Fig. 7. To create a stapled esophago-jejunostomy a 25 or 28 mm end-to-end anastomosis stapler is most commonly used. First, a full-thickness running suture is placed at the end of the esophagus as a purestring suture (*A*). The jejunal limb is placed cephalad in close approximation to the esophagus (*B*). The stapler is then introduced through the cut end of the jejunum (*C*). With the anvil placed in the esophagus, the purestring suture is tied, and the stapler is closed and fired (*D*). The enterotomy in the jejunum is then closed using a GIA stapler (*E*). It is important to ensure that two complete rings are retrieved from the stapler. The integrity of the anastomosis can be tested by insufflating air through the naso-gastric tube while clamping the jejunum. (*From* Weitz J, Brennan M. Total gastrectomy with reconstruction options. Operat Tech Gen Surg 2003;5(1):31; with permission.)

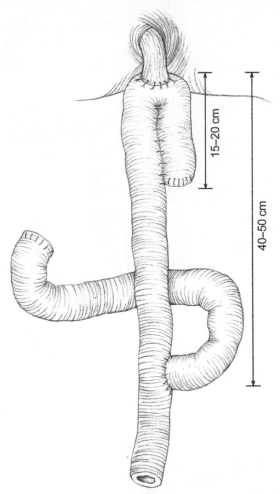

15–20 cm

40–50 cm

Fig. 8. The Hunt-Lawrence J pouch is felt to increase the capacity of the functional reservoir after a total gastrectomy.

gastric cancer typically have multifocal involvement of the entire stomach and should be strongly considered for a total gastrectomy.

Resection

The main difference in performing a distal versus a total gastrectomy is the delineation of the proximal resection margin (**Fig. 9**). This should be located at least 5 cm proximal to the proximal end of the tumor and at least 2 cm distal to the gastroesophageal junction. Irrespective, the left gastric artery should be ligated at its origin and its lymph nodes should be included with the distal gastrectomy specimen to enhance lymph node clearance.

Two additional points merit further consideration during a radical distal subtotal gastrectomy for adenocarcinoma:

- Preservation of some of the short gastric vessels is critical, because this operation entails division of all 4 main arteries supplying the stomach. Therefore, the

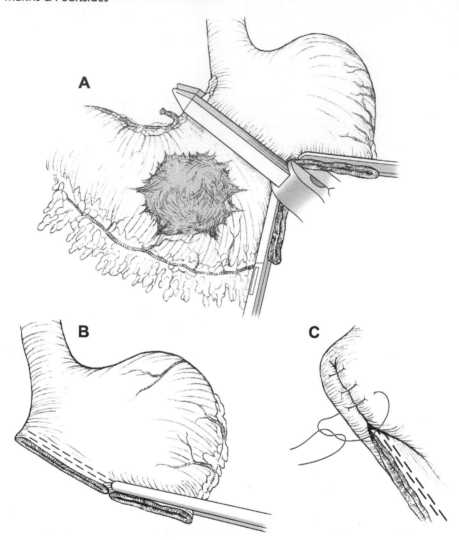

Fig. 9. Division of the proximal stomach for a distal gastrectomy with the stapler (A) or bowel clamps (B). The staple line may be imbricated for added strength (C).

perfusion of the gastric remnant might be solely dependent on some of the remaining short gastric vessels.

- Another important anatomic point is that the left gastric artery usually bifurcates high on the lesser curvature into cranial and caudal branches. Therefore, to adequately dissect the lymph nodes along the cranial branch of the left gastric artery, surgeons must be diligent in carrying the dissection proximally along the lesser curvature, often including the lower 2 cm to 3 cm of the intra-abdominal esophagus **(Fig. 10)**. This is particularly important in the resection of cancers located in the lesser curvature.

Reconstruction

Although there are several options for reconstruction after a distal subtotal gastrectomy, including various types of interposition loops and pouches, the 2 most common

A   **B**

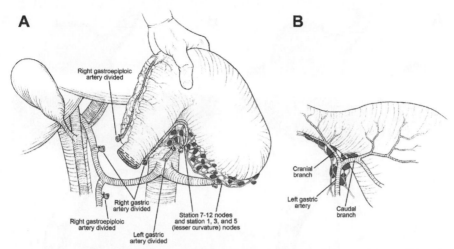

Fig. 10. (*A*) The left gastric artery is identified and suture-ligated at its origin and the adjacent nodal tissue is reflected toward the crura of the diaphragm. (*B*) The left gastric artery bifurcation into cranial and caudal branches at the proximal lesser curvature of the stomach. Both branches and surrounding lymphatic tissue should be dissected to ensure an adequate lymphadenectomy.

feasible types are the Billroth II loop gastrojejunostomy and the Roux-en-Y gastrojejunostomy. Although a Billroth I gastroduodenostomy is another possible reconstructive option after a distal gastrectomy, it is not a realistic option after a true subtotal gastrectomy in which at least 75% of the stomach is resected, because the duodenum simply does not reach the gastric stump in a majority of cases, even after an extensive Kocher maneuver.

A Billroth II gastrojejunostomy may be constructed by bringing a loop of jejunum to the gastric pouch either in front of the transverse colon (antecolic anastomosis) or through a defect in the transverse mesocolon (retrocolic anastomosis) (**Fig. 11**). In either case, a proximal loop of jejunum (just distal to the ligament of Treitz) that reaches the stomach without tension or angulation should be chosen. It is particularly important to avoid an excessively lengthy afferent limb draining the biliary and pancreatic secretions, because such a limb is prone to kinking and occlusion, with the resultant afferent loop syndrome. Alkaline reflux gastritis and some degree of dumping are commonly observed after the procedure. Due to the loss of duodenal continuity, some degree of fat-soluble vitamin malabsorption can also usually encountered.

The advantage of a Roux-en-Y gastrojejunostomy is the diversion of bilious and pancreatic secretions away from the gastric remnant (**Fig. 12**), although some degree of dumping is to be expected.[5] Roux syndrome, or Roux stasis syndrome, is a rare complication of Roux-en-Y reconstruction resulting from gastric atony combined with the adverse effects of jejunal transection. This syndrome is characterized by abdominal pain and vomiting and, in severe cases, may require completion gastrectomy. The goal is to create a Roux limb that is neither too short nor too long. In the former case, the risk of alkaline reflux gastritis is increased, whereas the latter situation may result in a higher risk of Roux stasis syndrome. Observational studies have found an approximately 40-cm to 50-cm long afferent limb strikes the best balance between these risk factors.[5,17,18]

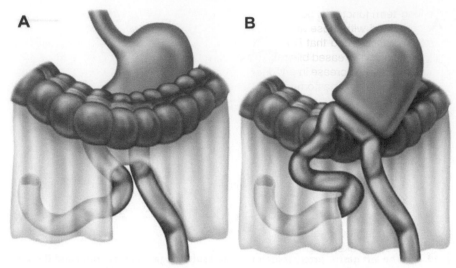

Fig. 11. (*A*) Retrocolic construction of the Billroth II gastrojejunostomy. The afferent limb is relatively short in this case. (*B*) Antecolic Billroth II gastrojejunostomy. The afferent limb is significantly longer than that in A. (*From* Lo SK. ERCP in surgically altered anatomy. In: Baron TH, editor. ERCP, 2nd edition. Philadelphia: Elsevier Saunders. p. 273; with permission.)

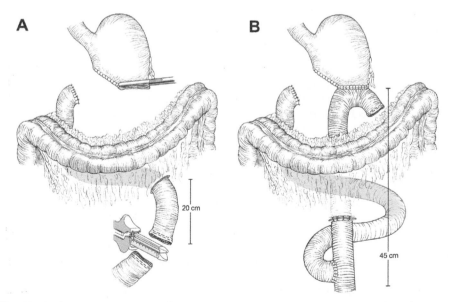

Fig. 12. Reconstruction by a retrocolic, Roux-en-Y gastrojejunostomy. (*A*) The jejunum is divided with the GIA stapler approximately 20 cm distal to the ligament of Treitz. (*B*) A retrocolic, end-to-side Roux-en-Y gastrojejunostomy is created with a Roux limb at least 40 cm in length.

The long-term functional outcomes after Roux-en-Y reconstruction are thought superior compared with those after a Billroth I or Billroth II. A meta-analysis of 15 randomized trials indicated that Roux-en-Y reconstruction is associated with improved quality of life and decreased bile reflux compared with Billroth I or Billroth II techniques without associated increase in perioperative morbidity, which might be expected as a result of an additional anastomosis.[19] The results of a randomized trial comparing Billroth I with Roux-en-Y reconstruction conducted subsequent to this meta-analysis suggest the same conclusion.[20] A separate comparative study, which followed patients up to 21 years postprocedure, indicated that patients randomly assigned to receive a Roux-en-Y gastrojejunostomy showed better clinical outcomes than those randomly assigned to Billroth II reconstruction.[21] For example, Roux-en-Y reconstruction patients had a significantly lower incidence of reflux esophagitis (3% vs 33%) and fewer abnormal upper endoscopy findings at the gastric remnant, distal esophagus, and the esophagogastric junction (10% vs 82%) as well as a lower incidence of Barrett esophagus (3% vs 21%). Roux limb length was preselected to 60 cm in this study. Symptoms suggestive of the Roux syndrome were not detected and the study investigators expressed skepticism regarding its potential occurrence.

Pylorus-Preserving Distal (Central) Gastrectomy

Because radical resection of the stomach with resulting loss of pyloric function can lead to postoperative conditions, such as dumping syndrome, bile reflux, and weight loss,[22] pylorus-preserving gastrectomy (PPG) has emerged as a function-sparing surgery for the treatment of early gastric cancer. According to the Japanese gastric cancer treatment guidelines 2014 (ver. 4),[23] PPG can be performed for cT1N0M0 gastric cancer located in the middle-third of the stomach, at least 4.0 cm away from the pylorus. Although the length of the antral cuff gradually increased from 1.5 cm at the initial description of the procedure[24–26] to 3.0 cm currently, its optimal length remains unclear. The preservation of pyloric function, infrapyloric vessels, and hepatic branch of the vagus nerve makes PPG technically more difficult and raises concerns about incomplete lymph node dissection.[27] To that end, Kong and colleagues[28] examined the metastasis rate to the infrapyloric and suprapyloric lymph node stations in 1802 patients with gastric cancer who underwent curative subtotal gastrectomy. Among patients with a distal resection margin (DRM) less than 6.0 cm, the metastasis rate to station 5 (suprapyloric) was 0.3% (1 of 317) for patients with T1a cancer, 2.7% (8 of 293) for patients with T1b cancer, and 8.0% (10 of 125) for patients with T2a cancer. For metastasis to lymph node station 6 (infrapyloric), the rate was 0.6% (2 of 330) for patients with T1a cancer, 9.5% (28 of 294) for patients with T1b cancer, and 25.4% (33 of 130) for patients with T2a cancer (**Fig. 13**). Therefore, the short-term oncological outcomes of PPG may be comparable to those for distal gastrectomy but with several advantages, such as lower incidence of dumping syndrome, bile reflux, and gallstone formation and improved nutritional status.[24,25] An ongoing Korean multicenter randomized controlled trial (KLASS-04),[29] which compares laparoscopy-assisted PPG and laparoscopy-assisted distal gastrectomy for T1N0 cancer in the middle-third of the stomach, will provide more clear evidence about the advantages and oncologic safety of PPG.

THE EXTENT OF LYMPHADENECTOMY

The optimal extent of lymphadenectomy during gastric cancer resection has been the subject of a long-standing and contentious debate. The Japanese Research Society for Gastric Cancer categorizes the draining lymph node basins of the stomach

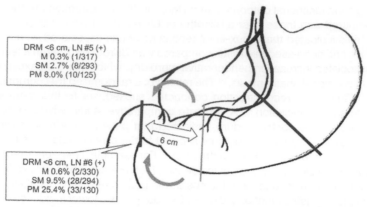

DRM <6 cm, LN #5 (+)
M 0.3% (1/317)
SM 2.7% (8/293)
PM 8.0% (10/125)

6 cm

DRM <6 cm, LN #6 (+)
M 0.6% (2/330)
SM 9.5% (28/294)
PM 25.4% (33/130)

Fig. 13. Station 5 (suprapyloric) and station 6 (infrapyloric) lymph node metastasis rate of gastric cancer in the middle third of the stomach among patients with a distal resection margin (DRM) less than 6.0 cm. LN, lymph node; M, mucosa (T1a); PM, proper muscle (T2a); SM, submucosa (T1b). (*From* Oh SY, Lee HJ, Yang HK. Pylorus-Preserving Gastrectomy for Gastric Cancer. J Gastric Cancer 2016;16(2):66; with permission.)

into 16 stations, including 6 perigastric stations and 10 regional stations along the major vessels and adjacent to the pancreas.[30] The extent of lymph node dissection is indicated by the designation D: a D1 dissection includes only the perigastric nodes (stations 1–6); a D2 dissection includes the lymph nodes along the common hepatic, left gastric, celiac, and splenic arteries (stations 7–11, with distal pancreatectomy and splenectomy advocated for proximal gastric tumors); and a D3 dissection includes additional nodes within the porta hepatis and adjacent to the aorta (stations 12–16).

In Asia, D2 lymphadenectomy has been traditionally regarded as the gold standard, yielding remarkable long-term survival rates with a perioperative mortality rate of less than 1% in single arm studies.[31] Two prospective randomized trials carried out in the United Kingdom and the Netherlands, however, in the early 1990s failed to identify a survival advantage of D2 over D1 lymphadenectomy.[32–35] The sizable perioperative mortality in the D2 arms of these trials (13% and 10%, as opposed to 6.5% and 4%, respectively, for the D1 arms), largely attributed to the routine performance of distal pancreatectomy and splenectomy for D2 dissections, was believed to perhaps offset any potential survival benefit provided by the more radical surgery. More recently, however, the Italian Gastric Cancer Study Group demonstrated that Western surgeons can perform D2 dissections with very low mortality (2.2%)[36] and Japanese surgeons have embraced pancreas-preserving D2 dissections as equally effective as pancreas-sacrificing ones.[37] Furthermore, a recent randomized trial from Taiwan demonstrated a statistically significant survival advantage associated with D3 versus D1 dissection,[38] and the most recent update of the Dutch D1D2 trial showed D2 dissections to be associated with improved disease-specific survival over D1 dissections (lower disease-related death rate, 37% vs 48%, respectively) after a median follow-up of 15 years.[39] A trial recently conducted by the Japan Clinical Oncology Group, in which patients undergoing an R0 resection were randomized at the time of surgery to either to a D2 lymphadenectomy alone or with a para-aortic (D3) nodal dissection, demonstrated no difference in survival between the 2 groups.[40]

The accurate staging of patients with gastric cancer, according to AJCC Cancer staging manual 8th edition,[41] demands the evaluation of at least 16 lymph nodes. The nodal staging is then based on the number of positive nodes, with N1 (1–2 positive nodes), N2 (3–6 positive nodes), N3a (7–15 positive nodes), and N3b ($\geq$16 positive nodes) categories. Retrospective studies have shown a correlation between improved patient survival and larger numbers of lymph nodes examined in the specimen.[42–46] This observation may simply reflect stage migration as opposed to a therapeutic benefit from the procedure. There is indirect and recent direct evidence, however, that a D2 lymph node dissection may result in lower rates of locoregional recurrence, and this may translate into a survival benefit for gastric adenocarcinoma patients.[39]

THE UTILITY FOR INTRAOPERATIVE FROZEN SECTION OF MARGINS

Intraoperative frozen section analysis of the proximal and distal margins during gastric cancer surgery has been traditionally recommended. With a diagnostic accuracy of 93% to 98%, frozen section has the potential to change operative management.[47–49] In addition to Japanese treatment guidelines, which endorse frozen section examination to optimize the chance of a negative margin resection,[50] this practice is also widely used in the United States. The hypothesis is that an R1 margin is associated with increased local recurrence, and, by re-excising an R1 margin to convert it to an R0 margin, patients would have better outcomes. The value of this suggested practice, although intuitive, is debatable.[51]

A positive frozen section margin has been independently associated with tumor location in the proximal stomach, presence of signet ring cells, larger tumors (>5 cm), increased T stage, and more infiltrative disease.[48,52,53] As such, it has been recommended to use frozen section analysis only in patients with the aforementioned risk factors. Predicting which patients might have positive margins on frozen section and identifying the patient subset that would most benefit from re-resection are 2 separate issues, however. The question inherently lies in the utility of further resection of the R1 frozen section margin.

Multiple studies have examined the value of extending the resection margin in response to an R1 margin on intraoperative frozen section analysis. In a US study from the late 1990s, Kim and colleagues[54] found that conversion from an R1 to R0 margin by re-excision of a positive frozen section margin compared with no re-excision of an R1 margin was associated with improved survival only in patients with less than 5 positive lymph nodes. In an updated study from the same institution, Bickenbach and colleagues[55] showed that margin status was an independent predictor of survival in patients with T1–T2 disease or less than or equal to 3 positive nodes but not in patients with T3–T4 disease or greater than 3 positive nodes. Along the same lines, a recent study from China showed that median survival was longer in patients with N0–N2 disease undergoing re-excision (44 vs 25 months; $P = .021$) but not in patients with N3 disease.[56] In a Korean study, 83 patients who had an R1 margin converted to an R0 margin after frozen section analysis were compared with patients who had R0 margins on frozen section. Although both groups ultimately had R0 margins, the cohort that initially had an R1 frozen section margin had decreased survival (41 vs 93 months; $P = .049$), suggesting that an R1 margin on frozen section analysis is really a surrogate for biologically aggressive disease.[53] Another large series from South Korea patients who had R0 margins on permanent section reported that when accounting for factors associated with recurrence, positive frozen section margins were not independently associated with local or peritoneal recurrence compared with negative margins; however, both tumor and nodal stage were associated with these events.[52] This again suggests that the clinical context in which the R1 frozen section occurs, rather than the R1 margin itself, is the major determinant of outcome.

In a large study of Western patients (n = 520), the US Gastric Cancer Collaborative compared 3 patient groups: patients who had R0 margins on frozen section and on permanent section, those who had R1 margins on frozen section and were then converted to a final permanent margin of R0 after additional resection, and those who had R1 frozen and final pathologic margins.[57] The mere occurrence of a positive frozen section was rare in patients with early stage disease (stage I: 6.2%). Patients who were converted to R0 margin after a positive frozen section had a decreased rate of local recurrence compared with patients with an R1 permanent margin (10 vs 32%; P = .01). In multivariate analysis accounting for other adverse pathologic factors related to local recurrence, however, margin status did not persist as an independent predictor of local recurrence. In survival analyses, recurrence-free survival and overall survival of patients who had R1 converted to R0 margins were in the middle ground between patients with R0 and R1 margins on permanent section, although these differences did not reach statistical significance (**Fig. 14**).[57] A positive frozen section margin seems to be a marker for other aggressive features, often encountered in late stage disease, which cannot always be overcome simply by converting that R1 margin to a negative R0 margin. Surgeons should strive to achieve negative margins during gastric cancer resection but they should keep in mind that the need to extend the resection proximally or distally is usually a sign of advanced disease and the outcomes are not as optimal as with an upfront R0 resection.

PALLIATIVE GASTRECTOMY

The palliation of symptoms caused by locally unresectable or metastatic gastric cancer (obstruction, bleeding, pain, and perforation) requires collaboration across disciplines, including surgery, radiation oncology, medical oncology, advanced endoscopy, interventional radiology, and palliative care. Surgical intervention is generally considered a last resort in these situations but has a role when these disciplines have failed to address the complication.

A variety of retrospective studies have attempted to examine the benefit of primary tumor resection in patients with incurable gastric cancer. As expected, these studies have produced conflicting results. Some studies showed no benefit related to palliative gastrectomy in terms of survival and/or quality of life,[58–62] whereas other studies have demonstrated a survival advantage.[63–71] The latter observation is heavily related to selection bias, because surgeons probably selected the more robust patients requiring the least radical operations for surgical palliation.

Thankfully, there are recent randomized controlled data to answer this question. The phase III REGATTA trial performed in Japan, South Korea, and Singapore enrolled 175 advanced gastric cancer patients with a single noncurable factor confined to the liver, peritoneum, or para-aortic lymph nodes between 2008 and 2013.[72] These patients were randomized to receive either chemotherapy (oral S-1 plus cisplatin) only or palliative D1 gastrectomy without metastasectomy followed by the same chemotherapy regimen. At the first interim analysis, no clinically meaningful difference in 2-year survival between the 3 arms was found (25% for gastrectomy plus chemotherapy vs 32% chemotherapy alone) and the study was closed on the basis of futility. Furthermore, the incidence of grade 3 to grade 4 chemotherapy-associated adverse effects, such as anorexia, hyponatremia, leukopenia, and nausea, was significantly higher in the gastrectomy group. Based on these results, the study concluded that palliative

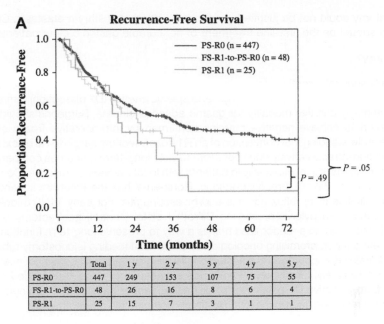

	Total	1 y	2 y	3 y	4 y	5 y
PS-R0	447	249	153	107	75	55
FS-R1-to-PS-R0	48	26	16	8	6	4
PS-R1	25	15	7	3	1	1

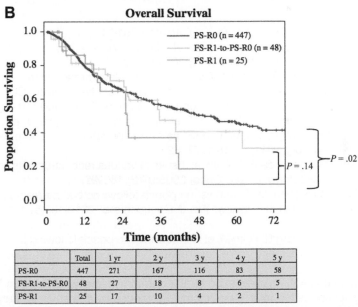

	Total	1 yr	2 y	3 y	4 y	5 y
PS-R0	447	271	167	116	83	58
FS-R1-to-PS-R0	48	27	18	8	6	5
PS-R1	25	17	10	4	2	1

Fig. 14. For gastric cancer resection, when a positive proximal frozen section margin (FS-R1) is converted to a negative permanent section margin (FS-R1-to-PS-R0), the (A) recurrence-free survival and (B) overall survival are in the middle between those of PS-R1 patients and PS-R0 patients. (*From* Squires MH 3rd, Kooby DA, Pawlik TM, et al. Utility of the proximal margin frozen section for resection of gastric adenocarcinoma: a 7-Institution Study of the US Gastric Cancer Collaborative. Ann Surg Oncol 2014;21(13):4208; with permission.)

gastrectomy could not be justified even in the setting of solitary metastasis. Chemotherapy should be the first-line treatment of noncurable gastric cancer patients.

SUMMARY

Complete surgical resection of the primary gastric tumor and regional lymph nodes along the common hepatic, left gastric, celiac, and splenic arteries (D2 dissection) remains the only potentially curative modality for gastric adenocarcinoma. Surgeons should make every effort to achieve negative margins confirmed by intraoperative frozen section, with the understanding that conversion of an R1 frozen section margin to R0 by extending the resection intraoperatively does not seem to yield long-term outcomes comparable to an upfront R0 resection, especially in patients with locally advanced disease. Compared with Billroth I or Billroth II reconstructions, Roux-en-Y has the theoretic advantage of avoiding alkaline (bile) reflux gastritis and/or esophagitis. For early T1N0 middle-third gastric cancers, a pylorus-preserving Billroth I distal (central) gastrectomy is being currently evaluated in a randomized trial as a way to preserve long-term functional outcomes without compromising oncologic benefit. Use of feeding jejunostomy tubes and external drains is encouraged in selected challenging situations but does not need to be performed routinely. Finally, level I evidence suggests that there is no added survival benefit from palliative D1 gastrectomy for gastric cancer patients with a single site of metastasis receiving fluoropyrimidine-platinum combination chemotherapy.

REFERENCES

1. Carcas LP. Gastric cancer review. J Carcinog 2014;13:14.
2. Kunisaki C, Shimada H, Nomura M, et al. Therapeutic strategy for signet ring cell carcinoma of the stomach. Br J Surg 2004;91(10):1319–24.
3. Bardram L, Hansen TV, Gerdes AM, et al. Prophylactic total gastrectomy in hereditary diffuse gastric cancer: identification of two novel CDH1 gene mutations-a clinical observational study. Fam Cancer 2014;13(2):231–42.
4. Tsujimoto H, Sakamoto N, Ichikura T, et al. Optimal size of jejunal pouch as a reservoir after total gastrectomy: a single-center prospective randomized study. J Gastrointest Surg 2011;15(10):1777–82.
5. El Halabi HM, Lawrence W Jr. Clinical results of various reconstructions employed after total gastrectomy. J Surg Oncol 2008;97(2):186–92.
6. Yang K, Chen XZ, Hu JK. Pouch vs. no pouch following total gastrectomy: meta-analysis and systematic review. Am J Gastroenterol 2010;105(5):1208 [author reply: 1208–9].
7. Gertler R, Rosenberg R, Feith M, et al. Pouch vs. no pouch following total gastrectomy: meta-analysis and systematic review. Am J Gastroenterol 2009;104(11):2838–51.
8. Fein M, Fuchs KH, Thalheimer A, et al. Long-term benefits of Roux-en-Y pouch reconstruction after total gastrectomy: a randomized trial. Ann Surg 2008;247(5):759–65.
9. Dann GC, Squires MH 3rd, Postlewait LM, et al. An assessment of feeding jejunostomy tube placement at the time of resection for gastric adenocarcinoma: a seven-institution analysis of 837 patients from the U.S. gastric cancer collaborative. J Surg Oncol 2015;112(2):195–202.
10. Sun Z, Shenoi MM, Nussbaum DP, et al. Feeding jejunostomy tube placement during resection of gastric cancers. J Surg Res 2016;200(1):189–94.
11. Kim J, Lee J, Hyung WJ, et al. Gastric cancer surgery without drains: a prospective randomized trial. J Gastrointest Surg 2004;8(6):727–32.

12. Alvarez Uslar R, Molina H, Torres O, et al. Total gastrectomy with or without abdominal drains. A prospective randomized trial. Rev Esp Enferm Dig 2005; 97(8):562–9.
13. Kumar M, Yang SB, Jaiswal VK, et al. Is prophylactic placement of drains necessary after subtotal gastrectomy? World J Gastroenterol 2007;13(27):3738–41.
14. Liu HP, Zhang YC, Zhang YL, et al. Drain versus no-drain after gastrectomy for patients with advanced gastric cancer: systematic review and meta-analysis. Dig Surg 2011;28(3):178–89.
15. Wang Z, Chen J, Su K, et al. Abdominal drainage versus no drainage post-gastrectomy for gastric cancer. Cochrane Database Syst Rev 2015;(5):CD008788.
16. Dann GC, Squires MH 3rd, Postlewait LM, et al. Value of peritoneal drain placement after total gastrectomy for gastric adenocarcinoma: a multi-institutional analysis from the US Gastric Cancer Collaborative. Ann Surg Oncol 2015; 22(Suppl 3):S888–97.
17. Burden WR, Hodges RP, Hsu M, et al. Alkaline reflux gastritis. Surg Clin North Am 1991;71(1):33–44.
18. Gustavsson S, Ilstrup DM, Morrison P, et al. Roux-Y stasis syndrome after gastrectomy. Am J Surg 1988;155(3):490–4.
19. Zong L, Chen P. Billroth I vs. Billroth II vs. Roux-en-Y following distal gastrectomy: a meta-analysis based on 15 studies. Hepatogastroenterology 2011;58(109): 1413–24.
20. Hirao M, Takiguchi S, Imamura H, et al. Comparison of Billroth I and Roux-en-Y reconstruction after distal gastrectomy for gastric cancer: one-year postoperative effects assessed by a multi-institutional RCT. Ann Surg Oncol 2013;20(5):1591–7.
21. Csendes A, Burgos AM, Smok G, et al. Latest results (12-21 years) of a prospective randomized study comparing Billroth II and Roux-en-Y anastomosis after a partial gastrectomy plus vagotomy in patients with duodenal ulcers. Ann Surg 2009;249(2):189–94.
22. Eagon JC, Miedema BW, Kelly KA. Postgastrectomy syndromes. Surg Clin North Am 1992;72(2):445–65.
23. Japanese Gastric Cancer Association. Japanese gastric cancer treatment guidelines 2014 (ver. 4). Gastric Cancer 2017;20:1–19.
24. Isozaki H, Okajima K, Momura E, et al. Postoperative evaluation of pylorus-preserving gastrectomy for early gastric cancer. Br J Surg 1996;83(2):266–9.
25. Imada T, Rino Y, Takahashi M, et al. Postoperative functional evaluation of pylorus-preserving gastrectomy for early gastric cancer compared with conventional distal gastrectomy. Surgery 1998;123(2):165–70.
26. Kodama M, Koyama K. Indications for pylorus preserving gastrectomy for early gastric cancer located in the middle third of the stomach. World J Surg 1991; 15(5):628–33 [discussion: 633–4].
27. Oh SY, Lee HJ, Yang HK. Pylorus-preserving gastrectomy for gastric cancer. J Gastric Cancer 2016;16(2):63–71.
28. Kong SH, Kim JW, Lee HJ, et al. The safety of the dissection of lymph node stations 5 and 6 in pylorus-preserving gastrectomy. Ann Surg Oncol 2009;16(12): 3252–8.
29. Comparison of Laparoscopic Pylorus Preserving Gastrectomy Versus Laparoscopic Distal Gastrectomy (KLASS-04). ClinicalTrials.gov. Available at: https://clinicaltrials.gov/ct2/show/NCT02595086.
30. Japanese Gastric Cancer Association. Japanese classification of gastric carcinoma: 3rd English edition. Gastric Cancer 2011;14:101–12.

31. Maruyama K, Okabayashi K, Kinoshita T. Progress in gastric cancer surgery in Japan and its limits of radicality. World J Surg 1987;11(4):418–25.
32. Cuschieri A, Fayers P, Fielding J, et al. Postoperative morbidity and mortality after D1 and D2 resections for gastric cancer: preliminary results of the MRC randomised controlled surgical trial. The Surgical Cooperative Group. Lancet 1996; 347(9007):995–9.
33. Cuschieri A, Weeden S, Fielding J, et al. Patient survival after D1 and D2 resections for gastric cancer: long-term results of the MRC randomized surgical trial. Surgical Co-operative Group. Br J Cancer 1999;79(9–10):1522–30.
34. Bonenkamp JJ, Hermans J, Sasako M, et al. Extended lymph-node dissection for gastric cancer. N Engl J Med 1999;340(12):908–14.
35. Hartgrink HH, van de Velde CJ, Putter H, et al. Extended lymph node dissection for gastric cancer: who may benefit? Final results of the randomized Dutch gastric cancer group trial. J Clin Oncol 2004;22(11):2069–77.
36. Degiuli M, Sasako M, Ponti A, Italian Gastric Cancer Study Group. Morbidity and mortality in the Italian Gastric Cancer Study Group randomized clinical trial of D1 versus D2 resection for gastric cancer. Br J Surg 2010;97(5):643–9.
37. Maruyama K, Sasako M, Kinoshita T, et al. Pancreas-preserving total gastrectomy for proximal gastric cancer. World J Surg 1995;19(4):532–6.
38. Wu CW, Hsiung CA, Lo SS, et al. Nodal dissection for patients with gastric cancer: a randomised controlled trial. Lancet Oncol 2006;7(4):309–15.
39. Songun I, Putter H, Kranenbarg EM, et al. Surgical treatment of gastric cancer: 15-year follow-up results of the randomised nationwide Dutch D1D2 trial. Lancet Oncol 2010;11(5):439–49.
40. Sasako M, Sano T, Yamamoto S, et al. D2 lymphadenectomy alone or with para-aortic nodal dissection for gastric cancer. N Engl J Med 2008;359(5):453–62.
41. Amin MB, Edge S, Greene F, et al. AJCC Cancer staging manual. 8th edition; 2017.
42. Bouvier AM, Haas O, Piard F, et al. How many nodes must be examined to accurately stage gastric carcinomas? Results from a population based study. Cancer 2002;94(11):2862–6.
43. Lee HK, Yang HK, Kim WH, et al. Influence of the number of lymph nodes examined on staging of gastric cancer. Br J Surg 2001;88(10):1408–12.
44. Siewert JR, Bottcher K, Stein HJ, et al. Relevant prognostic factors in gastric cancer: ten-year results of the German Gastric Cancer Study. Ann Surg 1998;228(4): 449–61.
45. Smith DD, Schwarz RR, Schwarz RE. Impact of total lymph node count on staging and survival after gastrectomy for gastric cancer: data from a large US-population database. J Clin Oncol 2005;23(28):7114–24.
46. Gholami S, Janson L, Worhunsky DJ, et al. Number of Lymph Nodes Removed and Survival after Gastric Cancer Resection: an analysis from the US Gastric Cancer Collaborative. J Am Coll Surg 2015;221(2):291–9.
47. Ferreiro JA, Myers JL, Bostwick DG. Accuracy of frozen section diagnosis in surgical pathology: review of a 1-year experience with 24,880 cases at Mayo Clinic Rochester. Mayo Clin Proc 1995;70(12):1137–41.
48. Shen JG, Cheong JH, Hyung WJ, et al. Intraoperative frozen section margin evaluation in gastric cancer of the cardia surgery. Hepatogastroenterology 2006; 53(72):976–8.
49. Spicer J, Benay C, Lee L, et al. Diagnostic accuracy and utility of intraoperative microscopic margin analysis of gastric and esophageal adenocarcinoma. Ann Surg Oncol 2014;21(8):2580–6.

50. Japanese Gastric Cancer Association. Japanese gastric cancer treatment guidelines 2010 (ver. 3). Gastric Cancer 2011;14(2):113–23.
51. Postlewait LM, Maithel SK. The importance of surgical margins in gastric cancer. J Surg Oncol 2016;113(3):277–82.
52. Lee JH, Ahn SH, Park do J, et al. Clinical impact of tumor infiltration at the transected surgical margin during gastric cancer surgery. J Surg Oncol 2012;106(6):772–6.
53. Kim SY, Hwang YS, Sohn TS, et al. The predictors and clinical impact of positive resection margins on frozen section in gastric cancer surgery. J Gastric Cancer 2012;12(2):113–9.
54. Kim SH, Karpeh MS, Klimstra DS, et al. Effect of microscopic resection line disease on gastric cancer survival. J Gastrointest Surg 1999;3(1):24–33.
55. Bickenbach KA, Gonen M, Strong V, et al. Association of positive transection margins with gastric cancer survival and local recurrence. Ann Surg Oncol 2013;20(8):2663–8.
56. Chen JD, Yang XP, Shen JG, et al. Prognostic improvement of reexcision for positive resection margins in patients with advanced gastric cancer. Eur J Surg Oncol 2013;39(3):229–34.
57. Squires MH 3rd, Kooby DA, Pawlik TM, et al. Utility of the proximal margin frozen section for resection of gastric adenocarcinoma: a 7-Institution Study of the US Gastric Cancer Collaborative. Ann Surg Oncol 2014;21(13):4202–10.
58. Kokkola A, Louhimo J, Puolakkainen P. Does non-curative gastrectomy improve survival in patients with metastatic gastric cancer? J Surg Oncol 2012;106(2):193–6.
59. Li C, Yan M, Chen J, et al. Survival benefit of non-curative gastrectomy for gastric cancer patients with synchronous distant metastasis. J Gastrointest Surg 2010;14(2):282–8.
60. Kahlke V, Bestmann B, Schmid A, et al. Palliation of metastatic gastric cancer: impact of preoperative symptoms and the type of operation on survival and quality of life. World J Surg 2004;28(4):369–75.
61. Ouchi K, Sugawara T, Ono H, et al. Therapeutic significance of palliative operations for gastric cancer for survival and quality of life. J Surg Oncol 1998;69(1):41–4.
62. Schmidt B, Look-Hong N, Maduekwe UN, et al. Noncurative gastrectomy for gastric adenocarcinoma should only be performed in highly selected patients. Ann Surg Oncol 2013;20(11):3512–8.
63. Chang YR, Han DS, Kong SH, et al. The value of palliative gastrectomy in gastric cancer with distant metastasis. Ann Surg Oncol 2012;19(4):1231–9.
64. Kulig P, Sierzega M, Kowalczyk T, et al. Non-curative gastrectomy for metastatic gastric cancer: rationale and long-term outcome in multicenter settings. Eur J Surg Oncol 2012;38(6):490–6.
65. Al-Amawi T, Swider-Al-Amawi M, Halczak M, et al. Advisability of palliative resections in incurable advanced gastric cancer. Pol Przegl Chir 2011;83(8):449–56.
66. Turanli S. The value of resection of primary tumor in gastric cancer patients with liver metastasis. Indian J Surg 2010;72(3):200–5.
67. Lin SZ, Tong HF, You T, et al. Palliative gastrectomy and chemotherapy for stage IV gastric cancer. J Cancer Res Clin Oncol 2008;134(2):187–92.
68. Zhang JZ, Lu HS, Huang CM, et al. Outcome of palliative total gastrectomy for stage IV proximal gastric cancer. Am J Surg 2011;202(1):91–6.

69. Mariette C, Bruyere E, Messager M, et al. Palliative resection for advanced gastric and junctional adenocarcinoma: which patients will benefit from surgery? Ann Surg Oncol 2013;20(4):1240–9.
70. Shridhar R, Almhanna K, Hoffe SE, et al. Increased survival associated with surgery and radiation therapy in metastatic gastric cancer: a Surveillance, Epidemiology, and End Results database analysis. Cancer 2013;119(9):1636–42.
71. Jeong O, Park YK, Choi WY, et al. Prognostic significance of non-curative gastrectomy for incurable gastric carcinoma. Ann Surg Oncol 2014;21(8):2587–93.
72. Fujitani K, Yang HK, Mizusawa J, et al. Gastrectomy plus chemotherapy versus chemotherapy alone for advanced gastric cancer with a single non-curable factor (REGATTA): a phase 3, randomised controlled trial. Lancet Oncol 2016;17(3):309–18.

Surveillance for Gastric Cancer

Shachar Laks, MD, Michael O. Meyers, MD, Hong Jin Kim, MD*

KEYWORDS

- Stomach neoplasms • Gastric cancer • Early gastric cancer • Adenocarcinoma
- Surveillance • Gastrectomy • Follow-up studies

KEY POINTS

- National Comprehensive Cancer Network guidelines for surveillance following resection of gastric adenocarcinoma emphasize clinical follow-up with further investigations based primarily on patient symptoms.
- Current trials studying the utility of surveillance following gastric cancer resection fail to show a survival improvement with intensive surveillance, but are limited because of their retrospective nature.
- Early gastric cancer has different treatment and recurrence patterns compared with advanced gastric cancer and as such requires consideration of different surveillance strategies.
- A variety of modalities are used in surveillance of gastric cancer, including computed tomography (CT), PET/CT, tumor markers, and endoscopy.

INTRODUCTION

Cancer surveillance has a variety of potential benefits and objectives. Primarily, the goal is to identify recurrent or metastatic disease early, and offer treatment that may potentially affect both survival and disease palliation. Other objectives include patient reassurance, psychological support, identification of treatment-related conditions and secondary cancers, and improvement in quality of life. The treatment of gastric cancer has evolved greatly over the last 2 decades with the increased use of endoscopic mucosal resection (EMR) and endoscopic submucosal dissection (ESD) for early gastric cancers; surgical advances in the management of local, regional, and metastatic disease; and improvement in multidrug chemotherapy and targeted therapies for both neoadjuvant and adjuvant therapy, as well as metastatic disease. These changes in treatment affect the timing, incidence, and type of recurrence, and require that surveillance regimens be continually reexamined.

Disclosure: The authors have nothing to disclose.
Division of Surgical Oncology, University of North Carolina, 170 Manning Drive, CB #7213, 1150 Physicians Office Building, Chapel Hill, NC 27599-7213, USA
* Corresponding author.
E-mail address: kimhj@med.unc.edu

This article evaluates currently published guidelines, and reviews the available literature detailing the utility of common surveillance strategies. It discusses the specific issues related to early gastric cancer and emerging endoscopic therapies as they apply to surveillance. It also discusses the various surveillance modalities, and their respective advantages and disadvantages for optimal cancer surveillance.

CURRENT NATIONAL GUIDELINES, SOCIETY RECOMMENDATIONS, AND GLOBAL CONSENSUS

At present, the National Comprehensive Cancer Network (NCCN) guidelines on follow-up and surveillance of gastric cancer recommends a history and physical (HP) every 3 to 6 months for 1 to 2 years, followed by every 6 to 12 months for 3 to 5 years, then annually. Complete blood count (CBC), complete metabolic profile (CMP), radiological imaging, or upper gastrointestinal endoscopy should only be ordered as clinically indicated per patient symptoms. In addition, the NCCN also recommends monitoring for nutritional deficiency (eg, B_{12}, and iron) in surgically resected patients.[1] Query of the other major international societies, including the Society of Surgical Oncology, American Society of Clinical Oncology, European Society of Medical Oncology, European Society of Surgical Oncology, Cancer Care Ontario, National Institute for Clinical Excellence, Cochrane Collaboration, and Society of the Alimentary Tract yielded no additional quantitative recommendations regarding gastric cancer surveillance.[2]

Contrary to the American and European minimalistic recommendations, the Japanese guidelines are: "Patients undergoing gastrectomy should be followed systematically for treatment of postoperative symptoms, lifestyle guidance, and early detection of recurrence or second cancer depending on risk of recurrence with endoscopy, US [ultrasonography], and CT [computed tomography] scan. At five years or later after surgery, basic checkups are recommended every year."[3] The Japanese guidelines further expound on surveillance specifically in resection of early gastric cancer with EMR or ESD and that *Helicobacter pylori* should be examined, and, if positive, should be eradicated. Follow-up with abdominal US or CT, as well as annual or biannual endoscopy, is recommended.[4] There are various potential explanations for the heightened surveillance recommended by Eastern agencies. These explanations include a markedly higher incidence of gastric cancer, a higher proportion of early-stage disease as related to aggressive screening protocols, differences in effectiveness of available adjuvant therapies, and potentially a different disease cause and biology.

The discrepancy between the Eastern and Western guidelines are marked and have led to attempts at reaching an international consensus. The conclusion of an international Web round-table of 32 experts from 12 countries discussing the rationale and limits of gastric cancer surveillance was published in 2014.[5] The experts were unable to reach conclusive and uniform recommendations for surveillance. The consensus forum revealed that even the experts practiced a wide variety of regimens, including some experts who practiced intensive surveillance with HPs every 3 months, CBC, CMP, serum markers combined with cross-sectional imaging every 6 months, and endoscopy compared with other experts who performed HPs alone at intervals of 3 to 6 months. However, all experts agree that the available data currently have not shown a survival improvement associated with intensive surveillance. Various reasons for using such intensive surveillance were cited, including patient reassurance, identification of secondary malignancies, symptomatic relief, and outcomes research. Given the lack of consensus, Hur and colleagues[6] examined the surveillance regimens that were being practiced by surgeons, oncologists, and other gastric cancer specialists. They published their survey results of 96 respondents from the Korean Gastric

Cancer Association in 2010. The most common frequency of surveillance in early gastric cancer was every 6 months (64.4%) for the first year, every 12 months (47.9%) for the next 4 years, and every 12 months (68.8%) beyond 5 years. In advanced gastric cancer, the most common frequencies were every 3 months (43.8%) for the first year, every 6 months (75%) for the next 4 years, and then every 12 months (75%) beyond 5 years. CT and PET were used routinely by 88.5% and 60.4%, respectively.[6] This study shows that, despite a lack of data proving any survival advantage, most respondents were very high users of intensive surveillance regimens. Note that this is an Eastern study treating a high-risk population of patients who are often diagnosed and treated at an earlier stage compared with Western populations.

STUDIES DETAILING THE UTILITY OF SURVEILLANCE

No prospective study of surveillance after curative treatment of gastric cancer has ever been performed. The recommendation of limited surveillance practiced by many Western institutions was initially based on 2 retrospective studies that have shown no survival improvement using more intensive regimens. The first report suggesting that early aggressive surveillance and early detection of recurrences did not improve overall survival of patients with gastric cancer was a German series by Bohner and colleagues.[7] They retrospectively evaluated 135 patients who had undergone potentially curative gastrectomies with 67 (49.6%) recurrences. The study differentiated the groups into asymptomatic recurrences (n = 15, 22.3%) and symptomatic recurrences (n = 52, 77.7%). No difference in overall survival (OS) was noted between the 2 groups. Another article, by Kodera and colleagues,[8] reported the results from 197 patients with recurrent gastric cancer, of whom 88 (45%) had asymptomatic recurrences and 109 (55%) had symptomatic recurrences. As is described by the Japanese guidelines, patients were surveilled every 3 months with HPs, CBC, CMPs, and US or CT every 6 months, and annual endoscopy. The asymptomatic group received more palliative chemotherapy than the symptomatic cohort. Local and regional recurrences made up slightly more than half of recurrences, although the asymptomatic group had a higher incidence of distant disease. Nonetheless, metastasectomy was performed in only 15 (7.6%) patients, and in a greater frequency in the asymptomatic group (n = 10, 11.4%), and patients who underwent resection of their recurrences had improved survival (P = .0017). The asymptomatic group had a longer postrecurrence detection survival, but a shorter disease-free survival. Ultimately, no OS difference was observed, pointing to a lead-time bias to explain the difference in disease-free survival (ie, the recurrences are identified earlier but this has no effect on ultimate outcome). Collectively, these studies have a few significant limitations. First, their retrospective nature and lack of a true control group makes interpreting these results difficult. Both studies used the symptomatic and asymptomatic groups as surrogates for intensive surveillance versus nonintensive surveillance. This surrogacy is problematic, because it is reasonable to question whether patients with symptomatic recurrences have a different disease biology in terms of location of recurrences, aggressiveness of the malignancy, doubling time of tumor, response to treatment, and potentially other differences in clinical behavior from patients with asymptomatic recurrences. Another issue is that most of the patients treated and surveilled in these studies were treated in the early to mid-1990s. The quality of cross-sectional imaging, US, and use of tumor markers for detection has dramatically improved diagnostic sensitivities. Because of the traditionally poor outcomes of patients with metastatic gastric cancer, only a small percentage of these patients received surgical treatment of their metastases, and none received biologic targeted therapy. Whether more of those patients would have been candidates for these approaches, or whether these therapies would have improved their survival, remains unknown.

In 2005, the Memorial Sloan Kettering Cancer Center published their institutional experience, adding a large United States cohort to existing data.[9] They reported their experience with 1172 curative-intent gastrectomies for gastric cancer and 561 (48%) recurrences from 1985 to 2000. The investigators adhered to the NCCN guidelines for follow-up and, like the studies discussed earlier, used asymptomatic and symptomatic recurrences to compare the groups as surrogates for nonintensive and intensive follow-up. Asymptomatic recurrences were found earlier at 10.8 months versus 12.4 months, but this was not statistically significant. Median postrecurrence survival was significantly longer in the asymptomatic group at 13.5 months as opposed to only 4.8 months in the symptomatic group ($P>.01$). Unlike the previous studies, this improvement did not depend on lead time bias because the initial time to recurrence from the time of surgery was not significantly different between the symptomatic and asymptomatic cohorts (10.8 vs 12.4 months, as stated earlier). The investigators were able to show an improvement in median disease-specific survival from the time of resection of 29.4 months versus 21.6 months favoring the asymptomatic group ($P<.05$). Multivariate analysis did show that symptomatic disease was associated with worse survival, as were 4 other biological factors (stage, poor differentiation, multiple recurrence sites, and disease-free interval). The investigators concluded that they could not separate the impact of symptomatic disease from the markers of biologically aggressive tumors, and that symptomatic recurrence was simply a marker of more aggressive disease biology and does not necessarily indicate improved survival with early detection. Again, the major limitation of the study is that asymptomatic recurrence was used as a surrogate for close follow-up, but no intensive regimen of follow-up was used in any of these patients. This finding could explain why there was no statistically significant difference in time to detection of the first recurrence between the two groups. Second, there is no mention of which, if any, additional therapies were used to treat locoregional or metastatic disease. The use of these modalities varies greatly between institutions and they have gained some popularity since the publication of that study.

A study from Singapore retrospectively assessed 102 patients with curative-intent gastrectomy and differentiated the groups into regular and intensive follow-up based on whether they had regular HPs, CBC, CMP, tumor markers, and CT scans more frequently or less frequently than once a year. Similar to previous studies, the investigators were able to show an earlier detection at 11.5 months compared with 19.2 months, but there was no survival difference noted.[10] The retrospective nature of the study leads to the question of whether patients in the intensive group were selected into this cohort because of more aggressive disease at the time of presentation. Furthermore, in the period from 1995 to 1998, little effective treatment was routinely offered, with only 1 patient reexplored to have potentially curative resection of locoregional disease, and none for metastatic disease.

In addition, 2 large studies from Korea by Eom and colleagues[11] and Park and colleagues[12] spanning the period from 2001 to 2008 described nearly 4500 patients treated with curative-intent surgery who underwent an intensive follow-up regimen including at least yearly (in some cases as frequent as every 3 months) laboratory work, cross-sectional imaging, tumor markers, and endoscopy. The investigators studied the OS of patients with symptomatic recurrences versus asymptomatic recurrences and failed to show a survival benefit despite earlier detection and prolonged postrecurrence survival.[11,12] Again, only a small percentage of patients were treated with surgical resection for locoregional recurrences, but how many additional patients would have been candidates for this approach is unknown. In addition, the study by Eom and colleagues[11] showed no difference in the use of chemotherapy for recurrence, which was 62.3% and 64.8% for the symptomatic and asymptomatic arms, respectively. Both studies showed that patients with symptomatic recurrence have significantly worse survival, corroborating the findings from multiple other studies.[9,13,14] Park and colleagues[12] also suggested that the every-3-month high-frequency surveillance did not lead to a higher proportion of asymptomatic patients at recurrence, and concluded that, if surveillance was beneficial, yearly investigations were equivalent to more frequent evaluation. Peixoto and colleagues[15] shared the Canadian experience in the follow-up of 292 patients who had curative-intent resection, and retrospectively assigned their surveillance to (1) discharge to general practitioner (30%), (2) follow-up by oncologist with clinical assessments only (6%), (3) specialist follow-up with laboratory investigations (11%), and (4) specialist follow-up with imaging/endoscopy (53%). No significant difference was found in OS or relapse-free survival.[15] However, the applicability of this study is limited because it targeted patients with both esophageal and gastric cancer, with both squamous cell and adenocarcinoma histologies; those patients treated with curative-intent chemoradiotherapy were followed more intensively. A summary of these studies is outlined in **Table 1**.

As discussed earlier, the currently available studies examining the utility of surveillance are severely limited. When symptoms at time of recurrence are used as a surrogate for intensity of surveillance, it seems that earlier detection of recurrences, such as those detected by active surveillance, does not independently yield a significant OS benefit compared with recurrences detected by patient symptoms, but the data are not conclusive and several questions remain. In addition to the potential impact on surgical management of local or regional recurrences if detected early enough, there are also questions about the impact of symptoms on the potential for other forms of therapy. Specifically, it remains unclear whether asymptomatic patients are more likely to be treated with chemotherapy and whether they may be more likely to be eligible for a clinical trial when they are asymptomatic given that they are more likely to have a better performance and nutritional status. This question has even greater implications in the era of targeted therapy and a growing number of drugs that may meaningfully affect postrecurrence survival. Prospective data examining this question, in particular a prospective randomized trial of intensive versus nonintensive surveillance for curative-intent gastrectomy, would provide much-needed guidance on this subject.

MODALITIES OF FOLLOW-UP

There are several modalities that are used to detect tumor recurrence. Routine HPs are an inexpensive and efficient way to discover recurrences and are an integral part of every published guideline for gastric cancer surveillance. In the setting of an intensive surveillance regimen, HPs are still the initial detection method for 24.8% of patients.[11] Patients who are detected through this method are more likely to have undifferentiated and Lauren diffuse-type tumors and to be detected later in follow-up, are less likely to have isolated locoregional recurrences, and are less likely to receive salvage resection.[8–11]

Cross-sectional imaging is perhaps the most sensitive early detection tool used as a part of surveillance strategies. Because most recurrences of gastric cancer occur in the abdominal cavity, CT of the abdomen and pelvis can be an efficient tool to detect

Table 1
Summary of studies of utilities of surveillance

Study, Year/Country	Study Years	Number of Recurrences	Surveillance Method	Results
Bohner et al,[7] 2000/Germany	1987–1996	52 symptomatic 15 asymptomatic	3 mo HPs∖labs 6 mo US 6 mo endoscopy	• No OS advantage • No OS advantage for chemotherapy
Kodera et al,[8] 2003/Japan	1985–1996	109 symptomatic 88 asymptomatic	3 mo HPs∖labs 6 mo CT 1 y endoscopy	• No OS advantage • DFS shorter in asymptomatic group but improved postrecurrence survival
Bennett et al,[9] 2005/United States	1985–2000	283 symptomatic 99 asymptomatic	NCCN guidelines, no routine surveillance	• No significant change in DFS but postrecurrence survival and DSS improved in asymptomatic group
Tan et al,[10] 2007/Singapore	1995–1998	23 nonintensive 24 intensive	Intensive surveillance defined as HPs∖labs∖CT >once per year	• No OS advantage • Earlier detection of recurrence in intensive surveillance group
Eom et al,[11] 2011/Korea	2001–2004	77 symptomatic 233 asymptomatic	6 mo HPs∖labs At least annual CT and endoscopy	• No OS advantage • Survival after recurrence improved in asymptomatic group
Park et al,[12] 2016/Korea	2006–2008	376 recurrences 101, <3 mo 137, 3–6 mo 108, 6–12 mo	CT or PET-CT at intervals of <3 mo, 3–6 mo, or 6–12 mo	• Surveillance intervals of <6–12 mo do not improve OS or postrecurrence survival

Abbreviations: DFS, disease-free survival; DSS, disease-specific survival; labs, laboratory tests.
Data from Refs.[7–12]

locoregional recurrences, hepatic metastases, and peritoneal disease with acceptable sensitivity.[16–18] Eom and colleagues,[11] among others, have shown that, as a part of a comprehensive multimodality intensive follow-up, CT of the abdomen and pelvis provides the earliest initial detection in 50% to 60% of patients.[10] PET and PET/CT have had an emerging role in surveilling gastric cancer. Nonetheless, their utility compared with conventional contrast-enhanced CT is not clear, with multiple studies and meta-analyses showing conflicting results.[19–26] Contrast-enhanced CT seems to have a discriminatory advantage in identifying peritoneal disease in advanced primary tumors, whereas PET/CT seems to be preferable in identifying new primary tumors in the surveillance of early gastric cancer.[19–21] The sensitivity and specificity of CT for detecting recurrences are from 64.3% to 89.4%, and 62.4% to 86.5%, respectively.[20,21,25] The sensitivity and specificity for PET/CT for detecting recurrences are from 53.6% to 95.8% and 63.5% to 87.7%, respectively.[19–25] As technology improves, the role of PET/CT may evolve, because the most recent meta-analysis shows the sensitivity and specificity of PET/CT to be 85% and 78%, respectively.[26] Other clinicians use PET/CT as an adjunct study in surveillance and have shown that, when suspicion for recurrence exists based on increased levels of tumor markers, PET/CT has a sensitivity of 73%, and affected management 42% of the time. When recurrence is suggested by other imaging studies, PET/CT has a sensitivity of 81% and affected management 48% of the time.[22]

Multiple tumor markers have been examined in the management of gastric cancer with varying levels of clinical utility, including carcinoembryonic antigen (CEA), carbohydrate antigen (CA) 19-9, CA50, sialyl Tn antigen, CA72-4, CA125, and alpha fetoprotein. Based on a meta-analysis, the 3 markers most clinically used are CEA, CA19-9, and CA72-4, with a sensitivity at time of diagnosis of 24%, 27%, and 29.9%, respectively.[27] Takahashi and colleagues[28] performed a nationwide, prospective observational study in 135 Japanese institutions evaluating CEA and CA19-9 preoperatively and every 3 months for 5 years in 321 patients. Sensitivity and specificity for recurrence using CEA and CA19-9 were 65.8% and 81.8%, and 55.0% and 93.7%, respectively. With the combination of CEA and CA19-9, the sensitivity for recurrence was 85.0%. If the levels of the markers were increased preoperatively, the sensitivity of each of the markers was more than 90%.[28] These results are congruent with other reports of the increasing sensitivity of CEA varying from 40.0% to 51.9% to 100% in patients with preoperative increases and advanced disease at the time of presentation.[29–31] Nonetheless, even patients who did not express CEA and CA19-9 preoperatively could have their recurrence detected by these tumor markers, with 54.7% of patients with CEA and 40.0% of patients with CA19-9 increases having initial increases only at recurrence.[28] With regard to site of disease recurrence, CEA and CA19-9 have lower sensitivity in detecting locoregional recurrence compared with their sensitivity for detecting distant disease, whereas CA72-4 has a slightly superior sensitivity for detecting locoregional recurrence of 51%, and specifically peritoneal disease with a sensitivity of 66.7%, which is significantly higher than the sensitivity of CEA and CA19-9 for peritoneal disease.[29,30] The studies suggest that tumor markers detect recurrences between 2 and 4 months before demonstration of recurrences by imaging modalities.[28,32] The impact of tumor markers in managing otherwise undetectable disease remains unclear. However, even if recurrence is not otherwise detected at the time of initial increase of tumor marker levels, this may be important in altering ongoing follow-up strategies, such as plans for subsequent imaging.

The utility of endoscopic surveillance as a tool in advanced gastric cancer varies. Routine endoscopy after total gastrectomy can successfully identify a small number of recurrences. Lee and colleagues[33] reported that, in a cohort of 622 patients with advanced gastric cancer treated with gastrectomy, 18 recurrences were identified by endoscopy. Of these, 10 were anastomotic recurrences, 4 small bowel, 4 within the regional lymph nodes, and all occurred in patients with advanced disease at presentation. They also reported 72 patients with anastomotic stenosis, of which 62 were symptomatic and 80% were benign. The benign recurrences occurred earlier, at a median of 6.3 months versus 11.9 months for the malignant recurrences.[33] The utility of routine endoscopic surveillance following total gastrectomy was also investigated by Park and colleagues[34] in an analysis of 197 patients with total gastrectomy and advanced disease who were followed by both CT and endoscopy. Only 6 local recurrences were identified, of which 3 were identified by both endoscopy and CT, 2 identified by CT alone, and 1 by endoscopy alone. The mean number of endoscopies was 4 per person. In this study, 788 endoscopies were required to identify 1 recurrence that would not have otherwise been identified by CT.[34] Thus, there is limited utility in routine surveillance endoscopies in asymptomatic patients with advanced gastric cancer treated by total gastrectomy.

Gastric stump cancer (GSC) is an ill-defined entity that refers to all cancers diagnosed in the remnant stomach after gastrectomy regardless of the indication for gastrectomy. GSC following distal gastrectomy represents 1% to 2% of all gastric cancers.[35] Komatsu and colleagues[35] retrospectively evaluated 14 patients treated for GSC after subtotal gastrectomy for gastric cancer and found that more than 50% had early-stage disease at GSC presentation and 78.8% underwent curative-intent resections. Moreover, as the endoscopic surveillance interval lengthened, so did the likelihood of more advanced disease, with mean endoscopic interval of 2.04 and 2.50 years for stage I and II, respectively, and 3.12 and 4.50 years for stage III and IV, respectively.[35] An evaluation of clinicopathologic characteristics of curative resection in 38 patients with GSC yielded annual endoscopic examination after the initial gastrectomy as the only independent factor for curative resection in multivariate analysis (odds ratio, 35.2; confidence interval, 1.94–641; $P = .016$).[36] Note that these are patient populations that have a significant risk of gastric cancer and it is difficult to discern in which patients recurrences are being identified and in which there are second primary gastric cancers. Nonetheless, there are enough data to suggest that, at least in these higher risk populations, and in patients with other underlying disorders that increase risk, like intestinal metaplasia or dysplasia, for whom surveillance would be used regardless, endoscopic surveillance at least every 2 years is warranted after distal gastrectomy. Similarly, patients with a close margin after subtotal gastrectomy may be well served by surveillance endoscopy because their local recurrence would be higher as well.

FOLLOW-UP OF EARLY GASTRIC CANCER AND ENDOSCOPIC RESECTIONS

Surveillance of early gastric cancer poses unique challenges and considerations in cancer surveillance that are not currently addressed by NCCN guidelines. Early gastric cancer is an important entity in Eastern populations in which screening has led to stage migration to earlier disease. Even in Western populations, screening programs of at-risk populations and increasing use of endoscopy and cross-sectional imaging are identifying disease at earlier stages than historically seen. The survival rate of early (stage I and II) gastric cancer is improving, and localized disease is associated with a 66.4% long-term survival.[37] Most Eastern databases estimate disease-specific mortality from stage I gastric cancer to be as low as 1.4% to 2.2%.[4,38] Long-term follow-up of these patients shows that between 3.3% and 10.3% develop extragastric new primary cancers, most commonly colorectal and lung cancer.[38–40] Further, metachronous gastric primaries in the remnant stomach develop in 2.9% to 4.8% of patients with early gastric cancer treated with partial gastrectomy.[41–43] Because this is significantly higher than the 0.7% remnant gastric carcinoma seen after partial gastrectomy for benign disease in Western series, it is tempting to attribute this incidence to the overall increased incidence of primary gastric cancer in Eastern populations; nonetheless, at least 1 large multicenter Italian study after partial gastrectomy for early gastric cancer showed a gastric remnant cancer rate of 2.6%, 3.2%, and 4% at 10, 15, and 20 years, respectively.[40,44] Ohashi and colleagues[45] showed that surgical resection of T2 to T4 gastric remnant carcinoma after previous distal gastrectomy for gastric cancer had 1-year, 3-year, and 5-year survivals of 90%, 66%, and 44%, respectively. The study included both tumors at the previous anastomosis and elsewhere in the remnant. These results suggest that, in patients with early gastric cancer, long-term endoscopic surveillance to identify new primary gastric cancers should be considered, because they are amenable to treatment. When early gastric cancer does recur, Ikeda and colleagues[39] showed that most recurrences occur with metastatic spread to the liver. Note that the 3-year survival after recurrence was 51%, and 23% of recurrences occurred after 5 years of follow-up, suggesting that early gastric cancer has a good prognosis even when recurrent, and that recurrences may present late in follow-up. Patients with early disease may preferentially benefit from follow-up and endoscopic surveillance should be continued beyond the usual 5-year point. A typical surveillance regimen for early-stage gastric cancer is outlined in **Table 2**.

Because of the favorable prognosis in early gastric cancers and low likelihood of lymphatic involvement, techniques such as EMR and ESD have gained significant popularity in the treatment of early gastric cancer. A systematic review of 11 retrospective cohort studies with more than 2301 patients with early gastric cancer treated with endoscopic resection versus gastrectomy showed no difference in 5-year OS, but a decrease in morbidity greatly favored the endoscopic approach.[46] The recurrence patterns of early gastric cancer treated with endoscopic resection differ significantly from those of advanced gastric cancer. Multiple studies have shown that metachronous recurrences occur after endoscopic surgery at a rate of between 3.4% and 15.2%, with lower rates seen after confirmed *Helicobacter* eradication and higher rates in studies with longer follow-up.[47–50] A systematic review confirmed a 2.7% to 14% rate of metachronous gastric cancers.[51] This systematic review further showed a local recurrence rate as high as 4.4% to 18% for EMR with expanded criteria, but as low as 0.40% in ESD with negative margins.[51] In addition, Min and colleagues[50] showed that rate of metachronous recurrence continue to increase even beyond 5 years, with 5-year, 7-year, and 10-year cumulative incidences of 9.5%, 13.1%, and 22.7%, respectively. Extragastric recurrences in the lymph nodes occurred at a rate of only 0.16% to 0.6%.[52,53] Two large studies of intensive follow-up after endoscopic resection have shown that all recurrences were identified by endoscopy

Table 2
Surveillance algorithm in stage I gastric cancer treated with either subtotal gastrectomy or endoscopic techniques

	6 mo	1 y	1.5 y	2 y	2.5 y	3 y	4 y	5 y	5+ y
HPs	X	X	X	X	X	X	X	X	X
CBC \ CMP \ Tumor Markers	X	X	X	X	X	X	X	X	—
Cross-sectional Imaging	—	X	—	X	—	X	X	X	—
Endoscopy	—	X	—	—	—	X	—	X	—[a]

[a] After 5 years, high-risk populations and patients with disorders, such as intestinal metaplasia/dysplasia, and familial gastric cancers should undergo endoscopic surveillance every 1 to 2 years indefinitely.

without additional benefit of CT, or tumor markers.[54,55] Hahn and colleagues[56] in 2016 reviewed 1347 patients who underwent ESD between 2007 and 2014 followed by endoscopy with a short surveillance period of less than 12 months or long surveillance greater than 12 months between endoscopies. Similar to previous studies, they showed a 2.48%/y rate of metachronous recurrence in the remnant stomach. This study showed that additional gastrectomy was necessary in only 7.1% in the short-surveillance group versus 46.2% in the long-surveillance group ($P = .033$). In contrast, 92.9% could have their metachronous recurrences managed with endoscopic techniques in the short-surveillance group versus only 53.8% in the long-surveillance group.[56] Other investigators have also shown a 97% rate of endoscopic management of metachronous gastric cancers with intensive surveillance.[57]

In summary, there is substantial evidence that metachronous and local recurrences occur after endoscopic resection of early gastric cancer. These recurrences are most likely to be identified by endoscopy. CT, PET/CT, and tumor markers add little value in the surveillance of early gastric cancer treated by endoscopic resection. Although the local recurrences generally occur within the first 3 years, metachronous recurrences may occur as late as 10 years and beyond, suggesting that the recommendation of surveillance should be for at least yearly endoscopic follow-up in these patients for a prolonged period. Note that all of these data arise from populations with a much higher incidence of gastric cancer, in which screening programs have already been found to be useful. The applicability of these standards to Western patients remains unclear, although an argument can be made that Western patients who have already developed gastric cancer are also at an increased risk, much like their Eastern counterparts. With a paucity of Western data on the topic, it seems appropriate to extend this surveillance recommendation to all patients treated for early gastric cancer regardless of geographic location.

ADVANCES IN THE MANAGEMENT OF METASTATIC DISEASE

For a surveillance regimen to confer a survival advantage, there must be effective treatment of recurrent or metastatic disease. Previously, there was little to offer patients with advanced recurrent and metastatic disease. However, in the last 2 decades, there has been increasing use of surgery for locoregional, peritoneal, and metastatic disease, as well as improvement in chemotherapy and targeted therapy for metastatic disease. The US Gastric Cancer Collaborative showed that, in patients treated with curative-intent gastrectomy and subsequent disease recurrence, 66.8% have recurrence at only a single site of disease. Of those, 23.4% had hematogenous-only disease (most commonly liver), 19.3% had peritoneal spread only, and 24.2% had locoregional spread.[58] In some patients with isolated recurrences, surgical therapy could potentially be used with curative intent and provide a survival advantage.[8,45]

In highly selected patients, surgical resection of recurrent disease has been shown to be associated with encouraging results, with 1-year, 3-year, and 5-year survival of 90%, 66%, and 44%, respectively.[45] Treatment options for peritoneal disease may also include cytoreduction and heated intraperitoneal chemotherapy (HIPEC), showing a median OS between 11 and 15.8 months, and a median 5-year survival between 10.7% and 15.8% in multiple studies.[59–63] In selected patients with complete cytoreduction treated with HIPEC, 5-year survival as high as 30% has been reported.[63] Resection for hepatic metastases has also show promising results. Two large meta-analyses and a large multi-institutional analysis have shown 5-year OS between 23.8% and 31.3%, and a median OS ranging from 8 to 48 months.[64–66] Resection of extrahepatic isolated metastases has also shown promising results, with one review of pulmonary metastasectomy for gastric cancer primary in 43 patients showing a 5-year OS of 33%.[67] These are highly selected patients with favorable biology of disease, but they do suggest that surgical resection for recurrent disease should be considered in selected patients and early detection may improve outcomes in these patients. The efficacy of chemotherapy and emergence of targeted therapy have also improved OS rates in metastatic gastric cancer in recent studies. A discussion of those advances is outside the scope of this article, but one of the biggest contributions in recent years is from the ToGA (Trastuzumab for Gastric Adenocarcinoma) trial, which showed an increase in survival by 4.3 months to 13.5 month median survival in highly overexpressed Her-2–positive gastric cancer treated with trastuzumab added to standard chemotherapy.[68] Many additional targeted therapies are being investigated and have the potential to significantly affect future systemic therapies for advanced gastric cancer.[69] Nevertheless, despite the advances in treatment of recurrent and metastatic disease, it remains unknown whether intensive surveillance strategies will affect the utility of these treatment modalities.

SUMMARY

Despite the minimalistic NCCN guidelines, practitioners still embrace a wide variety of surveillance patterns for a variety of reasons, including patient expectations, reassurance, and enrollment in clinical trials. All patients should be followed at minimum as recommended by the NCCN, with serial HPs and additional investigations based on patient-initiated findings. Furthermore, although early gastric cancers should be considered for intensive endoscopic follow-up, endoscopy is less likely to play a role in surveillance of advanced gastric cancer. Patients with advanced disease should only undergo intensive surveillance if they would be considered candidates for additional therapy, such as locoregional resection, cytoreduction and HIPEC, metastasectomy, or systemic chemotherapy and/or targeted therapy if recurrences or metastases are discovered. With regard to modalities of intensive follow-up, cross-sectional imaging in the form of contrast-enhanced CT is the most commonly used modality, although emerging data on the use of PET/CT exists, especially in the setting of increased levels of tumor markers or indeterminate imaging. In addition, tumor markers are a useful tool and generally detect recurrences 2 to 4 months before imaging modalities.[28,32] Of these, CEA, CA19-9, and CA72-4 are the most commonly used modalities. Preoperatively increased levels of markers are not a prerequisite for the utility of these markers, but sensitivity increases dramatically if they are increased. Ultimately, surveillance for gastric cancer should be individualized in each patient based on patient-related, tumor-related, and treatment-related factors, given the lack of standardized recommendations based on level I evidence.

REFERENCES

1. NCCN clinical practice guidelines in oncology (NCCN guidelines): gastric cancer. National Comprehensive Cancer Network. Available at: http://NCCN.org. Accessed June 7, 2016.
2. Wadhwa S, Johnson DY, Johnson FE. Stomach. In: Johnson FE, Maehara Y, Brownman GP, et al, editors. Patient Surveillance After Cancer Treatment. New York: Springer Science; 2013. p. 107–8.
3. Japanese Gastric Cancer Association. Guidelines for diagnosis and treatment of carcinoma of the stomach. Kyoto (Japan): Japanese Gastric Cancer Association; 2004. Available at: http://www.jgca.jp/pdf/Guidelines2004_eng.pdf. Accessed June 9, 2016.

4. Japanese Gastric Cancer Association. Japanese gastric cancer treatment guidelines 2010 (ver.3). Gastric Cancer 2011;14(2):113–23.
5. Baiocchi GL, Kodera Y, Marrelli D, et al. Follow-up after gastrectomy for cancer: results of an international web round table. World J Gastroenterol 2014;20(34): 119666–71.
6. Hur H, Song KY, Park CH, et al. Follow-up strategy after curative resection of gastric cancer: a nationwide survey in Korea. Ann Surg Oncol 2010;17(1):54–64.
7. Bohner H, Simmer T, Hopfenmuller W, et al. Detection and prognosis of recurrent gastric cancer – is routine follow-up after gastrectomy worthwhile. Hepatogastroenterology 2000;47(35):1489–94.
8. Kodera Y, Ito S, Yamamura Y, et al. Follow-up surveillance for recurrence after curative gastric cancer surgery lacks survival benefit. Ann Surg Oncol 2003; 10(8):898–902.
9. Bennett JJ, Gonen M, D'Angelica M, et al. Is detection of asymptomatic recurrence after curative gastric resection associated with improved survival in patients with gastric cancer? J Am Coll Surg 2005;201(4):503–10.
10. Tan IT, Jimmy BY. Value of intensive follow-up of patients after curative surgery for gastric carcinoma. J Surg Oncol 2007;96(6):503–6.
11. Eom BW, Ryu KW, Lee JH, et al. Oncologic effectiveness of regular follow-up to detect recurrence after curative resection of gastric cancer. Ann Surg Oncol 2011;18(2):358–64.
12. Park CH, Park JC, Chung H, et al. Impact of the surveillance interval on the survival of patients who undergo curative surgery for gastric cancer. Ann Surg Oncol 2016;23(2):539–45.
13. Bilci A, Salman T, Oven Ustaalioglu BB, et al. The prognostic value of detecting symptomatic or asymptomatic recurrence in patients with gastric cancer after a curative gastrectomy. J Surg Res 2013;180(1):e1–9.
14. Lee JH, Lim JK, Dwon SJ. The influence of post-operative surveillance on the prognosis after curative surgery for gastric cancer. Hepatogastroenterology 2014;61(135):2123–32.
15. Peixoto RD, Lim HJ, Kim H, et al. Patterns of surveillance following curative intent therapy for gastroesophageal cancer. J Gastrointest Cancer 2014;45(3):325–33.
16. Ha HK, Kim HH, Kim HS, et al. Local recurrence after surgery for gastric carcinoma. CT findings. Am J Roentgenol 1993;161(5):975–7.
17. Kim KW, Choi BI, Han JK, et al. Postoperative anatomic and pathologic findings at CT following gastrectomy. Radiographics 2002;22(2):326–36.
18. Mullin D, Shirkhoda A. Computed tomography after gastrectomy in primary gastric carcinoma. J Comput Assist Tomogr 1985;9(1):30–3.
19. Lee JW, Lee SM, Son MW, et al. Diagnostic performance of FDG PET/CT for surveillance in asymptomatic gastric cancer patients after curative surgical resection. Eur J Nucl Med Mol Imaging 2016;43(5):881–8.
20. Kim DW, Park SA, Kim CG. Detecting the recurrence of gastric cancer after curative resection: comparison of FDG PET/CT and contrast-enhanced abdominal CT. J Korean Med Sci 2011;26(7):875–80.
21. Sim SH, Kim YJ, Oh DY, et al. The role of PET/CT in detection of gastric cancer recurrence. BMC Cancer 2009;9:73.
22. Nakamoto Y, Togashi K, Fukda H, et al. Clinical value of whole-body FDG-PET fore recurrent gastric cancer: a multicenter study. Jpn J Clin Oncol 2009;39(5): 297–302.
23. Bilci A, Ustaalioglu BB, Seker M, et al. The role of 18F-FDG PET/CT in the assessment of suspected recurrent gastric cancer after initial surgical resection: can the

results of FDG PET/CT influence patients' treatment decision making. Eur J Nucl Med Mol Imaging 2011;38(1):64–73.

24. Park MJ, Lee WJ, Lim HK, et al. Detecting recurrence of gastric cancer: the value of FDG PET/CT. Abdom Imaging 2009;34(4):441–7.

25. Wu LM, Hu JN, Hua J, et al. 18 F-fluorodeoxyglucose positron emission tomography to evaluate recurrent gastric cancer after surgical resection: a systematic review and meta-analysis. J Gastroenterol Hepatol 2012;27(3):472–80.

26. Li P, Liu Q, Wang C, et al. Fluorine-18-fluorodeoxyglucose positron emission tomography to evaluate recurrent gastric cancer after surgical resection: a systematic review and meta-analysis. Ann Nucl Med 2016;30(3):179–87.

27. Shimada H, Noie T, Ohashi M, et al. Clinical significance of serum tumor markers for gastric cancer: a systematic review of literature by the Task Force of the Japanese Gastric Cancer Association. Gastric Cancer 2014;17(1):26–33.

28. Takahashi Y, Takeuchi T, Sakamoto J, et al, Tumor Marker Committee. The usefulness of CEA and/or CA19-9 in monitoring for recurrence in gastric cancer patients: a prospective clinical study. Gastric Cancer 2003;6(3):142–5.

29. Kim DH, Oh SJ, Oh CA, et al. The relationships between perioperative CEA, CA19-9, and CA72-4 and recurrence in gastric cancer patients after curative radical gastrectomy. J Surg Oncol 2011;104(6):585–91.

30. Marrelli D, Pinto E, De Stefano A, et al. Clinical utility of CEA, CA19-9, and CA72-4 in the follow-up of patients with resectable gastric cancer. Am J Surg 2001; 181(1):16–9.

31. Choi SR, Jang JS, Lee JH, et al. Role of serum tumor markers in monitoring for recurrence of gastric cancer following radical gastrectomy. Dig Dis Sci 2006; 51(11):2081–6.

32. Li Y, Yang Y, Lu M, et al. Predictive value of serum CEA, CA19-9 and CA72-4 in early diagnosis of recurrence after radical resection of gastric cancer. Hepatogastroenterology 2011;58(112):2166–70.

33. Lee S, Lee JH, Hwang NC, et al. The role of follow-up endoscopy after total gastrectomy for gastric cancer. Eur J Surg Oncol 2005;31(3):265–9.

34. Park YS, Park SJ, Jung I, et al. Mo1354 Is endoscopic surveillance necessary for patients who undergo total gastrectomy for gastric cancer? [abstract]. Gastrointest Endosc 2016;83(5S):AB466–7.

35. Komatsu S, Ichikawa D, Okamoto K, et al. Progression of remnant gastric cancer is associated with duration of follow-up following distal gastrectomy. World J Gastroenterol 2012;18(22):2832–6.

36. Ojima T, Iwahashi M, Nakamori M, et al. Clinicopathological characteristics of remnant gastric cancer after a distal gastrectomy. J Gastrointest Surg 2010;14: 277–81.

37. Howlader N, Noone AM, Krapcho M, et al. SEER cancer statistics review, 1975-2013. Bethesda (MD): National Cancer Institute; 2015. SEER Data. Available at: http://seer.cancer.gov/csr/1975_2013/. Accessed July 9, 2016.

38. Sano T, Sasako M, Knoshita T, et al. Recurrence of early gastric cancer: follow-up of 1475 patients and review of the Japanese literature. Cancer 1993;72(11): 3174–8.

39. Ikeda Y, Saku M, Kishihara F, et al. Effective follow-up for recurrence or a second primary cancer in patients with early gastric cancer. Br J Surg 2005;92(2):235–9.

40. Morgagni P, Gardini A, Marrelli D, et al, for the Italian Research Group for Gastric Cancer. Gastric stump carcinoma after distal subtotal gastrectomy for early gastric cancer: experience of 541 patients with long-term follow-up. Am J Surg 2015;209(6):1063–8.

41. Wu B, Wu D, Wang M, et al. Recurrence in patients following curative resection of early gastric carcinoma. J Surg Oncol 2008;98(6):411–4.

42. Nozaki I, Nasu J, Kubo Y, et al. Risk factors for metachronous gastric cancer in the remnant stomach after early cancer surgery. World J Surg 2010;34(7):1548–54.

43. Yamamoto M, Yamanaka T, Baba H, et al. The postoperative recurrence and the occurrence of second primary carcinomas in patients with early gastric carcinoma. J Surg Oncol 2008;97(3):231–5.

44. Lagergren J, Lindam A, Mason RM. Gastric stump cancer after distal gastrectomy for benign gastric ulcer in a population-based study. Int J Cancer 2012;131(6):E1048–52.

45. Ohashi M, Morita S, Fukagawa T, et al. Surgical treatment of non-early gastric remnant carcinoma developing after distal gastrectomy for gastric cancer. J Surg Oncol 2015;111(2):208–12.

46. Kondo A, Hourneaux de Moura EG, Bernardo WM, et al. Endoscopy vs surgery in the treatment of early gastric cancer: systematic review. World J Gastroenterol 2015;21(46):13177–87.

47. Gweon TG, Park JM, Lim CH, et al. Increased incidence of secondary gastric neoplasia in patients with early gastric cancer and coexisting gastric neoplasia at the initial endoscopic evaluation. Eur J Gastroeneterol Hepatol 2014;26(11):1209–16.

48. Fukase K, Kato M, Kikuchi S, et al, for Japan Gast Study Group. Effect of eradication of Helicobacter pylori on incidence of metachronous gastric carcinoma after endoscopic resection of early gastric cancer: an open-label, randomized controlled trial. Lancet 2008;372(9636):392–7.

49. Kikuchi S, Sato M, Katada N, et al. Efficacy of endoscopic surveillance of the upper gastrointestinal tract following distal gastrectomy for early gastric cancer. Hepatogastroenterology 2003;50(53):1704–7.

50. Min BH, Kim ER, Kim KM, et al. Surveillance strategy based on the incidence and patterns of recurrence after curative submucosal dissection for early gastric cancer. Endosocpy 2015;47(9):784–93.

51. Nishida T, Tsujii M, Kato M, et al. Endoscopic surveillance strategy after endoscopic resection for early gastric cancer. World J Gastrointest Pathophysiol 2014;5(2):100–6.

52. Abe S, Oda I, Suzuki H, et al. Long-term surveillance and treatment outcomes of metachronous gastric cancer occurring after endoscopic submucosal dissection. Endoscopy 2015;47(12):1113–8.

53. Choi J, Kim SG, Im JP, et al. Long-term clinical outcomes of endoscopic resection for early gastric cancer. Surg Endosc 2015;29(5):1223–30.

54. Park CH, Kim EH, Chung H, et al. Role of computed tomography scan for the primary surveillance of mucosal gastric cancer after complete resection by endoscopic submucosal dissection. Surg Endosc 2014;28(4):1307–13.

55. Sohn YJ, Jang JS, Choi SR, et al. Early detection of recurrence after endoscopic treatment for early gastric cancer. Scand J Gastroenterol 2009;44(9):1109–14.

56. Hahn KY, Park JC, Kim EH, et al. Incidence and impact of scheduled endoscopic surveillance on recurrence after curative endoscopic resection for early gastric cancer. Gastrointest Endosc 2016;84(4):628–38.e1.

57. Kato M, Nishida T, Yammoto K, et al. Scheduled endoscopic surveillance controls secondary cancer after curative endoscopic resection for early gastric cancer: a multicenter retrospective cohort study by Osaka University ESD study group. Gut 2013;62(10):1425–32.

58. Spolverato G, Ejaz A, Kim Y, et al. Rates and patterns of recurrence after curative intent resection for gastric cancer: a United States multi-institutional analysis. J Am Coll Surg 2014;219(4):664–75.

59. Rudlosff U, Langan RC, Mullinax JE, et al. Impact of maximal cytoreductive surgery plus regional heated intraperitoneal chemotherapy (HIPEC) on outcome of patients with peritoneal carcinomatosis of gastric origin: results of the GYMSSA trial. J Surg Oncol 2014;110(3):275–84.

60. Yang XJ, Huang CQ, Suo T, et al. Cytoreductive surgery and hyperthermic intraperitoneal chemotherapy improves survival of patients with peritoneal carcinomatosis from gastric cancer: final results of a phase III randomized clinical trial. Ann Surg Oncol 2011;18(6):1575–81.

61. Glehen O, Gilly FN, Arvieux C, et al, Association Francaise de Chirurgie. Peritoneal carcinomatosis from gastric cancer: a multi-institutional study of 159 patients treated by cytoreductive surgery combined with perioperative intraperitoneal chemotherapy. Ann Surg Oncol 2010;17(9):2370–7.

62. Canbay E, Mizumoto A, Ichinose M, et al. Outcome data of patients with peritoneal carcinomatosis from gastric origin treated by a strategy of bidirectional chemotherapy prior to cytoreductive surgery and hyperthermic intraperitoneal chemotherapy in a single specialized center in Japan. Ann Surg Oncol 2014; 21(4):1147–52.

63. Elias D, Goere D, Dumont F, et al. Role of hyperthermic intraoperative peritoneal chemotherapy in the management of peritoneal metastases. Eur J Cancer 2014; 50(2):332–40.

64. Petrelli F, Coinu A, Cabiddu M, et al. Hepatic resection for gastric cancer liver metastases: a systematic review and meta-analysis. J Surg Oncol 2015;111(8): 1021–7.

65. Gadde R, Tamariz L, Hanna M, et al. Metastatic gastric cancer (MGC) patients: can we improve survival by metastasectomy? A systematic review and meta-analysis. J Surg Oncol 2015;112(1):38–45.

66. Kinoshita T, Kinoshita T, Saiura A, et al. Multicenter analysis of long-term outcome after surgical resection for gastric cancer liver metastases. Br J Surg 2015; 102(1):102–7.

67. Kemp CD, Kitano M, Kerkar S, et al. Pulmonary resection for metastatic gastric cancer. J Thorac Oncol 2010;5(11):1796–805.

68. Bang YJ, Van Cutsem E, Feyereislova A, et al. Trastuzumab in combination with chemotherapy versus chemotherapy alone for treatment of Her-2-positive advanced gastric or gastroesophageal junction cancer (ToGA): a phase 3, open-label, randomized, controlled trial. Lancet 2010;376(9742):687–97.

69. Shah MA. Update on metastatic gastric and esophageal cancers. J Clin Oncol 2015;33(16):1760–9.

Neuroendocrine Tumors of the Stomach

Britney Corey, MD[a],*, Herbert Chen, MD[b]

KEYWORDS

- Gastric neuroendocrine tumor • Gastric carcinoid • Chronic atrophic gastritis
- Zollinger-Ellison syndrome • Sporadic carcinoid

KEY POINTS

- Gastric neuroendocrine tumors are increasing in incidence, possibly because of increased detection and better surveillance.
- Management strategies are based on the type of gastric neuroendocrine tumor.
- Type I gastric neuroendocrine tumors are associated with chronic atrophic gastritis and have a good prognosis. Endoscopic resection or surveillance is recommended.
- Type II gastric neuroendocrine tumors are associated with Zollinger-Ellison syndrome and multiple endocrine neoplasia type 1. Gastrinoma and neuroendocrine tumor resection is recommended.
- Type III gastric neuroendocrine tumors are sporadic, and have the worst prognosis, often presenting with metastatic disease. An oncologic resection is recommended if possible.

INTRODUCTION: GASTRIC NEUROENDOCRINE TUMORS

Gastric neuroendocrine tumors (NETs), commonly called carcinoids, are tumors that arise from neuroendocrine cells within the stomach. NETs can be located throughout the body, from solid endocrine organs to endocrine cells within other organs, such as the respiratory tract. This article focuses on a rare location, the stomach, which represents about 7% to 8% of all NETs.[1,2] However, the incidence of gastric NETs is increasing, possibly because of better surveillance or because of the widespread use of proton pump inhibitors.[2,3]

Disclosure: The authors have nothing to disclose.
[a] Department of Surgery, University of Alabama at Birmingham, KB 404, 1720 2nd Avenue South, Birmingham, AL 35294, USA; [b] Department of Surgery, UAB Hospital and Health System, UAB Comprehensive Cancer Center, University of Alabama at Birmingham, BDB 502, 1808 7th Avenue South, Birmingham, AL 35233, USA
* Corresponding author.
E-mail address: blprince@uabmc.edu

Surg Clin N Am 97 (2017) 333–343
http://dx.doi.org/10.1016/j.suc.2016.11.008
0039-6109/17/Published by Elsevier Inc.

The understanding of the behavior and pathophysiology of gastric NETs has developed and evolved since the 1970s, when it was noticed that patients with Zollinger-Ellison syndrome (ZES) had a proliferation of enterochromaffin-like (ECL) cells.[4] Clinicians now understand that gastric NETs develop from the histamine-secreting ECL cells of the stomach, although some NETs have been found to arise from serotonin-secreting enterochromaffin cells or ghrelin cells.[5] By the early 1990s, enough evidence was collected about gastric NETs to classify lesions into 3 distinct types (Table 1).[4,6]

TYPE I GASTRIC NEUROENDOCRINE TUMORS

Type I gastric NETs are the most common of the 3 types, comprising approximately 70% to 80% of cases of gastric NETs. They are associated with autoimmune atrophic gastritis, which causes achlorhydria and intrinsic factor deficiency.[4,7] As a result of the chronic achlorhydria, G-cell hyperplasia occurs, causing increased gastrin secretion, with subsequent hypergastrinemia.[7] Chronic proton pump inhibitors are thought to cause the development of gastric NETs in a similar fashion, although this has not been definitively established.[3,8] These tumors are more prevalent in women, and are usually small and multicentric. They tend to be confined to the mucosa or submucosa, and generally behave in a more benign fashion (Fig. 1).[8]

TYPE II GASTRIC NEUROENDOCRINE TUMORS

Type II gastric NETs are also associated with hypergastrinemia, in the setting of gastrinomas and ZES. Sporadic ZES rarely causes type II gastric NETs but they are common in the setting of multiple endocrine neoplasia type 1 (MEN-1).[7,9] They are the least frequently occurring, accounting for approximately 5% to 8%.[1,7,9] Although very similar to type I lesions, they tend to behave more aggressively, with an increased metastatic potential.[8] They occur equally in men and women (Fig. 2).[8,9]

Table 1
Characteristics of gastric neuroendocrine tumors

	Type 1	Type 2	Type 3
Percentage of Tumors	70–80	5–10	10–15
Associated Disease	Chronic atrophic gastritis, pernicious anemia	Multiple endocrine neoplasia type 1, ZES	None
Number of Tumors	>1	>1	1
Tumor Size (cm)	<1	<1	>1
Tumor Location	Fundus and body	Fundus, body, and occasionally antrum	Antrum or fundus
Gastric Acid Level	Low	High	Normal
Plasma Gastrin Level	High	High	Normal
Prognosis	Good	Moderately good	Poor

From Zhang L, Ozao J, Warner R, et al. Review of the pathogenesis, diagnosis, and management of type I gastric carcinoid tumor. World J Surg 2011;35(8):1880; with permission.

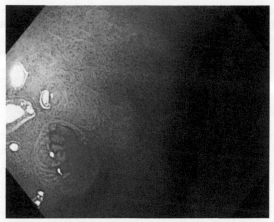

Fig. 1. A type I gastric NET seen on endoscopy in a patient with pernicious anemia. (*Courtesy of* Charles Wilcox, MD, University of Alabama at Birmingham, Birmingham, AL.)

TYPE III GASTRIC NEUROENDOCRINE TUMORS

Type III gastric NETs are considered sporadic because they do not occur with any associated condition, or in the setting of hypergastrinemia. They account for 15% to 20% of gastric NETs and have the most malignant potential. They predominate among men, and are usually large, solitary tumors ranging from 2 to 5 cm.[10]

NEUROENDOCRINE CARCINOMA

Although not originally identified in the classification system proposed by Rindi and colleagues,[6] a fourth type of gastric NET has been identified: the neuroendocrine carcinoma. These tumors are poorly differentiated with highly malignant behavior, typically presenting with advanced disease and widespread metastases.[11] In

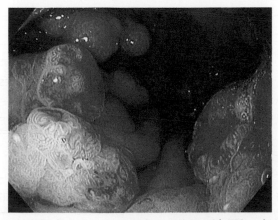

Fig. 2. Multiple gastric NETs during endoscopy in a patient with ZES and MEN-1. (*Courtesy of* Charles Wilcox, MD, University of Alabama at Birmingham, Birmingham, AL.)

general, a neuroendocrine carcinoma behaves more like an adenocarcinoma of the stomach but has an endocrine phenotype.[10] These patients are rarely candidates for oncologic resection, but may require surgical treatment of local symptoms of bleeding, perforation, or obstruction. Neuroendocrine carcinomas are occasionally classified as a type IV gastric NET, but this is not universally adopted.

PATHOPHYSIOLOGY

Gastric NETs arise from proliferating ECL cells. ECL cells are found in oxyntic gastric mucosa, typically located in the body of the stomach. ECL cells are acted on by gastrin, which causes the release of histamine.[10] Histamine then stimulates parietal cells to secrete acid. Gastrin also has a trophic effect on ECL cells, with hypergastrinemia causing ECL hypertrophy and hyperplasia. Gastric NETs then arise in the setting of this ECL hyperplasia, through a hyperplasia-dysplasia-neoplasia pathway.[1,7,9–11] In addition, patients with chronic atrophic gastritis are not able to suppress gastrin-producing G cells through the negative feedback of somatostatin, further promoting hypergastrinemia and its trophic effects on ECL cells (**Fig. 3**).[1]

Only a small percentage of patients with hypergastrinemia and ECL hyperplasia develop gastric NETs. Patients who have hypergastrinemia from other causes (eg, vagotomy) besides chronic atrophic gastritis and ZES do not develop gastric NETs. Patients with sporadic ZES not associated with MEN-1 are also far less likely to develop gastric NETs, which causes some clinicians to propose that an additional factor or influence is needed, such as a bacterial infection, genetic mutation, or local growth factor.[1] Type III gastric NETs arise sporadically, without any known evidence of a predisposing condition. There is no ECL hyperplasia as seen in type I and II.[11]

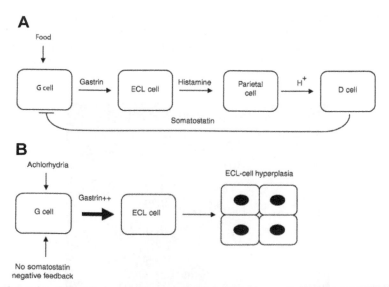

Fig. 3. The role of gastrin in (*A*) normal gastric epithelium and (*B*) gastric epithelium of patients with chronic atrophic gastritis. (*From* Burkitt MD, Pritchard DM. Review article: pathogenesis and management of gastric carcinoid tumours. Aliment Pharmacol Ther 2006;24:1306; with permission.)

GENETIC INFLUENCE

The MEN-1 gene has been studied the most extensively, because of its role in ZES. An autosomal dominant mutation located on chromosome 11q13 is associated with the development of gastric NETs, with all patients with type II having loss of heterozygosity, and 17% to 73% of patients with type I and 25% to 50% of patients with type III.[1,7] Mutated p53 is associated with type III gastric NETs. Other factors at the cellular level have possible contributions, such as the apoptosis-inhibiting protein BCL-2, extracellular matrix proteins matrix metalloproteinase (MMP)-7 and MMP-9, and growth factor Reg.[7]

CLINICAL PRESENTATION OF GASTRIC NEUROENDOCRINE TUMORS

Unlike other intestinal NETs, which may cause carcinoid syndrome, gastric NETs are typically nonfunctioning. Occasionally they become symptomatic when they become ulcerated, causing bleeding and/or anemia. For type I gastric NETs, the associated chronic atrophic gastritis can cause vitamin B_{12} and iron deficiency. Dyspepsia from slow gastric emptying may also be present.[12]

Type II gastric NETs arise in the setting of hypergastrinemia from a gastrinoma, which also causes increased acid secretion, with a high pH seen on 24-hour pH study or on aspiration of gastric secretions. Patients may therefore have the classic symptoms of peptic ulcer disease, and endoscopy often shows surrounding peptic ulcers. The gastric NET itself rarely causes the symptoms.[12]

The sporadic nature of type III gastric NETs means that there are no associated conditions to cause symptoms, and these lesions are usually discovered when they become symptomatic because of pain, bleeding, or weight loss. Rarely, these lesions are associated with an atypical form of carcinoid syndrome that causes itching, cutaneous wheals, and bronchospasms as a side effect of the release of high levels of histamine from ECL cells.[12]

DIAGNOSTIC PROCEDURES AND TECHNIQUES

The cornerstone of diagnostic procedures for gastric NETs remains esophagogastroduodenoscopy (EGD). In addition to directly observing the lesions, biopsies of the lesions should be performed, the number and size of the lesions noted, and biopsies of normal areas of gastric mucosa taken on the greater and lesser curve in order to have normal tissue for comparison of ECL density.[10,12] After a diagnosis of gastric NET is confirmed, endoscopic ultrasonography (EUS) may be warranted to determine the depth of invasion and the treatment strategy needed. Computed tomography (CT) or MRI scans are helpful if there is concern for metastatic disease or lymph node involvement. In addition, radiolabeled somatostatin analogues may assist in establishing location and extent of tumors, but are not routinely used.[10]

In addition to the diagnostic procedures mentioned earlier, serum biomarkers should be drawn, to include plasma chromogranin A (CgA), plasma histamine, plasma serotonin, and plasma gastrin. Increased gastrin levels are expected in type I and II, but should be normal in type III. CgA is a glycoprotein expressed in the secretory granules of ECL cells and released on stimulation along with other cells. CgA often has increased circulating levels in functional and nonfunctional NETs; however, increased levels can be found in other diseases as well, such as renal failure, cardiac disease, and in the setting of proton pump inhibitor use, so this must be taken into account.[13] In tumors with increased CgA levels, it is useful as a marker of response to treatment and to monitor for recurrence.[14] A study by Borch and colleagues[15] showed an increased plasma CgA concentration compared with patients without carcinoid, with a median plasma CgA concentration of 5.7 nmol/L (3.5–40).

HISTOLOGY AND GRADING OF GASTRIC NEUROENDOCRINE TUMORS

Histologic examination of gastric NETs can be difficult, and treatment in a large center with experience is recommended. Type I and type II gastric NETs show ECL cell lesions with neoplasia. They often stain for argyrophil and argentaffin, and CgA is identified in all tumors.[10] In comparison, type III gastric NETs have a more consistent histologic pattern, and usually stains for argyrophil but not argentaffin. In addition to immunoreactivity to CgA, they are also immunoreactive to neuron-specific enolase, synaptophysin, and s-100.[10]

Grading of gastric NETs is based on the World Health Organization 2010 classification system for neuroendocrine neoplasms. The rate of proliferation is determined by the number of mitoses per 10 high-power microscopic fields, and on the percentage of tumor cells positively immune labeled for Ki-67 antigen, called the Ki-67 index. Grade 1 tumors have a mitotic rate less than 2 and Ki-67 index less than 3%, whereas grade 2 tumors have a mitotic rate of 2 to 20, and Ki-67 index of 3% to 20%. Any mitotic rate greater than 20 or Ki-67 index greater than 20% is grade 3.[16] This grading system provides a common means for defining tumors pathologically. The National Comprehensive Cancer Network recommends staging gastric NETs according to the seventh edition of the American Joint Committee on Cancer manual, published in 2010. See the National Comprehensive Cancer Network Guidelines here: https://www.nccn.org/professionals/physician_gls/pdf/neuroendocrine.pdf.

DIAGNOSIS AND TREATMENT OF GASTRIC NEUROENDOCRINE TUMORS
Type I Gastric Neuroendocrine Tumors

Using the previously discussed diagnostic methods, type I gastric NETs are typically found in the fundus. They are usually polypoid, multicentric, and are in the 5-mm to 8-mm range. They may be irregularly shaped, erythematous, and have a depression or central ulcer.[11] Gastric secretions aspirated at the time of endoscopy show a pH greater than 4 because of the chronic atrophic gastritis and a lack of acid secretion from parietal cells.

Debate remains about the best treatment of type I gastric NETs less than 1 cm in size (**Fig. 4**). Some clinicians favor endoscopic polypectomy, whereas others argue that the favorable outcome of these lesions requires simple endoscopic surveillance. Whether removed or not, surveillance with endoscopy should be performed on a yearly basis. If the lesion is larger than 1 cm, EUS should be performed to assess the level of invasion. If the lesion is localized to the mucosa or submucosa, then an endoscopic mucosal resection or submucosal dissection with resection should be performed.[10] A surgical resection is recommended for any patient with 6 lesions, of which 3 to 4 of the lesions are larger than 1 cm, or if a single lesion is larger than 2 cm. If larger than 2 cm, CT or MRI is recommended to assess for invasion and nodal disease.[12] Medical management of type I gastric NETs includes intramuscular injections of a long-acting somatostatin analogue every month, with minimal side effects. This management is typically reserved for patients who are not candidates for surgical treatment.[14]

There remain a significant number of clinicians who favor a gastric antrectomy in the setting of type I gastric NET with multifocal lesions, invasive lesions, or for

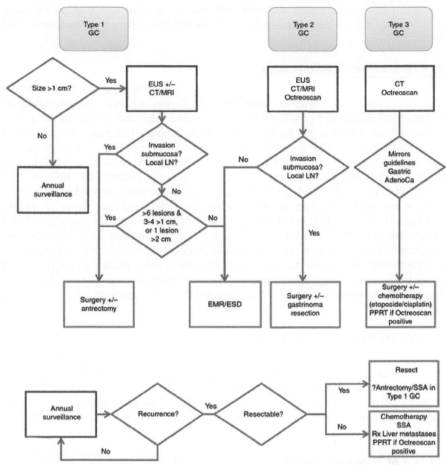

Fig. 4. Algorithm for treating gastric NETs based on type. SSA, somatostatin analogues. Adeno-CA, adenocarcinoma; EMR, endoscopic mucosal resection; ESD, endoscopic submucosal dissection; GC, gastric carcinoid; LN, lymph nodes; PPRT, Peptide Receptor Radionuclide Therapy; Rx, resect. (*From* Basuroy R, Srirajaskanthan R, Prachalias A, et al. Review article: the investigation and management of gastric neuroendocrine tumors. Aliment Pharmacol Ther 2014;39:1076; with permission.)

recurrent lesions, because antrectomy removes the G cells, thereby removing the source of hypergastrinemia.[17] There is evidence that more than 90% of gastric NETs regress once hypergastrinemia has resolved.[11] However, some lesions develop autonomy from gastrin secretion, and continue to progress even with normalized gastrin levels. In 2016, Jenny and colleagues[18] published a series of patients with type I gastric NETs who underwent laparoscopic antrectomy and had a lower recurrence risk and less postintervention monitoring with EGD compared with patients who underwent surveillance or polypectomy. Other investigators argue that these patients must be committed to lifelong surveillance regardless. Chen and colleagues[19] published the Mount Sinai experience with type I gastric NETs in 2014. In their series, 5.5% of patients with type I gastric NET later developed gastric adenocarcinoma, supporting continued endoscopic monitoring of patients.

This finding is in accordance with the National Comprehensive Cancer Network guidelines for EGD follow-up every 6 to 12 months following initial resection, then annually.[19,20]

Type II Gastric Neuroendocrine Tumors

Diagnosis and treatment of type II gastric NETs differs from type I because of the more malignant and invasive potential of these lesions. On endoscopy, multiple, small polypoid tumors are seen, and there may also be peptic ulcer disease visualized. Lesions are typically within the fundus, but may also be in the antrum. Gastric secretions are highly acidic, with a pH less than 2. Serum gastrin levels are increased in most patients, with levels greater than 1000 pg/mL.[12] In addition to endoscopy and serum gastrin, genetic testing for MEN-1 and localization of the associated gastrinomas should be pursued, as well as screening for other associated tumors in the parathyroid and pituitary. Type II gastric NETs should be resected; endoscopic resection is reserved for lesions without invasion beyond the submucosa. An oncologic resection is recommended for lesions that are invasive, as well as resection of the gastrinoma if possible. If the gastrinoma is unable to be resected, then acid hypersecretion should be controlled with high-dose proton pump inhibitors or serum serotonin antagonists. Surveillance should be continued on an annual basis following resection.

Type III Gastric Neuroendocrine Tumors

Type III gastric NETs are usually larger than 2 cm and solitary, and the surrounding gastric mucosa is normal. Invasion beyond the submucosa is typical and there are metastases in 50% to 100% of patients on presentation.[7,12] Staging with CT and/or MRI is required. If metastatic disease is present, then treatment with systemic therapy is first line. Resectable disease undergoes an oncologic resection with lymphadenectomy.

Treatment of Metastatic Disease

Metastatic liver disease from gastric NETs is managed using surgery, systemic therapy, and locoregional control methods. Somatostatin analogues (SSAs) can be used as antiproliferative agents or antisecretory agents if carcinoid syndrome is present.[12,16] In addition, SSAs may have a role in other types of gastric NETs by suppressing the gastrin secretion and decreasing the proliferative effect on the ECL cells. In general, treatment is well tolerated, with lesions showing regression or reduction in size; however, lesions recur once therapy is stopped. No improvement has yet been seen in outcomes using SSAs.[12] Chemotherapy in advanced disease can have a 20% to 40% response rate; commonly used agents include streptozotocin, 5-fluorouracil, cyclophosphamide, etoposide, and doxorubicin.[10,21]

A new therapy being developed is netazepide, an oral medication that is a selective antagonist of the gastrin/cholecystokinin (CCK)-2 receptor.[11] In a nonrandomized trial, it showed reduction in the number and size of type I gastric NETs, as well as normalization of CgA levels, but not of gastrin.[16] Further studies are needed to fully understand its potential therapeutic benefits for gastric NETs.

As more understanding is gained of the biochemical mechanisms behind gastric and other NET development, additional therapeutic targets can be developed. For example, Somnay and colleagues[22] recently showed that chrysin, an anticancer flavonoid, induces apoptosis and cell-cycle arrest in a gut NET line. This finding has important therapeutic possibilities across the spectrum of NETs.

CLINICAL OUTCOMES FOR GASTRIC NEUROENDOCRINE TUMORS

Outcomes for gastric NETs overall correlate well with the type of tumor, as well as with the grade, with type I tumors usually doing well and type III tumors behaving more poorly. Type I tumors are usually grade 1 and stage 1 tumors that have a low Ki67 are rarely invasive into the muscularis propria, and rarely metastasize when less than 1 cm. There is an excellent long-term prognosis, with a normal life expectancy, even on the rare occasion that metastases develop.[12,23–27]

Type II gastric NETs are usually well differentiated, with a grade of 1 or 2, but 5% to 35% have spread to regional lymph nodes. Overall, the prognosis remains good, with a mortality of less than 10%.[11,12,28] Most type III tumors are also grade 2, but grade 3 tumors are more common than in other types. Invasion beyond the submucosa is common and, as mentioned, metastatic disease is present in 50% to 100% of patients.[12] Survival is the poorest in this group, with a mortality of 25% to 30%.[28]

Postlewait and colleagues[29] published 15-year results of a cohort of patients at Emory Hospital. Three-year recurrence-free survival was 33% for type I versus 86% for type III, which is as expected because of the pathophysiology of type I tumors. Three-year disease-specific survival was 100% for type I and 75% for type III tumors. Similarly, Rappel and colleagues[23] showed that patients with type I gastric NETs had a normal life expectancy, whereas patients with type III gastric NETs had an age-corrected survival rate of 79%.

SUMMARY

There is much still to be learned about gastric NETs. A better understanding of the molecular genetic pathways that influence the development of all types of lesions is needed. Additional clinical studies are needed to delineate the best management strategies for type I and II gastric NETs. Further development of pharmacologic agents and randomized controlled trials of current agents are necessary. The increasing incidence of gastric NETs makes this all the more urgent.

REFERENCES

1. Nikou GC, Angelopoulos TP. Current concepts on gastric carcinoid tumors. Gastroenterol Res Pract 2012;2012:287825.
2. Modlin IM, Lye KD, Kidd M. A 5-decade analysis of 13,715 carcinoid tumors. Cancer 2003;97(4):934–59.
3. Nandy N, Hanson JA, Strickland RG, et al. Solitary gastric carcinoid tumor associated with long-term use of omeprazole: a case report and review of the literature. Dig Dis Sci 2016;61:708–12.
4. Bordi C. Neuroendocrine pathology of the stomach: the Parma contribution. Endocr Pathol 2014;25:171–80.
5. Latta E, Rotondo F, Leiter LA, et al. Ghrelin- and serotonin-producing gastric carcinoid. J Gastrointest Cancer 2012;43:319–23.
6. Rindi G, Petrone G, Inzani F. 25 Years of neuroendocrine neoplasms of the gastrointestinal tract. Endocr Pathol 2014;25:59–64.
7. Burkitt MD, Pritchard DM. Review article: pathogenesis and management of gastric carcinoid tumours. Aliment Pharmacol Ther 2006;24:1305–20.

8. Kidd M, Gustafsson B, Modlin IM. Gastric carcinoids (neuroendocrine neoplasms). Gastroenterol Clin North Am 2013;42:381–97.
9. Mulkeen A, Cha C. Gastric carcinoid. Curr Opin Oncol 2005;17(1):1–6.
10. Modlin IM, Kidd M, Lye KD. Biology and management of gastric carcinoid tumours: a review. Eur J Surg 2002;168:669–83.
11. Fendrich V, Bartsch DK. Surgical treatment of gastrointestinal neuroendocrine tumors. Langenbecks Arch Surg 2011;396:299–311.
12. Basuroy R, Srirajaskanthan R, Prachalias A, et al. Review article: the investigation and management of gastric neuroendocrine tumors. Aliment Pharmacol Ther 2014;39:1071–84.
13. Verbeek WH, Korse CM, Tesselaar MET. Secreting gastro-enteropancreatic neuroendocrine tumours and biomarkers. Eur J Endocrinol 2016;174:R1–7.
14. Zhang L, Ozao J, Warner R, et al. Review of the pathogenesis, diagnosis, and management of type I gastric carcinoid tumor. World J Surg 2011;35:1879–86.
15. Borch K, Stridsberg M, Burman P, et al. Basal chromogranin A and gastrin concentrations in circulation correlate to endocrine cell proliferation in type-A gastritis. Scand J Gastroenterol 1997;32(3):198–202.
16. Massironi S, Zilli A, Conte D. Somatostatin analogs for gastric carcinoids: for many, but not all. World J Gastroenterol 2015;21(22):6785–93.
17. Hirschowitz BI. Clinical aspects of ECL-cell abnormalities. Yale J Biol Med 1998; 71(3–4):303–10.
18. Jenny HE, Ogando PA, Fujitani K, et al. Laparoscopic antrectomy: a safe and definitive treatment in managing type 1 gastric carcinoids. Am J Surg 2016; 211:778–82.
19. Chen WC, Warner RRP, Ward SC, et al. Management and disease outcome of type I gastric neuroendocrine tumors: the Mount Sinai experience. Dig Dis Sci 2015;60:996–1003.
20. [Guideline] National Comprehensive Cancer Network. Available at: https://www.nccn.org/professionals/physician_gls/pdf/neuroendocrine.pdf. Accessed July 17, 2016.
21. Gilligan CJ, Lawton GP, Tang LH, et al. Gastric carcinoid tumors: the biology and therapy of an enigmatic and controversial lesion. Am J Gastroenterol 1995;90(3): 338–52.
22. Somnay YR, Dull BZ, Eide J, et al. Chrysin suppresses the achaete-scute complex-like 1 and alters the neuroendocrine phenotype of carcinoids. Cancer Gene Ther 2015;22(10):496–505.
23. Rappel S, Altendorf-Hofmann A, Stolte M. Prognosis of gastric carcinoid tumors. Digestion 1995;56(6):455–62.
24. Hosokawa O, Kaizaki Y, Hatoori M, et al. Long-term follow up of patients with multiple gastric carcinoids associated with type A gastritis. Gastric Cancer 2005; 8(1):42–6.
25. Kim BS, Park YS, Yook JH, et al. Differing clinical courses and prognoses in patients with gastric neuroendocrine tumors based on the 2010-WHO classification scheme. Medicine 2015;94(44):e1748.
26. La Rosa S, Inzani F, Vanoli A, et al. Histologic characterization and improved prognostic evaluation of 209 gastric neuroendocrine neoplasms. Hum Pathol 2011;42:1373–84.
27. Thomas D, Tsolakis AV, Grozinsky-Glasberg S, et al. Long term follow-up of a large series of patients with type 1 gastric carcinoid tumors: data from a multicenter study. Eur J Endocrinol 2013;168:185–93.

28. Ruszniewski P, Delle Fave G, Cadiot G, et al. Well-differentiated gastric tumors/carcinomas. Neuroendocrinology 2006;84:158–64.
29. Postlewait LM, Baptiste GG, Ethun CG, et al. A 15-year experience with gastric neuroendocrine tumors: does type make a difference? J Surg Oncol 2016; 114(5):576–80.

Genetics of Gastric Cancer

Matthew S. Strand, MD[a], Albert Craig Lockhart, MD, MHS[b],
Ryan C. Fields, MD[a],*

KEYWORDS

- Gastric adenocarcinoma • Gastric cancer • Hereditary gastric cancer syndromes
- Genetics • Targeted therapy • Immunotherapy • Prophylactic gastrectomy

KEY POINTS

- Gastric cancer carries a poor prognosis, is typically diagnosed at a late stage, and has significant geographic differences in incidence and mortality; environmental factors including *Helicobacter pylori* infection, smoking, and diet play a role in many cases.
- Next-generation sequencing has led to molecular classification systems that serve as adjuncts to traditional histologic schemes; these new systems are being used to design new targeted therapies and implement them in clinical trials.
- To date, most trials using targeted therapies against specific mutations have yielded disappointing results, with the notable exception of trastuzumab for HER2+ gastric cancers.
- Immunotherapy has demonstrated some benefit in select cases, with response rates correlating roughly with the mutational burden of the tumor.
- Hereditary syndromes recognized thus far account for about 1% to 3% of gastric cancer cases, but are associated with early onset and aggressive disease, making prophylactic gastrectomy the treatment of choice for many cases.

INTRODUCTION

Gastric cancer represents the third leading cause of cancer mortality worldwide, with an estimated incidence of 951,000 cases, causing 723,000 deaths annually.[1] The American Cancer Society estimates that in the United States in 2016, 26,370 cases of gastric cancer will be diagnosed and 10,730 will die from the disease.[2] More than 70% of new cases arise in the developing world, and despite an overall decline in age-adjusted incidence, the absolute incidence is increasing because of an aging population. Host risk factors in the United States include male gender, age, and nonwhite race.[3] Established environmental risk factors include *Helicobacter pylori* infection, smoking, consumption of foods high in salt or N-nitroso compounds such as processed or smoked meats, and Epstein-Barr virus (EBV) infection.[4] Interestingly,

[a] Department of Surgery, Barnes-Jewish Hospital and Washington University School of Medicine, 660 South Euclid Avenue, Campus Box 8109, St Louis, MO 63110, USA; [b] Department of Medicine, Barnes-Jewish Hospital and Washington University School of Medicine, 660 South Euclid Avenue, Campus Box 8056, St Louis, MO 63110, USA
* Corresponding author.
E-mail address: fieldsr@wudosis.wustl.edu

Surg Clin N Am 97 (2017) 345–370
http://dx.doi.org/10.1016/j.suc.2016.11.009
0039-6109/17/© 2016 Elsevier Inc. All rights reserved.

the incidence of gastric cancer seems to be increasing in younger age groups; however, the cause of this phenomenon is unknown.[5]

This article aims to cover the genetics of gastric cancer as it is currently understood, focusing first on recently developed molecular classification schemes that are useful adjuncts to older histopathological systems. After delving into the molecular subtypes and their defining features, the article discusses additional molecular alterations present across multiple subtypes that are actively being explored for targeted therapy. The results of clinical trials targeting these pathways are presented, followed by a brief review of immunotherapy in gastric cancer. Finally, hereditary gastric cancer and syndromes associated with gastric cancer are summarized.

CLASSIFICATION OF GASTRIC CANCER

The advent of next-generation sequencing and molecular characterization techniques has revolutionized the classification of gastric cancer from a histopathological system to a system based on molecular patterns. The Lauren system, developed in 1965, divides gastric cancer into diffuse and intestinal subtypes,[6] whereas the World Health Organization classification system uses 4 categories: papillary, tubular, mucinous, and poorly cohesive subtypes.[7] Although these older histopathological systems are useful for informing prognosis, they are poor predictors of response to therapy.[8] Modern molecular classification schemes developed within the last few years aim not only to inform prognosis but also to form a framework to predict treatment response, develop targeted therapies, and eventually guide clinical decisions. Two major cancer research groups, The Cancer Genome Atlas Research Group (TCGA) and the Asian Cancer Research Group (ACRG), have developed molecular classification systems based on gene expression profiling.[9,10]

The TCGA system classifies gastric cancer into 4 subtypes: EBV-positive (EBV), microsatellite unstable (MSI), chromosomally unstable (CIN), and genomically stable (GS). These subtypes were derived by subjecting chemotherapy-naive gastric cancers to 6 molecular analyses: whole exome sequencing, somatic copy number analysis, DNA methylation profiling, messenger and microRNA sequencing, and protein analysis. Cluster analysis for each of the 6 modalities was performed, and the results were integrated, yielding 4 distinct gastric cancer subtypes. Hallmarks of each subtype are demonstrated in **Fig. 1**; these molecular features may play a role in defining treatment groups. For example, EBV and MSI gastric cancers have been shown to exhibit significantly higher PD-L1 expression and a greater degree of T-lymphocyte infiltration compared with EBV-negative or GS tumors, suggesting a role for immunotherapy in these subtypes.[11]

EBV-subtype gastric cancers are defined by infection with EBV and comprise approximately 9% of all gastric cancers.[12] More than 75% of the EBV-positive gastric cancers occur in male patients, and most are located in the fundus or body of the stomach. Additional hallmarks of the EBV-subtype include extreme CpG island methylator phenotype, CDKN2A (p16INK4A) promoter hypermethylation, overexpression of PD-L1 and PD-L2, and a PIK3CA mutation rate exceeding 80%. These findings may indicate a role for immunotherapy and PI(3)-kinase inhibition in this subtype.

MSI tumors are characterized by elevated mutation rates, hypermethylation of MLH1 (in contrast to EBV tumors), and frequent mutations in PIK3CA, ERBB2, ERBB3, epidermal growth factor receptor (EGFR), and MHC class 1 genes. Unlike MSI colorectal cancers, gastric MSI tumors lack BRAFV600E mutations. These cancers tend be diagnosed in older patients, with a median age at diagnosis of 72 years. There is also a slight but significant female predominance (56%). In small, preliminary

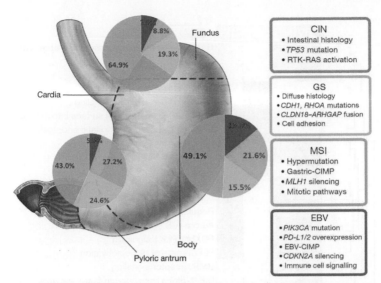

Fig. 1. Hallmarks of TCGA gastric cancer subtypes. CIMP, CpG island methylator phenotype. (*Adapted from* Cancer Genome Atlas Research Network. Comprehensive molecular characterization of gastric adenocarcinoma. Nature 2014;513(7517):206; with permission.)

studies, these tumors respond well to PD-1 blockade,[13] likely due to their tendency to have more robust T-cell infiltrates,[11] which in turn may be related to their high mutational burden.[9]

The GS and CIN subtypes are distinguished by low- versus high-somatic copy number variation. GS-subtype gastric cancers are enriched for the Lauren diffuse subtype; interestingly, elevated expression of cell adhesion pathways was observed in this group. Angiogenesis-related pathways also tend to be upregulated in these tumors, implying a potential role for vascular endothelial growth factor (VEGF) inhibitors. Additional key features include mutations in CDH1 and RHOA, a low frequency of p53 mutation, and CLDN18-ARHGAP fusions. Clinically, GS tumors are diagnosed at a significantly younger age than the other TCGA subtypes.

CIN tumors have a high degree of somatic copy number variation by definition. They are commonly p53-mutated and exhibit activation of the RTK-Ras pathway. The CIN subtype accounts for nearly half of all gastric cancers and comprises the predominant subtype of cancer of the gastroesophageal junction (GEJ) or cardia. These cancers are most commonly of the Lauren intestinal subtype.

Mutations seen across multiple subtypes include TP53, ARID1A, KRAS, PIK3CA, RNF43, ERBB2, as well as genes of the transforming growth factor-β and β-catenin pathways. Focal gene amplifications were seen in multiple known oncogenes, including ERBB2, CCNE1, KRAS, MYC, EGFR, CDK6, GATA4, GATA6, and ZNF217. Deletions were observed in several tumor suppressors, specifically PTEN, SMAD4, CDKN2A, and ARID1A. Integrated pathway analysis revealed a pattern of alterations in pathways involving mitosis, cell migration, and immune signaling (**Fig. 2**).

Similar to TCGA, the ACRG performed gene expression analysis to identify 4 clinically relevant molecular subtypes of gastric cancer: epithelial-to-mesenchymal transition (EMT), microsatellite-unstable (MSI), TP53-active (TP53+), and TP53 inactive (TP53−).[10] Principal component analysis was used to identify clusters of cancer cases with similar molecular traits; the association of these groups with predefined

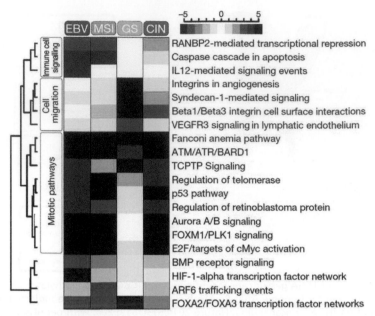

Fig. 2. Pathway alteration characteristics of TCGA gastric cancer subtypes. Red shading denotes upregulated pathways, while blue denotes downregulated pathways. IL-12, interleukin-12. (*From* Cancer Genome Atlas Research Network. Comprehensive molecular characterization of gastric adenocarcinoma. Nature 2014;513(7517):206; with permission.)

gene expression signatures was then determined. Two groups of cancer cases showed mutually exclusive associations with the epithelial-to-mesenchymal transition (EMT) signature and the MSI signature. Non-EMT, non-MSI cases were then divided into TP53-active and TP53-inactive groups. These molecular subtypes were then validated using the TCGA cohort and the Gastric Cancer Project '08 Singapore cohort, which confirmed the presence of these distinct groups.

As in the TCGA dataset, the MSI subtype was associated with hypermutation and mutations in KRAS, PI3K-PTEN-mTOR pathway, ALK, and ARID1A. The TP53+ subtype showed mutations in APC, ARID1A, KRAS, PIK3CA, and SMAD4. The ACRG also defined a genome instability index and found that this was significantly associated with the TP53− subtype. This group was also enriched for mutations in ERBB2, EGFR, CCNE1, CCND1, MDM2, ROBO2, GATA6, and MYC. Amplifications in ERBB2, EGFR, CCNE1, and CCND1 were also more common in this group.

Three major trends emerged from the ARCG molecular subtypes. The EMT subtype occurred in significantly younger patients and was enriched for Lauren diffuse gastric cancers, typically diagnosed at stage III or IV. MSI cancers were associated with the Lauren intestinal subtype, were typically located in the antrum, and were diagnosed at earlier stage (I/II). Most EBV-positive tumors were classified as TP53+. In contrast to the TCGA data, ACRG molecular subtypes did yield prognostic significance; moreover, this was validated when the ACRG classification was applied to the TCGA, SMC-2, and GSE14954 cohorts (**Fig. 3**). MSI carried the best prognosis, followed by TP53+ and TP53−, with EMT portending the worst prognosis.

A comparison of the TCGA and ACRG subtypes showed a strong correlation of the MSI groups in both studies, and some correlation of the TCGA GS, EBV+, and CIN subtypes with ACRG EMT, TP53+, and TP53− groups, respectively.

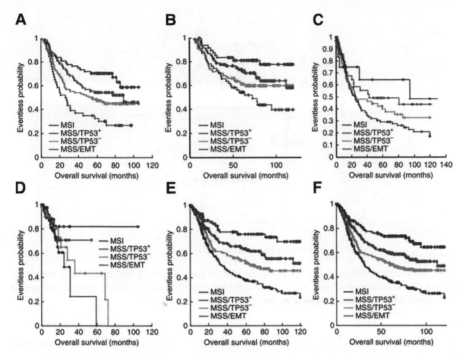

Fig. 3. Survival by ACRG gastric cancer subtype across multiple cohorts. (*A*) ACRG cohort. (*B*) SMC-2 cohort. (*C*) GSE14954 cohort. (*D*) TCGA cohort. (*E*) Merged SMC-2, GSE14954, and TCGA cohorts. (*F*) All 4 cohorts. Eventless probability indicates the likelihood of being alive (Y) at a given time (X) beginning from the time of diagnosis. (*From* Cristescu R, Lee J, Nebozhyn M, et al. Molecular analysis of gastric cancer identifies subtypes associated with distinct clinical outcomes. Nat Med 2015;21(5):452; with permission.)

PATHWAYS IMPLICATED IN GASTRIC CANCER AND RELEVANT TARGETED THERAPIES

A greater understanding of the molecular mechanisms of oncogenesis, progression, recurrence, and metastasis in gastric cancer has led to the development of targeted agents across a wide range of cellular pathways (**Fig. 4**). The following section reviews pathways known to play a role in gastric cancer, the targeted agents that have been developed to disrupt these pathways, and the results of corresponding clinical trials.

Human Epidermal Growth Factor Receptor 2

The human epidermal growth factor receptor 2 (HER2, also known as ERBB2) is a receptor tyrosine kinase involved in stimulating a variety of downstream pathways (MAPK, PI3K/PTEN/Akt/mTOR, PLC, STAT) involved in cell proliferation, differentiation, and migration.[14] Although its role as an oncogene first became relevant in breast cancer,[15] HER2 overexpression in gastric cancer was reported in 1986.[16] Across multiple studies, HER2 overexpression (as a result of mutation or amplification) ranges from 4.4% to 53.4%, with an average of 17.9% of all gastric cancers.[17] The prognostic significance of HER2 expression in gastric cancer is unclear, with some studies suggesting it is a poor prognostic marker,[18] and others finding no correlation with overall survival (OS).[19,20] HER2 does appear to have a stronger association with poor prognosis in younger patients (<60 years old),[19] low stage (stage I/II),[19] and Lauren

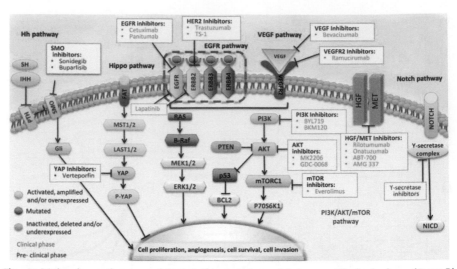

Fig. 4. Molecular pathways and targeted agents in gastric cancer. Hh, hedgehog. (*From* Riquelme I, Saavedra K, Espinoza JA, et al. Molecular classification of gastric cancer: towards a pathway-driven targeted therapy. Oncotarget 2015;6(28):24766.)

intestinal subtype cancers.[20] These observations spurred the use of HER2 inhibitors in gastric cancer in the form of monoclonal antibodies and small molecule inhibitors.

With the efficacy and safety of the anti-HER2 monoclonal antibody trastuzumab already established in HER2-positive breast cancer,[21] and evidence that HER2 was also a driver of tumor progression in gastric cancer, the Trastuzumab for Gastric Cancer (ToGA) trial was conducted to assess the efficacy of this agent.[22] Five hundred ninety-four patients with HER2-positive locally advanced, recurrent, or metastatic gastric or GEJ cancers were randomized to receive either chemotherapy alone or chemotherapy plus trastuzumab. Median OS was 13.8 months in the trastuzumab group, and 11.1 months in the chemotherapy-alone group ($P = .0049$) (**Fig. 5**). A subgroup of patients with especially high HER2 expression demonstrated a greater survival benefit, with a median survival of 16 months. This landmark study represents the major success of targeted therapy in gastric cancer to date, providing the best evidence for HER2 inhibition in gastric cancer. However, unlike for breast cancer, continuation of trastuzumab after failure of first-line therapy provides no additional benefit.

In a similar fashion, the Translational Research in Oncology/Lapatinib Optimization Study in HER2-Positive Gastric Cancer (TRIO-013/LOGiC) trial was conducted to assess the efficacy of lapatinib, a small molecule HER2 inhibitor approved for the treatment of HER2-positive breast cancer.[23] This study was a phase 3, double-blind, randomized controlled trial conducted across 186 centers in Asia, Europe, and North and South America, enrolling 545 patients with gastric, esophageal, or GEJ cancer to receive either capecitabine and oxaliplatin or lapatinib plus capecitabine and oxaliplatin. The primary endpoint of OS demonstrated no difference between the 2 groups, and an increased rate of adverse events (AEs) in the group receiving lapatinib. However, improved survival was seen in subgroup analyses of Asian patients and patients less than 60 years old.

The Tykerb with Taxol in Asian HER2-Positive Gastric Cancer (TyTAN) trial examined the efficacy of adding lapatinib to paclitaxel as second-line therapy for Asian

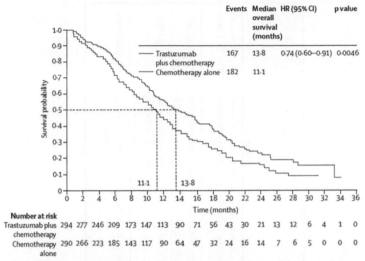

Fig. 5. Survival curves in the ToGA study. CI, confidence interval; HR, hazard ratio. *(From Bang YJ, Van Cutsem E, Feyereislova A, et al. Trastuzumab in combination with chemotherapy versus chemotherapy alone for treatment of HER2-positive advanced gastric or gastro-oesophageal junction cancer (ToGA): a phase 3, open-label, randomised controlled trial. Lancet 2010;376(9742):690; with permission.)*

patients with HER2+ gastric cancer.[24] OS trended toward favoring lapitinib plus paclitaxel versus paclitaxel alone (median OS 11.0 months vs 8.9 months), but this did not reach statistical significance. A secondary endpoint, response rate to therapy, did significantly favor the addition of lapatinib. Similar to the ToGA trial, increased efficacy was observed in the immunohistochemistry (IHC) 3+ group compared with lower levels of HER2 expression.

Despite efficacy in breast cancer,[25–27] there is currently no clear role for lapatinib in gastric cancer, although future clinical trials may eventually define a suitable subpopulation. The reasons for the differences in efficacy for anti-HER2 therapy between breast and gastric cancer are not clear, but could be related to changes in HER2 expression with first-line chemotherapy.[28] **Table 1** summarizes the major studies targeting HER2 in gastric cancer.

Epidermal Growth Factor Receptor

In addition to HER2, EGFR has been shown to be overexpressed in gastric cancer and is associated with a poor prognosis.[30] On the basis of this observation and the proven efficacy of EGFR inhibitors in multiple cancers,[31,32] 2 major phase 3 trials of EGFR inhibitors in gastric cancer were conducted: the Erbitux (cetuximab) in combination with Xeloda (capecitabine) and cisplatin in advanced esophagogastric cancer (EXPAND) trial, and the epirubicin, oxaliplatin, and capecitabine with or without panitumumab for patients with previously untreated advanced esophagogastric cancer (REAL3) trial. Unlike the HER2 trials discussed previously, neither study used molecular markers as an inclusion criterion. In both studies, patients in the intervention arm tended to fare worse than standard therapy, although these results were not statistically significant. There was also some evidence of increased AEs in the intervention groups. A few smaller trials have been conducted with other EGFR-targeting agents (**Table 2**), with largely similar results.

Table 1
Major clinical trials targeting human epidermal growth factor receptor 2 in gastric cancer

Investigator, Year, Trial Name, Ref.	Drug	Phase	Patient Population	Groups	Outcome
Bang et al,[22] 2010, ToGA	Trastuzumab	3	Inoperable or recurrent HER2+ GEJ or gastric cancer	Trastuzumab with capecitabine/cisplatin or fluorouracil/cisplatin vs chemo alone	Trastuzumab significantly improved median survival (13.8 vs 11.1 mo)
Hecht et al,[23] 2016, TRIO-013/LOGiC	Lapatinib	3	Unresectable HER2+ esophageal, GEJ, or gastric cancer	Lapatinib or placebo with capecitabine/oxaliplatin	No difference in OS, increased AEs in the lapatinib group
Satoh et al,[24] 2014, TyTAN	Lapatinib	3	Asians with HER2+ gastric cancer who progressed after first-line therapy	Lapatinib and paclitaxel or paclitaxel alone	Nonsignificant trend favoring OS in the lapatinib group; no difference in AEs
Kang et al,[29] 2016, GATSBY	T-DM1	2/3	HER2+ gastroesophageal cancer that progressed after first-line therapy	T-DM1 or paclitaxel or docetaxel	No benefit of T-DM1 over paclitaxel or docetaxel

Data from Refs.[22–24,29]

Table 2
Trials targeting epidermal growth factor receptor in gastric cancer

Investigator, Year, Trial Name, Ref.	Drug	Phase	Patient Population	Group	Outcome
Lordick et al,[33] 2013, EXPAND	Cetuximab	3	Previously untreated unresectable or metastatic GEJ or gastric cancer	Cetuximab with capecitabine/cisplatin, or capecitabine/cisplatin alone	Addition of cetuximab did not improve PFS
Waddell et al,[34] 2013, REAL3	Panitumumab	3	Inoperable gastroesophageal cancer	Panitumumab + EOC, or EOC alone	Addition of panitumumab did not improve OS
Trarbach et al,[35] 2013	Matuzumab	1	Inoperable EGFR+ gastroesophageal cancer	Matuzumab (400 or 800 mg) with chemotherapy	Acceptably safe; modest antitumor efficacy
Satoh et al,[36] 2015	Nimotuzumab	2	5-Fluorouracil (5-FU) refractory gastroesophageal cancer	Nimotuzumab with irinotecan or irinotecan alone	No increase in PFS with addition of nimotuzumab to irinotecan

Abbreviation: EOC, epirubicin, oxaliplatin, and capecitabine.
Data from Refs.[33-36]

A lack of efficacy and possible harm in some patient groups have contributed to waning enthusiasm for EGFR inhibitors for the treatment of gastroesophageal cancers, at least until molecular markers that improve patient selection can be identified and validated. Anlotinib, another EGFR inhibitor, is undergoing investigation in a phase 3 clinical trial (NCT02461407).

Hepatocyte Growth Factor and Hepatocyte Growth Factor Receptor

The tyrosine kinase receptor MET (also known as hepatocyte growth factor receptor) and its only known ligand, hepatocyte growth factor (HGF), have well-established roles in a variety of cellular functions, including proliferation and survival, motility, and EMT.[37] Known pathways activated by HGF/MET include MAPK, PI3K-Akt, and STAT.[38] Deranged signaling involving the MET-HGF pathway has been implicated in several cancers, including gastric cancer.[39] Furthermore, MET expression has been associated with disease progression and poor prognosis in gastric cancer,[40] making it an attractive target for intervention.

Iveson and colleagues[41] used rilotumumab, a monoclonal antibody to HGF, in a phase 2 trial of patients with MET-positive GEJ and gastric tumors, demonstrating its safety in combination with epirubicin, cisplatin, and capecitabine (ECX) and showing a trend for improved survival in the group receiving rilotumumab plus ECX over ECX alone. These results prompted 2 phase 3 trials, RILOMET-1 and RILOMET-2; however, both trials were stopped early because of a statistically significant increase in deaths in the intervention group in RILOMET-1.[42] Additional inhibitors of MET have been developed and are currently undergoing investigation (**Table 3**).

Fibroblast Growth Factor 2

Similar to MET, fibroblast growth factor receptors (FGFR) are transmembrane tyrosine kinase receptors involved in several important cellular functions, including cell proliferation, migration, and differentiation.[50] Aberrant FGFR signaling due to receptor overexpression, gene amplification or mutation, or polysomy has been implicated in multiple cancers, including gastric cancer.[51] Although the overall rate of FGFR2 gene amplification is just 4.2% to 11.5%,[52,53] it correlates significantly with lymph node metastasis and portends a worse prognosis.[52,53]

A selective inhibitor of FGFR(1–3), AZD4547, showed promise in preclinical studies in inhibiting tumor growth.[54] On this basis, the SHINE trial, a phase 2 study of AZD4547 versus paclitaxel in patients with FGFR2-overexpressing, inoperable gastric cancer who progressed on first-line therapy, was conducted.[55] Although AZD4547 was well tolerated, there was no improvement in progression-free survival (PFS) in patients receiving the drug.

Vascular Endothelial Growth Factor

Angiogenesis is considered a hallmark of tumor growth.[56] VEGF and its receptors (VEGFR-1 and VEGFR-2) have been shown to promote angiogenesis in the physiologic and pathologic settings.[57] Furthermore, VEGF appears to be involved in autocrine and paracrine signaling mechanisms within the tumor microenvironment and plays a role in the function of cancer stem cells.[58] In gastric cancer, VEGF expression is associated with tumor aggressiveness[59] and poor outcomes.[60] Bevacizumab, a monoclonal antibody targeting VEGF, has shown efficacy in the treatment of multiple cancers when combined with chemotherapy[61,62] and demonstrated efficacy in gastric cancer in preclinical studies.[63] Ohtsu and colleagues[64] conducted a randomized, double-blind, placebo-controlled phase 3 trial, Avastin in Gastric Cancer (AVAGAST), to assess the efficacy of bevacizumab in addition to capecitabine-cisplatin for patients with locally

Table 3
Completed and ongoing trials of hepatocyte growth factor/hepatocyte growth factor receptor inhibitors in gastric cancer

Investigator or NCT, Year, Trial Name, Ref.	Drug	Phase	Patient Population	Group	Outcome/Aim
Iveson et al,[41] 2014	Rilotumumab	1b/2	Unresectable or locally advanced GEJ or gastric cancer	ECX with either rilotumumab 15 mg/kg, rilotumumab 7.5 mg/kg, or placebo	Rilotumumab is safe and trends toward improved survival
Cunningham et al,[42] 2013, RILOMET-1	Rilotumumab	3	Advanced MET+ GEJ or gastric cancer	Rilotumumab or placebo with ECX	Discontinued due to higher death rate in intervention arm
NCT02137343 RILOMET-2[43]	Rilotumumab	3	Advanced MET+ GEJ or gastric cancer	Rilotumumab or placebo with cisplatin and capecitabine	Discontinued due to higher death rate in RILOMET-1
Cunningham et al,[44] 2013	Onartuzumab	3	HER2-negative and MET+ untreated GEJ and gastric cancer	mFOLFOX6 with either onartuzumab or placebo	No benefit from onartuzumab
Kang et al,[45] 2014	Tivantinib	2	Previously treated metastatic gastric cancer	Tivantinib monotherapy (single arm)	Modest efficacy; disease control rate 36.7%
Shah et al,[46] 2013	Foretinib	2	Unresectable or locally advanced GEJ or gastric cancer	Foretinib monotherapy, 240 mg/d for 5 d every 2 wk, or 80 mg/d during each 2-wk cycle	No efficacy in unselected patients, despite evidence of MET inhibition
Hong et al,[47] 2014	AMG-337	1a	Advanced solid tumors	AMG-337 single-arm dose escalation	Responses seen in MET-amplified tumors
Molife et al,[48] 2014	Golvatinib	1a	Advanced solid tumors	Golvatinib single-arm dose escalation	Well tolerated with evidence of c-Met target modulation
NCT00940225[49]	Cabozantinib	2	Advanced solid tumors	Cabozantinib at various doses or placebo	Evaluate safety and efficacy; results pending

Data from Refs.[41–49]

advanced or metastatic GEJ or gastric cancer. Seven hundred seventy-four patients were randomized to receive a fluoropyrimidine-cisplatin regimen plus Bevacizumab or placebo with a primary endpoint of OS. Median OS for the intervention arm was 12.1 months compared with 10.1 months in the placebo group. Although this difference did not reach statistical significance ($P = .1$), the estimated 1-year OS was significantly higher in the bevacizumab group (50.2% vs 42.3%). Secondary endpoints including PFS and objective response rate (ORR) were significantly improved in the treatment arm.

In contrast to bevacizumab, ramucirumab targets the VEGF receptor on endothelial cells, VEGFR-2, rather than VEGF itself. Preclinical studies demonstrated that inhibition of VEGFR-2 with ramucirumab could decrease gastric tumor size and reduce peritumoral angiogenesis.[65] The Ramucirumab monotherapy for previously treated advanced gastric or gastro-oesophageal junction adenocarcinoma (REGARD) trial was conducted as an international, randomized, double-blind, placebo-controlled phase 3 trial that enrolled 355 patients with locally advanced, recurrent, or metastatic gastric or GEJ cancer who had progressed after first-line therapy.[66] Patients received either ramucirumab or placebo; the primary outcome was OS. Median OS was significantly longer in the ramucirumab group versus the treatment group (5.2 vs 3.8 months).

The Ramucirumab plus paclitaxel versus placebo plus paclitaxel in patients with previously treated advanced gastric or gastro-oesophageal junction adenocarcinoma (RAINBOW) trial also assessed the efficacy of ramucirumab in patients with previously treated gastric cancer.[67] This randomized, double-blind, placebo-controlled, phase 3 study treated 665 patients with gastric or GEJ cancers with paclitaxel plus either ramucirumab or placebo. The study largely confirmed the results of the REGARD trial, with an improved median survival of 9.6 months in the group receiving ramucirumab and paclitaxel, compared with 7.4 months in patients receiving paclitaxel alone.

Li and colleagues[68] tested the VEGFR2 inhibitor apatinib in a phase 3 trial of patients with advanced gastric or GEJ cancer who had progressive or nonresponsive disease after 2 chemotherapy regimens. Patients in the apatinib groups experienced improved OS (6.5 months vs 4.7 months) and PFS (2.6 months vs 1.8 months) compared with placebo. **Table 4** summarizes studies of VEGF inhibitors in gastric cancer.

On the basis of these studies, ramucirumab should be considered in patients with inoperable or progressive gastric cancer, especially as second-line therapy. No predictive biomarkers are currently known for response to therapy, but the indications for ramucirumab could expand to the neoadjuvant, adjuvant, or maintenance settings if such biomarkers could be established. Bevacizumab shows promise, and apatinib appears to be effective as a third-line agent.

Phosphoinositide 3-Kinase, AKT, and Mammalian Target of Rapamycin

Phosphoinositide 3-kinase (PI3K), AKT, and mammalian target of rapamycin (mTOR) comprise a signaling network that is known to control a wide range of cellular functions, including several hallmarks of cancer, such as cell cycle, metabolism, survival, and genomic instability.[56] This pathway has been implicated in supporting angiogenesis and inflammation within the tumor microenvironment,[71] and overexpression of PI3KCA, the gene encoding PI3K, has been demonstrated in up to 80% of gastric cancers.[72] Overexpression of PI3KCA has been shown to portend poor prognosis and has been linked to metastasis.[73] In the TCGA analysis, PIK3CA alterations occurred in 80% and 42% of EBV and MSI subtypes, respectively.[9] Multiple PI3K inhibitors are undergoing investigation, including BKM120, a pan-PI3K inhibitor, as well as BYL719, BEZ235, XL765, GDC-0980, GDC0084, SF1126, and PF-46915.[74] Multiple AKT inhibitors have been developed and have recently undergone or are currently undergoing investigation: MK2206, AZ6535, and GDC0068.[75]

Table 4
Trials targeting vascular endothelial growth factor in gastroesophageal cancers

Investigator, Year, Trial Name, Ref.	Drug	Phase	Patient Population	Group	Outcome
Ohtsu et al,[64] 2011, AVAGAST	Bevacizumab	3	Untreated inoperable gastroesophageal cancer	Bevacizumab or placebo with fluoropyrimidine-cisplatin	Improved PFS and ORR with addition of bevacizumab
Fuchs et al,[66] 2014, REGARD	Ramucirumab	3	Inoperable GEJ or gastric cancer and progression after first-line therapy	Ramucirumab or placebo	Improved OS with ramucirumab
Wilke et al,[67] 2014, RAINBOW	Ramucirumab	3	Inoperable GEJ or gastric cancer and progression after first-line therapy	Ramucirumab or placebo with paclitaxel	Improved OS with ramucirumab when added to paclitaxel
Li et al,[68] 2016	Apatinib	3	Inoperable GEJ or gastric cancer and progression after 2 lines of therapy	Apatinib or placebo	Improved OS with apatinib
Xu et al,[69] 2013	Endostar	3	Stage IV gastric cancer	Endostar with SOX chemotherapy or SOX alone	Endostar improved PFS but not OS
Pavlakis et al,[70] 2015, INTEGRATE	Regorafenib	2	Advanced gastric cancer and progression after 1 or 2 lines of therapy	Regorafenib or placebo with best supportive care	Regorafenib improved PFS, and although OS favored regorafenib, it was not statistically significant

Abbreviations: S-1, tegafur, gimeracil, oteracil; SOX, S-1 and oxaliplatin.
Data from Refs.[64,66–70]

Everolimus, an inhibitor of the mTOR complex-1, has been the most extensively studied mTOR inhibitor to date. It has proven efficacy in several cancers, including metastatic breast cancer and advanced renal cell carcinoma.[76,77] Several studies have also demonstrated that mTOR dysregulation is relevant in gastric cancer and that mTOR inhibition can reduce gastric cancer proliferation.[73] Consequently, the Everolimus for Previously Treated Gastric Cancer study was conducted, a phase 3 clinical trial to evaluate the efficacy of everolimus in patients with advanced gastric cancer.[78] The primary end point, OS, was not met, although there was a trend toward benefit in the everolimus group (OS 5.4 vs 4.3 months).

Hedgehog Pathway

The Hedgehog pathway is involved in embryogenesis and stem cell activity, although the details of the pathway are still under investigation.[79] Recent studies have demonstrated the role of the Hedgehog pathway in the development, progression, aggressiveness, and metastasis of gastric cancer.[80] In addition, expression of members of the pathway was noted to be independently associated with poor survival in gastric cancer.[81] The most developed inhibitors of the hedgehog pathway target smoothened, a protein in the Hedgehog pathway, including vismodegib, IPI-926, LDE-225, BMS-833923, and PF-04449913. At present, little clinical data exist on the use of this emerging therapeutic class.

IMMUNOTHERAPY IN GASTRIC CANCER

The characterization of the interplay between the immune system and cancer cells has led to the discovery of several pathways with therapeutic relevance in oncology. Chief among these are molecules involved in regulating cytotoxic T-lymphocyte (CTL) activity and the so-called immune checkpoints: cytotoxic T-lymphocyte–associated protein 4 (CTLA-4) and programmed cell death protein-1 (PD-1). Findings from the TCGA appear to confirm long-standing hypotheses that immunotherapies might work best in cancers with high mutational burden; the EBV and MSI subtypes, which have significantly higher mutation rates,[9] have been noted to harbor larger T-cell infiltrates,[11] and early data suggest that they respond more robustly to immunotherapy.[13]

CTLA-4 is expressed by activated cytotoxic T-lymphocytes (CTLs); it competes with the costimulatory molecule CD28 for binding with B7 molecules.[82] The CTLA-4/B7 interaction dampens the immune response. Thus, preventing CTL inactivation by interfering with the CTLA-4/B7 interaction promotes a more robust, durable anti-tumor response.

Ipilimumab, a monoclonal antibody against CTLA-4, was the first checkpoint therapy to reach the clinical arena, demonstrating clear efficacy in patients with unresectable or metastatic melanoma.[83] Multiple trials are currently underway to examine the efficacy of CTLA-4 blockade in gastric cancer. NCT01585987 is an ongoing randomized, phase 2 clinical trial that compares the efficacy of ipilimumab over best supportive care after first-line chemotherapy in patients with advanced or metastatic gastric cancer.[84] Tremelimumab, another antibody against CTLA-4, is currently being studied in a phase 1/2B trial in conjunction with the PD-L1 antibody durvalumab (NCT02340975) for patients with gastric cancer.[85]

PD-1 is expressed by CTLs; when stimulated by PD-L1 or PD-L2, this causes CTL apoptosis. Expression of PD-L1 and/or PD-L2 has been demonstrated in gastric cancer in up to 50.8% of cases.[86] In addition, PD-L1 and PD-L2 expression has been shown to correlate with larger tumor size, invasion, metastasis, and poorer OS.[87,88]

Pembrolizumab is a monoclonal antibody for PD-1 that blocks the interaction between PD-1 and its ligands, thus preventing apoptosis in CTLs and enabling a more durable and robust antitumor response. KEYNOTE-012 was conducted as a phase 1b trial to establish the safety and activity of pembrolizumab in patients with recurrent or metastatic gastric or GEJ cancers.[89] Twenty-two percent of the patients enrolled had a partial response, and just 13% experienced grade 3 or 4 AEs. Phase 3 clinical trials are currently ongoing (KEYNOTE-061 and KEYNOTE-062).[90,91]

The PD-1 antibody nivolumab and PD-L1 antibodies atezolizumab and avelumab are also undergoing clinical trials in a wide range of cancers, including gastric cancer (NCT02471846, NCT01633970, NCT01928394, NCT01772004, NCT02625610). Tables 5 and 6 summarize completed and ongoing immunotherapy trials in gastric cancer, respectively.

HEREDITARY GASTRIC CANCER

Hereditary gastric cancer accounts for about 1% to 3% of all cases of gastric adeno-carcinomas.[102] There are 3 recognized syndromes: hereditary diffuse gastric cancer (HDGC), gastric adenocarcinoma and proximal polyposis of the stomach (GAPPS), and familial intestinal gastric cancer (FIGC).[103] Additional cancer-associated syndromes that also predispose to gastric cancer include Lynch, Li-Fraumeni, Peutz-Jeghers, familial adenomatous polyposis, juvenile polyposis, and the BRCA breast-ovarian cancer syndromes.

Among gastric-specific syndromes, HDGC is the only syndrome for which known mutations exist, and even within HDGC, only 40% carry the hallmark mutation. Germline mutation in the CDH1 gene, which encodes E-cadherin, was the first HDGC mutation discovered.[104] Loss of E-cadherin expression has been linked to tumor progression, invasion, and metastasis.[105] The mechanisms of genetic inactivation of E-cadherin in HDGC are diverse, including rearrangements and frameshift, splice site, missense, and nonsense mutations.[102] Promoter hypermethylation is the most common cause of a second hit that inactivates the wild-type allele and initiates tumorigenesis.[106]

Clinical criteria for HDGC include a personal or family history of at least one of the following conditions: (i) 2 or more cases of gastric cancer, with at least one case of diffuse gastric cancer (in first- or second-degree relatives); (ii) diffuse gastric cancer before 40 years of age; (iii) personal or family history of diffuse gastric cancer and lobular breast cancer, with one diagnosis before 50 years of age.[107] Patients fulfilling any of these criteria should undergo genetic counseling and CDH1 testing. Because of the poor prognosis of diffuse gastric cancer, the low sensitivity of endoscopic surveillance, and the high penetrance of disease, the risk of diffuse gastric cancer exceeds 80% by 80 years.[108] Prophylactic total gastrectomy has gained clinical acceptance for those who have CDH1 mutations. Patients who refuse or wish to delay gastrectomy should be monitored with regular endoscopies, as outlined in the Cambridge protocol.[108] Current consensus guidelines recommend gastrectomy (without the need for D2 lymphadenectomy) between 20 and 30 years of age[109]; however, given the clinical heterogeneity of the disease, family history of disease onset should be considered when choosing when to operate. Prophylactic gastrectomy is a very safe operation, and long-term health-related quality of life is excellent.[110] Nearly all patients who undergo prophylactic gastrectomy are found to have invasive cancer or carcinoma in situ upon pathologic examination.[111,112] In addition, women who carry CDH1 mutation should undergo clinical breast examination and bilateral breast MRI every 6 months beginning at age 35 due to the increased risk of lobular breast carcinoma. Asymptomatic patients who do not have a CDH1 mutation are candidates for clinical research studies as well as regular surveillance.

GAPPS is a hereditary gastric cancer syndrome with an unknown genetic cause.[113] Clinical criteria for diagnosis include the following: (i) polyposis of the proximal

Table 5
Trials of immunotherapeutic agents in gastric cancer

Investigator, Year, Ref.	Drug	Phase	Patient Population	Group	Outcome/Aim
Ralph et al,[92] 2010	Tremelimumab	2	Metastatic gastroesophageal cancer	Tremelimumab 15 mg/kg every 90 d	4 of 18 achieved stable disease, 1 had partial response
Moehler et al,[93] 2013	Ipilimumab	2	Unresectable or metastatic GEJ or gastric cancer without progression after first-line chemotherapy	Ipilimumab 10 mg/kg for 4 doses followed by ipilimumab 10 mg/kg every 12 wk vs best supportive care	Worse PFS in the ipilimumab group but no difference in OS
Segal et al,[94] 2014	Durvalumab	1	Inoperable solid tumors, including gastroesophageal cancers	Durvalumab 10 mg/kg every 2 wk for 12 mo	Shrinkage in multiple tumor types, including gastroesophageal cancer
Muro et al,[95] 2015	Pembrolizumab	1	Inoperable solid tumors, including gastroesophageal cancers	Pembrolizumab 10 mg/kg every 2 wk for 24 mo	ORR: 22%
Le et al,[96] 2016	Nivolumab	1/2	Inoperable solid tumors, including gastroesophageal cancers	Nivolumab 3 mg/kg every 2 wk until progression or intolerable toxicity	ORR: 12%

Data from Refs.[92–96]

Table 6
Ongoing phase 3 trials of immunotherapeutic agents in gastric cancer

NCT ID, Name, Ref.	Drug	Patient Population	Group	Estimated Completion	Primary Endpoint
NCT02267343[97]	Nivolumab	Unresectable advanced or recurrent GEJ or gastric cancer refractory to or intolerant of first-line therapy	Nivolumab 3 mg/kg vs placebo	Aug. 2017	OS
NCT02370498 KEYNOTE-061[98]	Pembrolizumab	Advanced HER2-negative, PD-L1-positive GEJ, or gastric cancer without progression after first-line therapy	Pembrolizumab 200 mg every 3 wk vs paclitaxel	Dec. 2017	PFS
NCT02494583 KEYNOTE-062[82]	Pembrolizumab	Advanced HER2-negative, PD-L1 positive GEJ or gastric cancer without prior treatment	Pembrolizumab vs Pembrolizumab + cisplatin + 5-FU vs placebo + cisplatin + 5-FU	July 2019	PFS
NCT02564263 KEYNOTE-181[99]	Pembrolizumab	Esophageal or GEJ cancer with progression on first-line therapy	Pembrolizumab or standard therapy (paclitaxel, docetaxel, or irinotecan)	May 2018	PFS
NCT02625610 JAVELIN Gastric 100[100]	Avelumab	Advanced or metastatic GEJ or gastric cancer without prior therapy	Avelumab vs oxaliplatin-fluoropyrimidine doublet	Nov. 2023	OS
NCT02625623 JAVELIN Gastric 300[101]	Avelumab	Advanced or metastatic GEJ or gastric cancer with progression after 2 lines of chemotherapy	Avelumab vs paclitaxel or irinotecan or best supportive care	Sept. 2022	OS

Data from Refs.[97–101]

stomach, without evidence of colorectal or duodenal polyposis; (ii) more than 100 polyps carpeting the proximal stomach in an index case or greater than 30 polyps in a first-degree relative of a known case; (iii) a predominance of fundic gland polyps with some dysplasia, or a family member with fundic gland polyposis or gastric cancer; and (iv) an autosomal-dominant pattern of inheritance. Although management should be approached on a case-by-case basis, accepted clinical practice includes endoscopic surveillance and strong consideration for prophylactic gastrectomy.[114]

FIGC is characterized by an autosomal-dominant pattern of inheritance of intestinal subtype gastric cancer, in the absence of gastric polyposis. No genetic alterations have yet been linked to FIGC. Clinical criteria for diagnosis include either (i) 2 or more cases of gastric cancer in first-degree or second-degree relatives, with at least one case of intestinal-type gastric cancer occurring before 50 years of age; or (ii) 3 or more confirmed cases of intestinal-type gastric cancer, regardless of age of onset.[115] Yearly endoscopies beginning at age 60 with random biopsies have been suggested as a surveillance strategy.[116]

CURRENT RECOMMENDATIONS FOR GASTRIC CANCER TESTING

Current recommendations for the routine molecular characterization of gastric cancer are limited to the assessment of HER2 status, as determined by IHC and fluorescence in situ hybridization, for patients who would be candidates for trastuzumab.[116] At the present time, there is no role for routine EGFR, VEGF, FGFR2, MET or other expression analysis, except in the setting of clinical trials or other research. As new, more effective targeted therapies emerge, the characterization of individual gastric cancers at the molecular level will likely expand beyond HER2 analysis in the near future.

SUMMARY

Despite a decline in the age-adjusted incidence of gastric cancer worldwide, gastric cancer will likely continue to be a major global health problem due to an aging population, the recent increase in the incidence of gastric cancer in young patients, and a lack of cost-effective screening measures.

Gastric cancers exhibit a wide range of molecular alterations, including pathways involved in mitosis, immune signaling, cell adhesion and migration, and more. New molecular classification systems have laid the groundwork for many recent and ongoing clinical trials of targeted agents aimed at specific gastric cancer molecular phenotypes. Although these systems have revealed druggable targets, clinical efficacy of targeted therapy has been limited. At present, trastuzumab for the treatment of HER2-positive gastric cancer remains the most successful example. Ramucirumab has also shown efficacy as second-line therapy, albeit in an unselected population. Shortcomings of targeted therapy may be related to intratumoral heterogeneity, escape pathways or molecular redundancy within cancers, or alternative drivers of carcinogenesis. With molecular expression analysis in its infancy, the true heterogeneity of gastric cancer is emerging. Further efforts to discover additional molecular markers that might predict response to targeted therapy are needed not only to identify new targets but also to maximize benefit from current targeted therapies.

Early reports of immunotherapy are promising, and molecular and genomic profiling indicates that GEJ and gastric cancers are good candidates for immunotherapy, based on a relatively high mutational burden compared with many cancers. Ongoing and future studies will optimize candidacy for these treatments, perhaps based on known molecular markers such as PD-L1 expression or MSI status, or markers yet to be discovered. Efficacy will likely improve as patient selection is refined and combinatorial strategies involving multiple immunotherapies with or without conventional chemotherapy are developed.

ACKNOWLEDGMENTS

M.S. Strand would like to acknowledge funding from NCI grant T32 CA 009621.

REFERENCES

1. Ferlay J, Soerjomataram I, Dikshit R, et al. Cancer incidence and mortality worldwide: sources, methods and major patterns in GLOBOCAN 2012. Int J Cancer 2015;136(5):E359–86.
2. Siegel RL, Miller KD, Jemal A. Cancer statistics, 2016. CA Cancer J Clin 2016; 66(1):7–30.
3. Schlansky B, Sonnenberg A. Epidemiology of noncardia gastric adenocarcinoma in the United States. Am J Gastroenterol 2011;106(11):1978–85.
4. Fang X, Wei J, He X, et al. Landscape of dietary factors associated with risk of gastric cancer: a systematic review and dose-response meta-analysis of prospective cohort studies. Eur J Cancer 2015;51(18):2820–32.
5. Correa P. Gastric cancer: two epidemics? Dig Dis Sci 2011;56(5):1585–6 [author reply: 1586].
6. Lauren P. The two histological main types of gastric carcinoma: diffuse and so-called intestinal-type carcinoma. An attempt at a histo-clinical classification. Acta Pathol Microbiol Scand 1965;64:31–49.
7. Bosman FT. WHO classification of tumours of the digestive system. Lyon: International Agency for Research on Cancer, 2010. Lyon (France): International Agency for Research on Cancer; 2010.
8. Ott K, Fink U, Becker K, et al. Prediction of response to preoperative chemotherapy in gastric carcinoma by metabolic imaging: results of a prospective trial. J Clin Oncol 2003;21(24):4604–10.
9. Cancer Genome Atlas Research Network. Comprehensive molecular characterization of gastric adenocarcinoma. Nature 2014;513(7517):202–9.
10. Cristescu R, Lee J, Nebozhyn M, et al. Molecular analysis of gastric cancer identifies subtypes associated with distinct clinical outcomes. Nat Med 2015; 21(5):449–56.
11. Ma C, Patel K, Shaikh F, et al. Frequent programmed death-ligand 1 expression in gastric cancer associated with Epstein-Barr virus or microsatellite instability: implications for predictive biomarker development [Meeting Abstracts]. J Clin Oncol 2016;34(15 Suppl):e15579.
12. Murphy G, Pfeiffer R, Camargo MC, et al. Meta-analysis shows that prevalence of Epstein-Barr virus-positive gastric cancer differs based on sex and anatomic location. Gastroenterology 2009;137(3):824–33.
13. Le DT, Uram JN, Wang H, et al. PD-1 blockade in tumors with mismatch-repair deficiency. N Engl J Med 2015;372(26):2509–20.
14. Menard S, Pupa SM, Campiglio M, et al. Biologic and therapeutic role of HER2 in cancer. Oncogene 2003;22(42):6570–8.
15. Slamon DJ, Clark GM, Wong SG, et al. Human breast cancer: correlation of relapse and survival with amplification of the HER-2/neu oncogene. Science 1987;235(4785):177–82.
16. Sakai K, Mori S, Kawamoto T, et al. Expression of epidermal growth factor receptors on normal human gastric epithelia and gastric carcinomas. J Natl Cancer Inst 1986;77(5):1047–52.

17. Abrahao-Machado LF, Scapulatempo-Neto C. HER2 testing in gastric cancer: an update. World J Gastroenterol 2016;22(19):4619–25.

18. Liu X, Xu P, Qiu H, et al. Clinical utility of HER2 assessed by immunohistochemistry in patients undergoing curative resection for gastric cancer. Onco Targets Ther 2016;9:949–58.

19. Shen GS, Zhao JD, Zhao JH, et al. Association of HER2 status with prognosis in gastric cancer patients undergoing R0 resection: a large-scale multicenter study in China. World J Gastroenterol 2016;22(23):5406–14.

20. He C, Bian XY, Ni XZ, et al. Correlation of human epidermal growth factor receptor 2 expression with clinicopathological characteristics and prognosis in gastric cancer. World J Gastroenterol 2013;19(14):2171–8.

21. Piccart-Gebhart MJ, Procter M, Leyland-Jones B, et al. Trastuzumab after adjuvant chemotherapy in HER2-positive breast cancer. N Engl J Med 2005;353(16):1659–72.

22. Bang YJ, Van Cutsem E, Feyereislova A, et al. Trastuzumab in combination with chemotherapy versus chemotherapy alone for treatment of HER2-positive advanced gastric or gastro-oesophageal junction cancer (ToGA): a phase 3, open-label, randomised controlled trial. Lancet 2010;376(9742):687–97.

23. Hecht JR, Bang YJ, Qin SK, et al. Lapatinib in combination with capecitabine plus oxaliplatin in human epidermal growth factor receptor 2-positive advanced or metastatic gastric, esophageal, or gastroesophageal adenocarcinoma: TRIO-013/LOGiC–A randomized phase III trial. J Clin Oncol 2016;34(5):443–51.

24. Satoh T, Xu RH, Chung HC, et al. Lapatinib plus paclitaxel versus paclitaxel alone in the second-line treatment of HER2-amplified advanced gastric cancer in Asian populations: TyTAN–a randomized, phase III study. J Clin Oncol 2014;32(19):2039–49.

25. Robidoux A, Tang G, Rastogi P, et al. Lapatinib as a component of neoadjuvant therapy for HER2-positive operable breast cancer (NSABP protocol B-41): an open-label, randomised phase 3 trial. Lancet Oncol 2013;14(12):1183–92.

26. Geyer CE, Forster J, Lindquist D, et al. Lapatinib plus capecitabine for HER2-positive advanced breast cancer. N Engl J Med 2006;355(26):2733–43.

27. Baselga J, Bradbury I, Eidtmann H, et al. Lapatinib with trastuzumab for HER2-positive early breast cancer (NeoALTTO): a randomised, open-label, multicentre, phase 3 trial. Lancet 2012;379(9816):633–40.

28. Ishimine Y, Goto A, Watanabe Y, et al. Loss of HER2 positivity after trastuzumab in HER2-positive gastric cancer: is change in HER2 status significantly frequent? Case Rep Gastrointest Med 2015;2015:132030.

29. Kang Y, Shah M, Ohtsu A, et al. A randomized, open-label, multicenter, adaptive phase 2/3 study of trastuzumab emtansine (T-DM1) versus a taxane (TAX) in patients (pts) with previously treated HER2-positive locally advanced or metastatic gastric/gastroesophageal junction adenocarcinoma (LA/MGC/GEJC). J Clin Oncol 2016;34(Suppl 4S) [abstract: 5].

30. Kim MA, Lee HS, Lee HE, et al. EGFR in gastric carcinomas: prognostic significance of protein overexpression and high gene copy number. Histopathology 2008;52(6):738–46.

31. Vermorken JB, Mesia R, Rivera F, et al. Platinum-based chemotherapy plus cetuximab in head and neck cancer. N Engl J Med 2008;359(11):1116–27.

32. Pirker R, Pereira JR, Szczesna A, et al. Cetuximab plus chemotherapy in patients with advanced non-small-cell lung cancer (FLEX): an open-label randomised phase III trial. Lancet 2009;373(9674):1525–31.

33. Lordick F, Kang YK, Chung HC, et al. Capecitabine and cisplatin with or without cetuximab for patients with previously untreated advanced gastric cancer (EXPAND): a randomised, open-label phase 3 trial. Lancet Oncol 2013;14(6): 490–9.

34. Waddell T, Chau I, Cunningham D, et al. Epirubicin, oxaliplatin, and capecitabine with or without panitumumab for patients with previously untreated advanced oesophagogastric cancer (REAL3): a randomised, open-label phase 3 trial. Lancet Oncol 2013;14(6):481–9.

35. Trarbach T, Przyborek M, Schleucher N, et al. Phase I study of matuzumab in combination with 5-fluorouracil, leucovorin and cisplatin (PLF) in patients with advanced gastric and esophagogastric adenocarcinomas. Invest New Drugs 2013;31(3):642–52.

36. Satoh T, Lee KH, Rha SY, et al. Randomized phase II trial of nimotuzumab plus irinotecan versus irinotecan alone as second-line therapy for patients with advanced gastric cancer. Gastric Cancer 2015;18(4):824–32.

37. Birchmeier C, Birchmeier W, Gherardi E. Vande Woude GF. Met, metastasis, motility and more. Nat Rev Mol Cell Biol 2003;4(12):915–25.

38. Comoglio PM, Giordano S, Trusolino L. Drug development of MET inhibitors: targeting oncogene addiction and expedience. Nat Rev Drug Discov 2008;7(6): 504–16.

39. Hara T, Ooi A, Kobayashi M, et al. Amplification of c-myc, K-sam, and c-met in gastric cancers: detection by fluorescence in situ hybridization. Lab Invest 1998;78(9):1143–53.

40. Drebber U, Baldus SE, Nolden B, et al. The overexpression of c-met as a prognostic indicator for gastric carcinoma compared to p53 and p21 nuclear accumulation. Oncol Rep 2008;19(6):1477–83.

41. Iveson T, Donehower RC, Davidenko I, et al. Rilotumumab in combination with epirubicin, cisplatin, and capecitabine as first-line treatment for gastric or oesophagogastric junction adenocarcinoma: an open-label, dose de-escalation phase 1b study and a double-blind, randomised phase 2 study. Lancet Oncol 2014;15(9):1007–18.

42. Cunningham D, Tebbutt NC, Davidenko I, et al. Phase III, randomized, double-blind, multicenter, placebo (P)-controlled trial of rilotumumab (R) plus epirubicin, cisplatin and capecitabine (ECX) as first-line therapy in patients (pts) with advanced MET-positive (pos) gastric or gastroesophageal junction (G/GEJ) cancer: RILOMET-1 study [Meeting Abstracts]. J Clin Oncol 2013; 33(Suppl 15):4000.

43. A Phase 3 Study of Rilotumumab (AMG 102) with Cisplatin and Capecitabine (CX) as First-line Therapy in Gastric Cancer (RILOMET-2). 2014. Available at: https://clinicaltrials.gov/ct2/show/NCT02137343. Accessed July 31, 2016.

44. Cunningham D, Tabernero J, Shah M, et al. A randomized phase III study of onartuzumab (MetMAb) in combination with mFOLFOX6 in patients with metastatic HER2-negative and MET-positive adenocarcinoma of the stomach or gastroesophageal junction. J Clin Oncol 2013 [abstract: TPS4155]. Available at: http://meetinglibrary.asco.org/content/114845-132.

45. Kang YK, Muro K, Ryu MH, et al. A phase II trial of a selective c-Met inhibitor tivantinib (ARQ 197) monotherapy as a second- or third-line therapy in the patients with metastatic gastric cancer. Invest New Drugs 2014;32(2):355–61.

46. Shah MA, Wainberg ZA, Catenacci DV, et al. Phase II study evaluating 2 dosing schedules of oral foretinib (GSK1363089), cMET/VEGFR2 inhibitor, in patients with metastatic gastric cancer. PLoS One 2013;8(3):e54014.

47. Hong D, Lorusso P, Hamid O, et al. First-in-human study of AMG 337, a highly selective oral inhibitor of MET, in adult patients (pts) with advanced solid tumors. J Clin Oncol 2014;32(suppl):5s [abstract: 2508].

48. Molife LR, Dean EJ, Blanco-Codesido M, et al. A phase I, dose-escalation study of the multitargeted receptor tyrosine kinase inhibitor, golvatinib, in patients with advanced solid tumors. Clin Cancer Res 2014;20(24):6284–94.

49. Study of Cabozantinib (XL184) in Adults with Advanced Malignancies. Clinical-Trials.gov. A service of the U.S. National Insititutes of Health. 2016. Available at: https://clinicaltrials.gov/ct2/show/NCT00940225. Accessed July 29, 2016.

50. Turner N, Grose R. Fibroblast growth factor signalling: from development to cancer. Nat Rev Cancer 2010;10(2):116–29.

51. Katoh M. Genetic alterations of FGF receptors: an emerging field in clinical cancer diagnostics and therapeutics. Expert Rev Anticancer Ther 2010;10(9): 1375–9.

52. Su X, Zhan P, Gavine PR, et al. FGFR2 amplification has prognostic significance in gastric cancer: results from a large international multicentre study. Br J Cancer 2014;110(4):967–75.

53. Shoji H, Yamada Y, Okita N, et al. Amplification of FGFR2 gene in patients with advanced gastric cancer receiving chemotherapy: prevalence and prognostic significance. Anticancer Res 2015;35(9):5055–61.

54. Xie L, Su X, Zhang L, et al. FGFR2 gene amplification in gastric cancer predicts sensitivity to the selective FGFR inhibitor AZD4547. Clin Cancer Res 2013;19(9): 2572–83.

55. Bang YJ. A randomized, open-label phase II study of AZD4547 (AZD) versus paclitaxel (P) in previously treated patients with advanced gastric cancer (AGC) with fibroblast growth factor receptor 2 (FGFR2) polysomy or gene amplification (amp): SHINE study. J Clin Oncol 2015;33(Suppl) [abstract: 4014].

56. Hanahan D, Weinberg RA. Hallmarks of cancer: the next generation. Cell 2011; 144(5):646–74.

57. Ferrara N, Gerber HP, LeCouter J. The biology of VEGF and its receptors. Nat Med 2003;9(6):669–76.

58. Goel HL, Mercurio AM. VEGF targets the tumour cell. Nat Rev Cancer 2013; 13(12):871–82.

59. Kim SE, Shim KN, Jung SA, et al. The clinicopathological significance of tissue levels of hypoxia-inducible factor-1alpha and vascular endothelial growth factor in gastric cancer. Gut Liver 2009;3(2):88–94.

60. Lieto E, Ferraraccio F, Orditura M, et al. Expression of vascular endothelial growth factor (VEGF) and epidermal growth factor receptor (EGFR) is an independent prognostic indicator of worse outcome in gastric cancer patients. Ann Surg Oncol 2008;15(1):69–79.

61. Hurwitz H, Fehrenbacher L, Novotny W, et al. Bevacizumab plus irinotecan, fluorouracil, and leucovorin for metastatic colorectal cancer. N Engl J Med 2004; 350(23):2335–42.

62. Miller K, Wang M, Gralow J, et al. Paclitaxel plus bevacizumab versus paclitaxel alone for metastatic breast cancer. N Engl J Med 2007;357(26):2666–76.

63. Gerber HP, Ferrara N. Pharmacology and pharmacodynamics of bevacizumab as monotherapy or in combination with cytotoxic therapy in preclinical studies. Cancer Res 2005;65(3):671–80.

64. Ohtsu A, Shah MA, Van Cutsem E, et al. Bevacizumab in combination with chemotherapy as first-line therapy in advanced gastric cancer: a randomized,

double-blind, placebo-controlled phase III study. J Clin Oncol 2011;29(30): 3968–76.

65. Jung YD, Mansfield PF, Akagi M, et al. Effects of combination anti-vascular endothelial growth factor receptor and anti-epidermal growth factor receptor therapies on the growth of gastric cancer in a nude mouse model. Eur J Cancer 2002;38(8):1133–40.

66. Fuchs CS, Tomasek J, Yong CJ, et al. Ramucirumab monotherapy for previously treated advanced gastric or gastro-oesophageal junction adenocarcinoma (REGARD): an international, randomised, multicentre, placebo-controlled, phase 3 trial. Lancet 2014;383(9911):31–9.

67. Wilke H, Muro K, Van Cutsem E, et al. Ramucirumab plus paclitaxel versus placebo plus paclitaxel in patients with previously treated advanced gastric or gastro-oesophageal junction adenocarcinoma (RAINBOW): a double-blind, randomised phase 3 trial. Lancet Oncol 2014;15(11):1224–35.

68. Li J, Qin S, Xu J, et al. Randomized, double-blind, placebo-controlled phase III trial of apatinib in patients with chemotherapy-refractory advanced or metastatic adenocarcinoma of the stomach or gastroesophageal junction. J Clin Oncol 2016;34(13):1448–54.

69. Xu R, Ma N, Wang F, et al. Results of a randomized and controlled clinical trial evaluating the efficacy and safety of combination therapy with Endostar and S-1 combined with oxaliplatin in advanced gastric cancer. Onco Targets Ther 2013; 6:925–9.

70. Pavlakis N, Sjoquist K, Tsobanis E, et al. INTEGRATE: a randomized, phase II, double-blind, placebo-controlled study of regorafenib in refractory advanced oesophagogastric cancer (AOGC): a study by the Australasian Gastrointestinal Trials Group (AGITG)—final overall and subgroup results. J Clin Oncol 2015; 33(Suppl) [abstract: 4003].

71. Hirsch E, Ciraolo E, Franco I, et al. PI3K in cancer-stroma interactions: bad in seed and ugly in soil. Oncogene 2014;33(24):3083–90.

72. Tapia O, Riquelme I, Leal P, et al. The PI3K/AKT/mTOR pathway is activated in gastric cancer with potential prognostic and predictive significance. Virchows Arch 2014;465(1):25–33.

73. Ye B, Jiang LL, Xu HT, et al. Expression of PI3K/AKT pathway in gastric cancer and its blockade suppresses tumor growth and metastasis. Int J Immunopathol Pharmacol 2012;25(3):627–36.

74. Brana I, Siu LL. Clinical development of phosphatidylinositol 3-kinase inhibitors for cancer treatment. BMC Med 2012;10:161.

75. Ramanathan R, McDonough S, Kennecke H, et al. A phase II study of MK-2206, an allosteric inhibitor of AKT as second-line therapy for advanced gastric and gastroesophageal junction (GEJ) cancer: a SWOG Cooperative Group trial (S1005). J Clin Oncol 2014;32(Suppl):5s [abstract: 4041].

76. Motzer RJ, Escudier B, Oudard S, et al. Efficacy of everolimus in advanced renal cell carcinoma: a double-blind, randomised, placebo-controlled phase III trial. Lancet 2008;372(9637):449–56.

77. Beaver JA, Park BH. The BOLERO-2 trial: the addition of everolimus to exemestane in the treatment of postmenopausal hormone receptor-positive advanced breast cancer. Future Oncol 2012;8(6):651–7.

78. Ohtsu A, Ajani JA, Bai YX, et al. Everolimus for previously treated advanced gastric cancer: results of the randomized, double-blind, phase III GRANITE-1 study. J Clin Oncol 2013;31(31):3935–43.

79. Ingham PW, Nakano Y, Seger C. Mechanisms and functions of Hedgehog signalling across the metazoa. Nat Rev Genet 2011;12(6):393–406.

80. Yoo YA, Kang MH, Lee HJ, et al. Sonic hedgehog pathway promotes metastasis and lymphangiogenesis via activation of Akt, EMT, and MMP-9 pathway in gastric cancer. Cancer Res 2011;71(22):7061–70.

81. Kim JY, Ko GH, Lee YJ, et al. Prognostic value of sonic hedgehog protein expression in gastric cancer. Jpn J Clin Oncol 2012;42(11):1054–9.

82. Study of pembrolizumab (MK-3475) as first-line monotherapy and combination therapy for treatment of advanced gastric or gastroesophageal junction adenocarcinoma (MK-3475-062/KEYNOTE-062). 2015. Available at: https://clinicaltrials.gov/ct2/show/NCT02494583. Accessed July 31, 2016.

83. Hodi FS, O'Day SJ, McDermott DF, et al. Improved survival with ipilimumab in patients with metastatic melanoma. N Engl J Med 2010;363(8):711–23.

84. An Efficacy Study in Gastric and Gastroesophageal Junction Cancer Comparing Ipilimumab Versus Standard of Care Immediately Following First Line Chemotherapy. 2012, 2016. Available at: https://clinicaltrials.gov/ct2/show/results/NCT01585987.

85. A Phase 1b/2 Study of MEDI4736 with Tremelimumab, MEDI4736 or Tremelimumab Monotherapy in Gastric or GEJ Adenocarcinoma. 2015, 2016. Available at: https://clinicaltrials.gov/ct2/show/NCT02340975.

86. Zhang L, Qiu M, Jin Y, et al. Programmed cell death ligand 1 (PD-L1) expression on gastric cancer and its relationship with clinicopathologic factors. Int J Clin Exp Pathol 2015;8(9):11084–91.

87. Wu C, Zhu Y, Jiang J, et al. Immunohistochemical localization of programmed death-1 ligand-1 (PD-L1) in gastric carcinoma and its clinical significance. Acta Histochem 2006;108(1):19–24.

88. Tamura T, Ohira M, Tanaka H, et al. Programmed death-1 ligand-1 (PDL1) expression is associated with the prognosis of patients with stage II/III gastric cancer. Anticancer Res 2015;35(10):5369–76.

89. Muro K, Chung HC, Shankaran V, et al. Pembrolizumab for patients with PD-L1-positive advanced gastric cancer (KEYNOTE-012): a multicentre, open-label, phase 1b trial. Lancet Oncol 2016;17(6):717–26.

90. Ohtsu A, Tabernero J, Bang YJ, et al. Pembrolizumab versus paclitaxel as second-line therapy for advanced gastric or gastroesophageal junction (GEJ) adenocarcinoma: phase 3 KEYNOTE-061 study. J Clin Oncol 2016;34(Suppl) [abstract: TPS4137].

91. Tabernero J, Bang YJ, Fuchs CS, et al. KEYNOTE-062: phase III study of pembrolizumab (MK-3475) alone or in combination with chemotherapy versus chemotherapy alone as first-line therapy for advanced gastric or gastroesophageal junction (GEJ) adenocarcinoma. J Clin Oncol 2016;34(Suppl 4S) [abstract: TPS185].

92. Ralph C, Elkord E, Burt DJ, et al. Modulation of lymphocyte regulation for cancer therapy: a phase II trial of tremelimumab in advanced gastric and esophageal adenocarcinoma. Clin Cancer Res 2010;16(5):1662–72.

93. Moehler M, Kim YH, Tan IB, et al. Sequential ipilimumab (Ipi) versus best supportive care (BSC) following first-line chemotherapy (Ctx) in patients (pts) with unresectable locally advanced or metastatic gastric or gastro-esophageal junction (GEJ) cancer: a randomized, open-label, two-arm, phase II trial (CA184-162) of immunotherapy as a maintenance concept. J Clin Oncol 2013;31(Suppl) [abstract: TPS4151].

94. Segal N, Antonia SJ, Brahmer JR, et al. Preliminary data from a multi-arm expansion study of MEDI4736, an anti-PD-L1 antibody. J Clin Oncol 2014;32(Suppl):5s [abstract: 3002].

95. Muro K, Bang YJ, Shankaran V, et al. Relationship between PD-L1 expression and clinical outcomes in patients (Pts) with advanced gastric cancer treated with the anti-PD-1 monoclonal antibody pembrolizumab (Pembro; MK-3475) in KEYNOTE-012. J Clin Oncol 2015;33(Suppl 3) [abstract: 3].

96. Le DT, Bendell JC, Calvo E, et al. Safety and activity of nivolumab monotherapy in advanced and metastatic (A/M) gastric or gastroesophageal junction cancer (GC/GEC): results from the CheckMate-032 study. J Clin Oncol 2016; 34(Suppl 4S) [abstract: 6].

97. Study of ONO-4538 in unresectable advanced or recurrent gastric cancer. 2014. Available at: https://clinicaltrials.gov/ct2/show/NCT02267343. Accessed July 31, 2016.

98. A study of pembrolizumab (MK-3475) Versus paclitaxel for participants with advanced gastric/gastroesophageal junction adenocarcinoma that progressed after therapy with platinum and fluoropyrimidine (MK-3475–061/KEYNOTE-061). 2015. Available at: https://clinicaltrials.gov/ct2/show/NCT02370498. Accessed July 31, 2016.

99. Study of pembrolizumab (MK-3475) versus investigator's choice standard therapy for participants with advanced esophageal/esophagogastric junction carcinoma that progressed after first-line therapy (MK-3475-181/KEYNOTE-181). 2015. Available at: https://clinicaltrials.gov/ct2/show/NCT02564263. Accessed July 31, 2016.

100. Avelumab in first-line gastric cancer (JAVELIN Gastric 100). 2015. Available at: https://clinicaltrials.gov/ct2/show/NCT02625610. Accessed July 31, 2016.

101. Avelumab in third-line gastric cancer (JAVELIN Gastric 300). 2015. Available at: https://clinicaltrials.gov/ct2/show/NCT02625623. Accessed July 31, 2016.

102. Oliveira C, Pinheiro H, Figueiredo J, et al. Familial gastric cancer: genetic susceptibility, pathology, and implications for management. Lancet Oncol 2015; 16(2):e60–70.

103. Colvin H, Yamamoto K, Wada N, et al. Hereditary gastric cancer syndromes. Surg Oncol Clin N Am 2015;24(4):765–77.

104. Guilford P, Hopkins J, Harraway J, et al. E-cadherin germline mutations in familial gastric cancer. Nature 1998;392(6674):402–5.

105. Vleminckx K, Vakaet L Jr, Mareel M, et al. Genetic manipulation of E-cadherin expression by epithelial tumor cells reveals an invasion suppressor role. Cell 1991;66(1):107–19.

106. Oliveira C, Sousa S, Pinheiro H, et al. Quantification of epigenetic and genetic 2nd hits in CDH1 during hereditary diffuse gastric cancer syndrome progression. Gastroenterology 2009;136(7):2137–48.

107. van der Post RS, Vogelaar IP, Carneiro F, et al. Hereditary diffuse gastric cancer: updated clinical guidelines with an emphasis on germline CDH1 mutation carriers. J Med Genet 2015;52(6):361–74.

108. Fitzgerald RC, Hardwick R, Huntsman D, et al. Hereditary diffuse gastric cancer: updated consensus guidelines for clinical management and directions for future research. J Med Genet 2010;47(7):436–44.

109. Syngal S, Brand RE, Church JM, et al. ACG clinical guideline: genetic testing and management of hereditary gastrointestinal cancer syndromes. Am J Gastroenterol 2015;110(2):223–62 [quiz: 263].

110. Worster E, Liu X, Richardson S, et al. The impact of prophylactic total gastrectomy on health-related quality of life: a prospective cohort study. Ann Surg 2014; 260(1):87–93.
111. Huntsman DG, Carneiro F, Lewis FR, et al. Early gastric cancer in young, asymptomatic carriers of germ-line E-cadherin mutations. N Engl J Med 2001;344(25): 1904–9.
112. Norton JA, Ham CM, Van Dam J, et al. CDH1 truncating mutations in the E-cadherin gene: an indication for total gastrectomy to treat hereditary diffuse gastric cancer. Ann Surg 2007;245(6):873–9.
113. Worthley DL, Phillips KD, Wayte N, et al. Gastric adenocarcinoma and proximal polyposis of the stomach (GAPPS): a new autosomal dominant syndrome. Gut 2012;61(5):774–9.
114. Majewski IJ, Kluijt I, Cats A, et al. An alpha-E-catenin (CTNNA1) mutation in hereditary diffuse gastric cancer. J Pathol 2013;229(4):621–9.
115. Caldas C, Carneiro F, Lynch HT, et al. Familial gastric cancer: overview and guidelines for management. J Med Genet 1999;36(12):873–80.
116. Corso G, Roncalli F, Marrelli D, et al. History, pathogenesis, and management of familial gastric cancer: original study of John XXIII's family. Biomed Res Int 2013; 2013:385132.

Endoscopic Management of Early Gastric Adenocarcinoma and Preinvasive Gastric Lesions

CrossMark

Saowanee Ngamruengphong, MD[a],*, Seiichiro Abe, MD[b],
Ichiro Oda, MD[b]

KEYWORDS

- Gastric cancer • Stomach neoplasms • Narrow band imaging • Screening
- Detection • Early gastric cancer • Endoscopic submucosal dissection

KEY POINTS

- Early gastric cancer (ECG) can be difficult to diagnosis endoscopically. Endoscopists should be familiar with subtle changes and endoscopic features of EGC.
- Chromoendoscopy and image-enhanced endoscopy improve diagnostic accuracy and facilitate endoscopic resection.
- Endoscopic submucosal dissection is a preferred endoscopic technique for resection of EGC and offers a comparable overall survival to surgical resection.
- Given the risk of metachronous gastric cancer, endoscopic surveillance after endoscopic resection is required.
- Most benign gastric epithelial polyps (fundic gland polyps, hyperplastic polyps, and gastric adenoma) are found incidentally during routine endoscopy. Endoscopic management of these lesions depends on patient symptomatology, a patient's comorbidities (eg, familial syndromes), a lesion's characteristics, and risk of malignant transformation.

INTRODUCTION

With advanced endoscopic imaging technology and widespread use of upper endoscopy, more gastrointestinal abnormalities, including gastric mucosal lesions, are encountered during routine examination. Most benign gastric epithelial lesions and

Disclosures: No relevant financial disclosures. No commercial or financial conflicts of interest. Dr S. Ngamruengphong received the ASGE Cook Medical Don Wilson Award for international training at National Cancer Center, Tokyo, Japan.
[a] Division of Gastroenterology and Hepatology, Johns Hopkins Medicine, Johns Hopkins Medical Institutions, 4940 Eastern Avenue, A Building, 5th Floor, Baltimore, MD 21224, USA;
[b] Endoscopy Division, National Cancer Center Hospital, 5-1-1, Tsukiji, Chuo-ku, Tokyo 104-0045, Japan
* Corresponding author.
E-mail address: sngamru1@jh.edu

Surg Clin N Am 97 (2017) 371–385
http://dx.doi.org/10.1016/j.suc.2016.11.010
0039-6109/17/© 2017 Elsevier Inc. All rights reserved.

surgical.theclinics.com

early gastric cancer (EGC) are asymptomatic, but in very rare cases, they present with abdominal pain, gastric outlet obstruction, and bleeding. It is essential for clinicians to become familiar with the endoscopic management of these lesions. In this article, the authors provide an overview of endoscopic management of EGC and common premalignant gastric lesions (fundic gland polyps, hyperplastic polyps, and gastric adenoma).

EARLY GASTRIC CANCER

EGC is defined as a lesion confined to the mucosa or submucosa, regardless of lymph node status. Endoscopic resection offers a comparable long-term overall survival rate to surgical resection in patients with EGCs that have a negligible risk of lymph node metastasis.[1–3]

The Paris classification has been used to describe the macroscopic morphology of gastrointestinal lesions: (a) type 0-I (protruded type: 0-Ip, pedunculated; or 0-Is, sessile); (b) type 0-IIa (superficial and elevated type); (c) type 0-IIb (flat type); (d) type 0-IIc (superficial and depressed type); and (e) type III (excavated type).[4] Type 0-IIc is the most common type of EGCs and accounts for greater than 65% of cases, whereas type III (ulcerlike) is the least common type (<10%).[5]

Difference in classification systems used for gastrointestinal lesions results in discrepancies in the diagnosis of adenoma/dysplasia versus carcinoma between Western and Japanese pathologists. The difference in classification systems can be resolved by adopting the proposed terminology (Vienna classification): (1) negative for neoplasia/dysplasia; (2) indefinite for neoplasia/dysplasia; (3) noninvasive low-grade neoplasia (low-grade adenoma/dysplasia); (4) noninvasive high-grade neoplasia (high-grade adenoma/dysplasia, noninvasive carcinoma, and suspicion of invasive carcinoma); and (5) invasive neoplasia (intramucosal carcinoma, submucosal carcinoma, or beyond).[6]

Endoscopic Screening for Early Gastric Cancer

In Japan, because of national screening programs, approximately 50% of gastric cancer cases are diagnosed at early stage.[7] In western countries, early-stage cancer accounts for about 20% of cases.[8,9] A more favorable outcome noted for gastric carcinoma patients in Japan primarily is explained by the differences in a greater frequency of early-stage disease compared with gastric carcinoma patients in the United States.[9]

Endoscopy is the gold standard in detection of EGC; however, it is not a perfect test with a possibility of missing lesions, particularly for small or flat types. Overall sensitivity of endoscopy in detecting gastric cancer ranges from 77% to 93%.[10,11] In a retrospective analysis of 2727 patients in England, in 8.3% of patients with gastric cancer, their cancer was missed at endoscopy within the 3 previous years.[12]

Mass screening for gastric cancer has been implemented in countries with a high prevalence of gastric cancer, such as Japan and Korea.[13,14] On the contrary, in countries with a low prevalence of gastric cancer such as the United States, population-based screening is not cost-effective. However, endoscopy for gastric cancer screening should be considered in individuals at high risk for gastric cancer.[15] Currently, there are no guidelines regarding screening for gastric cancer in the United States. Experts recommend endoscopic screening (1) at age 50 for individuals who are first- or second-generation immigrants from high-incidence regions (East Asia, Russia, and South America); (2) for individuals with a family history of gastric cancer (begin endoscopic screening 10 years before diagnosis in the affected relative); and (3) those with atrophic gastritis or intestinal metaplasia. In addition, those with

Helicobacter pylori infection alone should be treated for *H pylori* eradication therapy with confirmation of eradication and then undergo endoscopic examination in 3 to 5 years to evaluate for progression to atrophic gastritis or intestinal metaplasia.[15]

Endoscopic Diagnosis of Early Gastric Cancer

Conventional white light imaging

Conventional white light imaging (WLI) is the first step for detection and characterization of gastric lesions. Some EGCs can be very subtle and difficult to identify. Findings suggestive of superficial mucosal lesions, including color changes in the mucosa (redness or pale faded), loss of visibility of underlying epithelial vessels, thinning and interruptions in mucosal folds, and spontaneous bleeding, should be carefully examined.[16] The key signs to differentiate cancerous and noncancerous lesions are surface and color change. Well-demarcated border or irregularity in color/surface pattern is suggestive of cancerous rather than noncancerous lesions.[17]

After detecting suspicious lesions during WLI, further characterization and determination of the extent of disease are warranted, commonly with dye-based image-enhanced endoscopy (chromoendoscopy) and equipment-based image-enhanced endoscopy using narrow band imaging (NBI; Olympus Corporation, Tokyo, Japan).

Chromoendoscopy

When a suspicious gastric lesion is detected using conventional WLI, chromoendoscopy using dye, such as indigo carmine and acetic acid, can facilitate visualization and effectively aid diagnosis. Dye staining can also improve determination of tumor margins before endoscopic resection, which is particularly important to ensure a negative horizontal margin.

The staining substances that have been commonly used in clinical practice include indigo carmine and acetic acid (**Fig. 1**). Indigo carmine is not absorbed by the mucosa; it simply pools in the mucosal crevices and grooves and allows better mucosal architecture definition.[18] Acetic acid causes transient changes of cellular proteins as well as congestion in the capillaries, which lead to enhancement of the surface architecture.[19] Studies using indigo carmine dye added to acetic acid demonstrated improvement in diagnostic accuracy and margin determination of the EGC compared with conventional WLI or chromoendoscopy with indigo carmine.[20,21] However, acetic acid–indigo

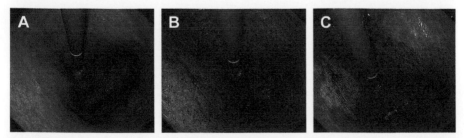

Fig. 1. Chromoendoscopy for EGC. (*A*) A depressed lesion with slightly elevated component (Paris 0-IIc + IIa) without ulceration at the posterior wall of the middle body of the stomach. The lesion border is unclear. (*B*) Endoscopic view after indigo carmine was sprinkled. The lesion's border is still unclear. (*C*) Endoscopic view after indigo carmine and acetic acid spray. The lesion's border became distinct, and the clarity of the endoscopic image is high. The lesion was 3.8 cm × 2.6 cm in size. The lesion was resected by ESD, and pathology revealed intramucosal well-differentiated adenocarcinoma without evidence of lymphovascular invasion. Horizontal and vertical margins were clear of the tumor.

carmine chromoendoscopy does not improve the border differentiation for undifferentiated adenocarcinomas.[21] In the authors' experience, addition of acetic acid is particularly useful for delineating the margins of slightly elevated lesions that are not clearly determined with chromoendoscopy with indigo carmine.

Magnifying endoscopy with narrow band imaging

NBI is digital technology integrated into standard endoscopy that involves the use of interference filters to illuminate the target in narrowed red, green, and blue bands of the spectrum. NBI technology results in different images at distinct levels of the mucosa and increases the contrast between the epithelial surface and the subjacent vascular network.[22] The advantages of NBI technology include ease of use without the application of contrast or absorptive dyes, and its wide availability. NBI can also be used with or without magnifying endoscopy. NBI aids differentiation between gastric neoplasia from nonneoplasia[23–25] and is useful for determining tumor margins. Whether NBI improves detection of EGCs remains unclear, and randomized trials of NBI compared with conventional WLI for detection of EGCs is ongoing.

In a multicenter study using nonmagnifying NBI (EVIS EXERA II video system center GIF-180; Olympus) for classification with gastric lesions, 85 patients (33% with dysplasia) were included in the study. In total, 224 different areas were biopsied, and histopathologic assessment was considered to be the gold standard. Proposed classification for gastric lesions on NBI using mucosal or vascular patterns was stratified into 3 groups: (1) pattern A: "regular vessels with circular mucosa" was associated with normal histology (accuracy 83%; 95% confidence interval [CI]: 75%–90%); (2) pattern B" "tubulovillous mucosa" was associated with intestinal metaplasia (accuracy 84%; 95% CI: 77%–91%; positive likelihood ratio = 4.75); and (3) pattern C: "irregular vessels and mucosa" was associated with dysplasia (accuracy 95% CI: 90%–99%; positive likelihood = 44.33).[26]

The benefit of NBI for diagnostic accuracy is maximized by using magnifying (zoom) endoscopy. Optical magnification by zoom endoscopy enables detailed examination of mucosal surface and vascular pattern, which are not observable by nonmagnifying observation.[27] Magnification endoscopy with NBI (M-NBI) has been proven to be an effective endoscopic tool in EGC diagnosis and had a better diagnostic performance than conventional WLI alone (**Figs. 2** and **3**). A proposed diagnostic system for EGC

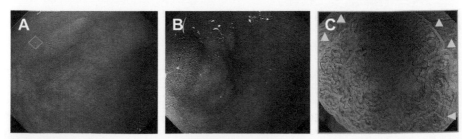

Fig. 2. Endoscopic findings of superficial elevated type EGC. (*A*) WLI demonstrates a superficial elevated type (Paris 0-IIa), poorly demarcated lesion with an irregular margin at the lesser curvature of the antrum of the stomach. (*B*) Near focus mode with NBI. Surface pattern could be visualized, but vascular pattern was hardly seen. (*C*) Magnifying endoscopy with NBI. A high magnification image of the region depicted by the blue square in (*A*) demonstrates an irregular microvascular pattern and irregular microsurface pattern with a clear demarcation line (*arrowheads*). These findings meet the criteria for a cancerous lesion. Histopathologic examination revealed well-differentiated adenocarcinoma.

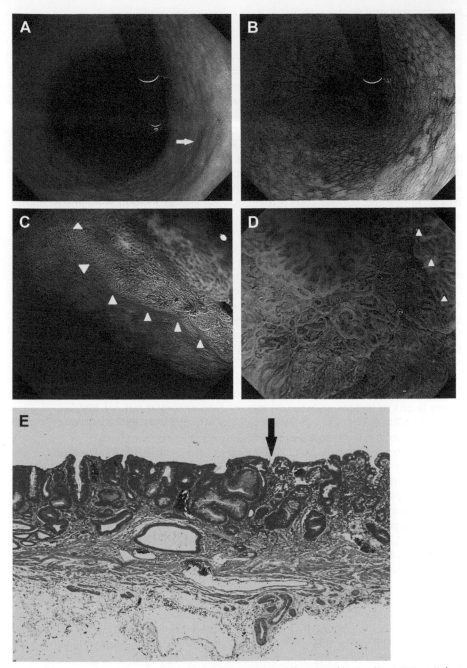

Fig. 3. Demonstrable case of EGC. (*A*) WLI demonstrates a depressed lesion (Paris 0-IIc + IIa) at the lesser curvature of the lower body of the stomach. The lesion's border was poorly defined. (*B*) Chromoendoscopy with indigo carmine dye. The lesion's border became clear. (*C*) Near focus mode with NBI. Vascular and surface pattern were irregular. A demarcation line (*arrowheads*) between the background mucosa and cancerous lesion was clearly seen. (*D*) Magnifying (full zoom) endoscopy with NBI clearly demonstrates an irregular microvascular pattern and irregular microsurface pattern with a clear demarcation line (*arrowheads*). These findings meet the criteria for a cancerous lesion. (*E*) Histopathologic examination of endoscopically resected specimen reveals a well-differentiated adenocarcinoma limited to the mucosa. Black arrow indicates the horizontal extent of the cancerous lesion (hematoxylin-eosin, original magnification ×40).

using M-NBI findings called the "VS (vessel plus surface)" has been applied in practice to simplify the process of diagnosis and improve accuracy. M-NBI findings of EGC comprise a clear demarcation line between the background noncancerous mucosa and the cancerous mucosa, and an irregular microvascular pattern and/or irregular microsurface pattern within the demarcation line. If the endoscopic findings fulfill either or both, the lesions are considered cancerous. Diagnosis of noncancerous lesions is made if neither is fulfilled. Up to 97% of EGCs fit the above criteria.[17,28] A randomized controlled trial that investigated differential diagnosis of small (<10 mm) depressed gastric cancer versus noncancerous lesions showed that the accuracy with combined M-NBI (80-fold optical magnification) surpassed that with conventional WLI or M-NBI alone. Two criteria (demarcation line and irregular microvascular or microsurface pattern) in the target lesion were examined. If findings fulfilled both criteria, endoscopic diagnosis of EGC is made with accuracy, sensitivity, and specificity of greater than 95%.[25]

Diagnosis of minute ($\leq$5 mm in diameter) gastric cancers is challenging. Chromoendoscopy is relatively ineffective for the minute gastric cancers at identifying the cancer-specific morphologic characteristics and on its own is insufficient to make an accurate diagnosis. M-NBI has an important application in this setting. A study demonstrated that M-NBI had greater sensitivity, specificity, and accuracy (78% vs 43%; 93% vs 81%; and 88% vs 70%, respectively) and higher reproducibility than chromoendoscopy with indigo carmine dye for the diagnosis of minute (<5 mm) gastric cancers.[29]

In about 20% of cases with EGC, lateral margins cannot be clearly determined by both conventional WLI and chromoendoscopy.[30,31] Accurate identification of lateral extent is crucial before endoscopic resection to ensure curative resection. In such cases, M-NBI also allows reliable delineation of the horizontal extent of EGC up to 72% of cases that the margins are unclear using chromoendoscopy.[30]

Magnifying endoscopy (EVIS LUCERA ELITE; Olympus) with 200 series endoscopes is capable of approximately 80 times optical magnification. This processor is sold in Japan, United Kingdom, and parts of Asia. Newer Olympus endoscopes (EVIS EXERA III/190 series systems) have a feature called near-focus imaging (low-powered optical zoom), allowing a maximum magnification of 65 times by simply pushing a button on the endoscope; it is available in the United States (see **Figs. 2** and **3**). Electronic or digital zoom ($\times$1.5) solely expands the central pixels on the screen and does not improve resolution of the image. The authors recommend using this endoscope, when available, with near focus function for detailed examination and characterization of suspicious gastric lesions.

Undifferentiated-type EGC often extends subepithelially and is covered with non-neoplastic foveolar epithelium. Thus, endoscopic diagnosis, even with enhanced imaging techniques, is inadequate for undifferentiated lesions.[23] Endoscopic delineation also remains difficult for this type of lesions with M-NBI.[30] Therefore, it is sometimes necessary to obtain a biopsy of the surrounding mucosa to diagnose undetectable tumor extent.[27]

Endoscopic Therapy and Its Indications for Early Gastric Cancer

Endoscopic resection is a minimally invasive technique developed to allow excision of lesions as a safe alternative to radical surgery for treatment of EGC. It should only be performed in patients with a negligible risk of lymph node metastasis, because it is a local therapy without lymph node dissection.[32] When the risk of lymph node metastasis is less than 1% in pT1a and less than 3% in pT1b (pathologic ["p"] stage), it is considered that endoscopic resection can achieve similar outcomes as surgical resection for EGC.[32]

Two main techniques of endoscopic resection are endoscopic mucosal resection (EMR) and endoscopic submucosal dissection (ESD). EMR involves separating the mucosal lesion from the underlying submucosa by injection and/or suction and subsequent removal of the mucosal lesions with snare resection. Several variations of EMR have been described, including injection-assisted, cap-assisted, and ligation-assisted techniques. ESD is a method whereby the mucosa surrounding the lesion is resected using an electrosurgical knife, followed by dissection of the submucosa beneath the lesion.[32] This approach allows en bloc resection of mucosal lesions regardless of the size. ESD is also feasible for locally recurrent EGC after previous endoscopic resection and lesions with ulcer scarring.[16,33,34]

The ESD procedure can be split into 4 consecutive steps: (1) accurately defining margins; (2) marking mucosal borders about 5 mm away from the borders of the lesion for gastric lesions; (3) mucosal incision made 5 mm outside of the marking, that is, at least 10 mm of normal tissue between the incision and the tumor; and (4) submucosal dissection (**Fig. 4**).[35]

Endoscopic submucosal dissection is superior to endoscopic mucosal resection for early gastric cancer

There have been no randomized trials comparing therapeutic outcomes of EMR and ESD for ECG. In 3 meta-analyses of retrospective studies, comparing ESD with EMR for EGC, ESD showed considerable advantages regarding higher en bloc resection rate (92% vs 52%; odds ratio [OR] 9.69, 95% CI 7.74 to 12.13), histologically complete resection rate (82% vs 42%; OR 5.66, 95% CI 2.92–10.96), and lower local recurrence (1% vs 6%; OR 0.10, 95% CI 0.06–0.18), even for lesions smaller than 10 mm. ESD had the disadvantage of higher complication rates for perforation (4% vs 1%; OR 4.67, 95% CI 2.77–7.87). The bleeding incidences were similar between the 2 groups (9% in both groups).[2,36,37]

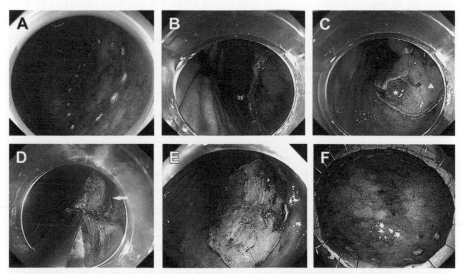

Fig. 4. Early gastric adenocarcinoma ESD. (*A*) Marking. (*B*) Mucosal circumferential incision. (*C, D*) Submucosal dissection. Submucosal layer beneath the lesion (*star* and *arrow*) and muscle layer (*triangle*) are clearly seen. (*E*) ESD mucosal defect. (*F*) Resected specimen.

According to 2015 European Society of Gastrointestinal Endoscopy guidelines, EMR is an acceptable option for lesions smaller than 10 to 15 mm with a very low probability of advanced histology (Paris 0-IIa). However, ESD is considered the treatment of choice for most gastric superficial neoplastic lesions.[38]

Indications of endoscopic submucosal dissection for early gastric cancer
In the past, patients with EGC could be considered for endoscopic resection only for small intramucosal cancers measuring 2 cm or less in diameter, differentiated histopathologic type, and without ulcerative findings (absolute indication).[39]

Following development of ESD to achieve en bloc resection even for larger and ulcerative lesions, efforts to expand its indications have been made. Gotoda and colleagues[40] and Hirasawa and colleagues[41] reviewed surgical pathologic specimens of patients (n = 5265 and 3843, respectively) who underwent gastrectomy with lymph node dissection for early-stage gastric adenocarcinoma and identified clinicopathologic factors that were associated with a negligible risk of lymph node metastasis,[32,42] as follows (Table 1):

1. Differentiated type, intramucosal cancer, greater than 2 cm in diameter, without ulceration
2. Differentiated type, intramucosal cancer, 3 cm in diameter or less, with ulceration
3. Undifferentiated type, intramucosal cancer, 2 cm in diameter or less, without ulceration

Mixed histologic types on a biopsy specimen, for example, moderately to poorly differentiated adenocarcinoma were defined as undifferentiated type.

In the absence of lymphovascular infiltration, none of the patients with lesions that fulfilled these criteria had lymph node metastases. Thus, the indications for ESD have been expanded to include these lesions (expanded indication).

Evaluation of curability of early gastric cancer after endoscopic submucosal dissection
Following ESD, histologic evaluation of curability and risk of lymph node metastasis according to tumor-related factors is performed when the lesion is resected en bloc with the following findings:

1. Differentiated type, intramucosal cancer, greater than 2 cm in diameter, without ulceration
2. Differentiated type, intramucosal cancer, 3 cm in diameter or less, with ulceration

Table 1
Indication of endoscopic submucosal dissection for early gastric cancer

Abnormality	Mucosal			
	Ulcer (−)		Ulcer (+)	
Pathology	≤2 cm	>2 cm	≤3 cm	>3 cm
Differentiated type[a]	A	E	E	X
Undifferentiated type[b]	E	X	X	X

Abbreviations: A, absolute indication lesion; E, expanded indication lesion; X, ESD is not recommended.
[a] Differentiated type includes papillary adenocarcinoma and tubular adenocarcinoma (well and moderately differentiated).
[b] Undifferentiated type includes poorly differentiated adenocarcinoma, signet-ring cell carcinoma, and mucinous adenocarcinoma.
Data from Ono H, Yao K, Fujishiro M, et al. Guidelines for endoscopic submucosal dissection and endoscopic mucosal resection for early gastric cancer. Dig Endosc 2016;28(1):3–15.

3. Undifferentiated type, intramucosal cancer, 2 cm in diameter or less, without ulceration
4. Differentiated type, 3 cm in diameter or less, minute submucosal (sm1) cancer (<500 μm below the muscularis mucosa)

Mixed histologic types in the resected specimens were determined by the major histologic features in the resected specimen.

In addition to the findings mentioned, in a lesion that is resected with negative surgical margins and without evidence of lymphovascular invasion, the risk of lymph node metastasis is exceedingly low and it is considered to be a curative resection.[32]

When ESD is considered noncurative at pathologic evaluation, additional surgical resection is indicated because of the clear risk of lymph node metastasis. After noncurative ESD, overall mortality and gastric cancer recurrence are higher in patients who did not undergo additional surgery than patients who underwent additional surgery (5-year mortality, 26%; 95% CI: 13.5% to 49.9%; 5-year recurrence, 17%; 95% CI, 7.6% to 37.8% in the former group).[43]

Long-term outcomes after endoscopic submucosal dissection for early gastric cancer
Studies that evaluated long-term outcomes of patients with EGC underwent ESD for absolute and expanded indications and achieved curative resections. After a median follow-up period of at least 5 years, risk of local recurrence was 0.2% to 1.1%,[44,45] and 5-year rates of overall survival and disease-specific survival were 92% and 99.9%, respectively.[46]

In comparison to surgery, ESD likely causes less postprocedural pain, earlier recovery, and shorter hospital stays. It is considered a safe and effective alternative to surgical resection. A noninferiority study by Pyo and colleagues[3] compared the long-term outcomes of endoscopic resection with those of surgery for EGC. In a propensity-matched analysis, 10-year overall survival after endoscopic resection was not inferior to that of surgery (97% vs 95%, respectively). However, 10-year recurrence-free survival might be lower after endoscopic resection than after surgery (93% vs 98%, respectively, risk difference 4.7%, 95% CI 2.50–6.97, P noninferiority = 0.820), mainly because of metachronous gastric cancer in the endoscopic resection group. Given the risk of metachronous gastric cancer, endoscopic surveillance after endoscopic resection is required.

Complications of endoscopic submucosal dissection
The 2 major complications of ESD are bleeding and perforation. ESD-related bleeding is classified into 2 groups, based on the time of onset: intraoperative bleeding and delayed bleeding. Intraoperative bleeding is defined as bleeding occurring during the ESD procedure. Management of immediate bleeding plays a critical role in the successful completion of ESD. Electrocautery is highly effective for hemostasis occurring during ESD.[42] Endoscopic clips may sometimes be necessary for bleeding control, but it can interfere with the subsequent resection procedure. Delayed bleeding is generally defined as clinical evidence of bleeding manifested by melena or hematochezia. It occurs in 1.8% to 15% of patients after gastric ESD.[3,47–49] Risk factors for delayed bleeding include age 80 years and older, antiplatelet drugs, lower and middle third of the stomach compared with the upper third of the stomach, lengthier procedure time, and resected specimens 40 mm in size or larger.[50] Several endoscopic treatment modalities can be used individually or in combination for hemostasis of delayed bleeding after endoscopic resection.[50] Postprocedure acid-suppressing drugs should be administered to reduce risk of delayed bleeding. Proton pump inhibitor therapy is

more effective to prevent delayed bleeding from the ulcer created after ESD than H2-receptor antagonists.[51]

Most perforations occur during the ESD procedure with rates ranging between 1.2% and 4.5% of gastric ESD cases.[3,47–49] Factors associated with perforation are larger size lesions, lesions with ulcer findings, and lesions in the upper and middle thirds of the stomach (as compared with the lower third of the stomach).[50] Endoscopic closure with endoclips is successful in greater than 98% of cases.[52] Gastric perforation following endoscopic resection for EGC does not lead to peritoneal seeding or dissemination.[53] Delayed perforation is rare and reported in 0.07% to 0.45% of procedures.[3,54] Patients who present with symptoms of peritoneal irritation with rebound tenderness require emergency surgery, whereas patients with mild symptoms can be managed with endoscopic closure of delayed perforation.[55]

BENIGN GASTRIC EPITHELIAL POLYPS

The prevalence of gastric polyps discovered during upper endoscopy in the US population is 6%. The most common lesion is fundic gland polyps (77%), followed by hyperplastic polyps (17%). Gastric adenomas are detected in 0.69% of cases.[56] Gastric adenoma is usually asymptomatic but can cause dyspepsia, heartburn, abdominal pain, and rarely, gastrointestinal bleeding and gastric outlet obstruction.

Hyperplastic Polyps

Hyperplastic polyps result from chronic inflammation. They are usually found in the setting of autoimmune gastritis (12%–51%) and chronic active H pylori gastritis (35%–37%). Thus, in the presence of hyperplastic polyps in the stomach, additional biopsies obtained from the antrum and body should always be performed.[57,58] On upper endoscopy, hyperplastic polyps are generally seen as reddish, smooth, domeshaped, sessile or pedunculated polyps and mostly are less than 1 cm in maximal diameter.[59] Endoscopic appearance may be similar to gastric adenomas; therefore, biopsy should be obtained.

Malignant changes develop via hyperplasia-dysplasia-carcinoma sequence. Dysplastic transformation is noted in about 2% to 19%.[60,61] Size greater than 1 cm and pedunculated type are associated with increased risk of malignancy in hyperplastic polyps.[60,62] Thus, endoscopic polypectomy should be considered for asymmetric gastric hyperplastic polyps greater than 1 cm.[62]

Fundic Gland polyps

Fundic gland polyps occur in 2 clinical settings: (1) sporadic and (2) familial syndrome in association with familial adenomatous polyposis, MUTYH-associated polyposis, and gastric adenocarcinoma and proximal polyposis of the stomach.[63–65]

Long-term use of proton pump inhibitors ($\geq$12 months) is associated with an increased risk of sporadic fundic gland polyps.[66] In addition, fundic gland polyps are associated with gastroesophageal reflux disease symptoms, gastric heterotopia, hyperplastic colonic polyps (only in men), and colonic adenomas (only in women, especially those greater than 60 years of age). The presence of fundic gland polyps is inversely correlated with H pylori infection and active gastritis.[67] They typically appear as small, sessile lesions with a smooth surface in the body of stomach. Biopsy of probable fundic gland polyps is recommended to exclude dysplasia and adenocarcinoma and to exclude the need for polypectomy as required for other types of polyp. Sporadic fundic gland polyps rarely progress to gastric cancer. In contrast, dysplasia is present in fundic gland polyps in familial adenomatous polyposis in about 40% of patients,[68–70] and progression to gastric adenocarcinoma has been reported.[65,71,72] Endoscopic polypectomy is not required for small sporadic fundic gland polyps.[73] Endoscopic resection of fundic gland polyps should be considered in lesions 1 cm in size or greater, high-grade dysplasia, or early adenocarcinoma.[62]

Gastric Adenomas

Gastric adenomas frequently occur in a background of chronic atrophic gastritis and intestinal metaplasia and are frequently found in the patients with familial adenomatous polyposis syndrome.[74] They are typically pale, flat, or slightly elevated. Depressed-type gastric adenomas are uncommon (12%).[75] Most adenomas locate in the antrum, but they can occur anywhere in the stomach. Microscopically, most gastric adenomas are tubular or tubulovillous types. The annual incidence of gastric cancer is 0.6% for mild to moderate dysplasia and 6% for severe dysplasia within 5 years after diagnosis.[76] Risk of carcinoma is higher in men, with increasing age and severe dysplasia, and in polyps larger than 2 cm in size.[76,77]

Endoscopic resection can be considered for gastric adenomas, which have potential risks of developing into adenocarcinoma, and biopsy of the surrounding mucosa is essential to evaluate the presence of underlying chronic inflammation and assess baseline risk of gastric malignancy. Endoscopic follow-up is recommended 1 year after polyp resection; however, the time interval can be modified based on the degree of dysplasia or completeness of polyp resection.[62,73]

In summary, endoscopic diagnosis and early treatment are crucial to improve outcomes of patients with EGC. Endoscopists should be familiar with endoscopic features of EGC because many of these lesions are subtle and difficult to diagnose. In addition, the use of chromoendoscopy and image-enhanced endoscopy improves diagnostic accuracy and facilitates endoscopic resection. ESD is a preferred endoscopic technique for resection of EGC and offers a comparable overall survival to surgical resection. Long-term outcomes of patients after ESD are excellent. Given the risk of metachronous gastric cancer, endoscopic surveillance after endoscopic resection is required. Further studies should evaluate new technologies to improve early detection and increase efficiency and safety of endoscopic resection techniques. Most benign gastric epithelial polyps are found incidentally during routine endoscopy. Endoscopic management of these lesions depends on patient symptomatology, patient's comorbidities (eg, familial syndromes), lesions characteristics, and risk of malignant transformation.

REFERENCES

1. Kim YI, Kim YW, Choi IJ, et al. Long-term survival after endoscopic resection versus surgery in early gastric cancers. Endoscopy 2015;47(4):293–301.
2. Park CH, Lee H, Kim DW, et al. Clinical safety of endoscopic submucosal dissection compared with surgery in elderly patients with early gastric cancer: a propensity-matched analysis. Gastrointest Endosc 2014;80(4):599–609.
3. Pyo JH, Lee H, Min BH, et al. Long-term outcome of endoscopic resection vs. surgery for early gastric cancer: a non-inferiority-matched cohort study. Am J Gastroenterol 2016;111(2):240–9.
4. The Paris endoscopic classification of superficial neoplastic lesions: esophagus, stomach, and colon: November 30 to December 1, 2002. Gastrointest Endosc 2003;58(6 Suppl):S3–43.
5. Katai H, Sano T. Early gastric cancer: concepts, diagnosis, and management. Int J Clin Oncol 2005;10(6):375–83.

6. Schlemper RJ, Riddell RH, Kato Y, et al. The Vienna classification of gastrointestinal epithelial neoplasia. Gut 2000;47(2):251–5.

7. Nashimoto A, Akazawa K, Isobe Y, et al. Gastric cancer treated in 2002 in Japan: 2009 annual report of the JGCA nationwide registry. Gastric Cancer 2013;16(1): 1–27.

8. Eckardt VF, Giessler W, Kanzler G, et al. Clinical and morphological characteristics of early gastric cancer. A case-control study. Gastroenterology 1990;98(3): 708–14.

9. Noguchi Y, Yoshikawa T, Tsuburaya A, et al. Is gastric carcinoma different between Japan and the United States? Cancer 2000;89(11):2237–46.

10. Gonzalez S. Red-flag technologies in gastric neoplasia. Gastrointest Endosc Clin N Am 2013;23(3):581–95.

11. Hosokawa O, Tsuda S, Kidani E, et al. Diagnosis of gastric cancer up to three years after negative upper gastrointestinal endoscopy. Endoscopy 1998;30(8): 669–74.

12. Chadwick G, Groene O, Riley S, et al. Gastric cancers missed during endoscopy in England. Clin Gastroenterol Hepatol 2015;13(7):1264–70.e1.

13. Hamashima C, Shibuya D, Yamazaki H, et al. The Japanese guidelines for gastric cancer screening. Jpn J Clin Oncol 2008;38(4):259–67.

14. Lee KS, Oh DK, Han MA, et al. Gastric cancer screening in Korea: report on the national cancer screening program in 2008. Cancer Res Treat 2011;43(2):83–8.

15. Kim GH, Liang PS, Bang SJ, et al. Screening and surveillance for gastric cancer in the United States: Is it needed? Gastrointest Endosc 2016;84(1):18–28.

16. Yada T, Yokoi C, Uemura N. The current state of diagnosis and treatment for early gastric cancer. Diagn Ther Endosc 2013;2013:241320.

17. Yao K. The endoscopic diagnosis of early gastric cancer. Ann Gastroenterol 2013;26(1):11–22.

18. Trivedi PJ, Braden B. Indications, stains and techniques in chromoendoscopy. QJM Feb 2013;106(2):117–31.

19. Deutsch J, Banks M. Gastrointestinal endoscopy in the cancer patient, vol. 1. Oxford (United Kingdom): John Wiley & Sons; 2013.

20. Sakai Y, Eto R, Kasanuki J, et al. Chromoendoscopy with indigo carmine dye added to acetic acid in the diagnosis of gastric neoplasia: a prospective comparative study. Gastrointest Endosc 2008;68(4):635–41.

21. Lee BE, Kim GH, Park DY, et al. Acetic acid-indigo carmine chromoendoscopy for delineating early gastric cancers: its usefulness according to histological type. BMC Gastroenterol 2010;10:97.

22. Kuznetsov K, Lambert R, Rey JF. Narrow-band imaging: potential and limitations. Endoscopy 2006;38(1):76–81.

23. Yao K, Doyama H, Gotoda T, et al. Diagnostic performance and limitations of magnifying narrow-band imaging in screening endoscopy of early gastric cancer: a prospective multicenter feasibility study. Gastric Cancer 2014;17(4): 669–79.

24. Zhang Q, Wang F, Chen ZY, et al. Comparison of the diagnostic efficacy of white light endoscopy and magnifying endoscopy with narrow band imaging for early gastric cancer: a meta-analysis. Gastric Cancer 2016;19(2):543–52.

25. Ezoe Y, Muto M, Uedo N, et al. Magnifying narrowband imaging is more accurate than conventional white-light imaging in diagnosis of gastric mucosal cancer. Gastroenterology 2011;141(6):2017–25.e3.

26. Pimentel-Nunes P, Dinis-Ribeiro M, Soares JB, et al. A multicenter validation of an endoscopic classification with narrow band imaging for gastric precancerous and cancerous lesions. Endoscopy 2012;44(3):236–46.
27. Uedo N, Fujishiro M, Goda K, et al. Role of narrow band imaging for diagnosis of early-stage esophagogastric cancer: current consensus of experienced endoscopists in Asia-Pacific region. Dig Endosc 2011;23(Suppl 1):58–71.
28. Muto M, Yao K, Kaise M, et al. Magnifying endoscopy simple diagnostic algorithm for early gastric cancer (MESDA-G). Dig Endosc 2016;28(4):379–93.
29. Fujiwara S, Yao K, Nagahama T, et al. Can we accurately diagnose minute gastric cancers ($\leq$5 mm)? Chromoendoscopy (CE) vs magnifying endoscopy with narrow band imaging (M-NBI). Gastric Cancer 2015;18(3):590–6.
30. Nagahama T, Yao K, Maki S, et al. Usefulness of magnifying endoscopy with narrow-band imaging for determining the horizontal extent of early gastric cancer when there is an unclear margin by chromoendoscopy (with video). Gastrointest Endosc 2011;74(6):1259–67.
31. Kiyotoki S, Nishikawa J, Satake M, et al. Usefulness of magnifying endoscopy with narrow-band imaging for determining gastric tumor margin. J Gastroenterol Hepatol 2010;25(10):1636–41.
32. Ono H, Yao K, Fujishiro M, et al. Guidelines for endoscopic submucosal dissection and endoscopic mucosal resection for early gastric cancer. Dig Endosc 2016;28(1):3–15.
33. Yokoi C, Gotoda T, Hamanaka H, et al. Endoscopic submucosal dissection allows curative resection of locally recurrent early gastric cancer after prior endoscopic mucosal resection. Gastrointest Endosc 2006;64(2):212–8.
34. Yamamoto H, Kawata H, Sunada K, et al. Successful en-bloc resection of large superficial tumors in the stomach and colon using sodium hyaluronate and small-caliber-tip transparent hood. Endoscopy 2003;35(8):690–4.
35. Bhatt A, Abe S, Kumaravel A, et al. Indications and techniques for endoscopic submucosal dissection. Am J Gastroenterol 2015;110(6):784–91.
36. Lian J, Chen S, Zhang Y, et al. A meta-analysis of endoscopic submucosal dissection and EMR for early gastric cancer. Gastrointest Endosc 2012;76(4): 763–70.
37. Facciorusso A, Antonino M, Di Maso M, et al. Endoscopic submucosal dissection vs endoscopic mucosal resection for early gastric cancer: a meta-analysis. World J Gastrointest Endosc 2014;6(11):555–63.
38. Pimentel-Nunes P, Dinis-Ribeiro M, Ponchon T, et al. Endoscopic submucosal dissection: European Society of Gastrointestinal Endoscopy (ESGE) Guideline. Endoscopy 2015;47(9):829–54.
39. Japanese Gastric Cancer Association. Japanese gastric cancer treatment guidelines 2010 (ver. 3). Gastric Cancer 2011;14(2):113–23.
40. Gotoda T, Yanagisawa A, Sasako M, et al. Incidence of lymph node metastasis from early gastric cancer: estimation with a large number of cases at two large centers. Gastric Cancer 2000;3(4):219–25.
41. Hirasawa T, Gotoda T, Miyata S, et al. Incidence of lymph node metastasis and the feasibility of endoscopic resection for undifferentiated-type early gastric cancer. Gastric Cancer 2009;12(3):148–52.
42. Jansen M, Wright NA. Stem cells, pre-neoplasia, and early cancer of the upper gastrointestinal tract. Vol 1. Springer International Publishing; 2016.
43. Eom BW, Kim YI, Kim KH, et al. Survival benefit of additional surgery after noncurative endoscopic resection in patients with early gastric cancer. Gastrointest Endosc 2017;85(1):155–63.

44. Kosaka T, Endo M, Toya Y, et al. Long-term outcomes of endoscopic submucosal dissection for early gastric cancer: a single-center retrospective study. Dig Endosc 2014;26(2):183–91.
45. Oda I, Oyama T, Abe S, et al. Preliminary results of multicenter questionnaire study on long-term outcomes of curative endoscopic submucosal dissection for early gastric cancer. Dig Endosc 2014;26(2):214–9.
46. Suzuki H, Oda I, Abe S, et al. High rate of 5-year survival among patients with early gastric cancer undergoing curative endoscopic submucosal dissection. Gastric Cancer 2016;19(1):198–205.
47. Oda I, Saito D, Tada M, et al. A multicenter retrospective study of endoscopic resection for early gastric cancer. Gastric Cancer 2006;9(4):262–70.
48. Chung IK, Lee JH, Lee SH, et al. Therapeutic outcomes in 1000 cases of endoscopic submucosal dissection for early gastric neoplasms: Korean ESD Study Group multicenter study. Gastrointest Endosc 2009;69(7):1228–35.
49. Isomoto H, Shikuwa S, Yamaguchi N, et al. Endoscopic submucosal dissection for early gastric cancer: a large-scale feasibility study. Gut 2009;58(3):331–6.
50. Oda I, Suzuki H, Nonaka S, et al. Complications of gastric endoscopic submucosal dissection. Dig Endosc 2013;25(Suppl 1):71–8.
51. Uedo N, Takeuchi Y, Yamada T, et al. Effect of a proton pump inhibitor or an H2-receptor antagonist on prevention of bleeding from ulcer after endoscopic submucosal dissection of early gastric cancer: a prospective randomized controlled trial. Am J Gastroenterol 2007;102(8):1610–6.
52. Minami S, Gotoda T, Ono H, et al. Complete endoscopic closure of gastric perforation induced by endoscopic resection of early gastric cancer using endoclips can prevent surgery (with video). Gastrointest Endosc 2006;63(4):596–601.
53. Ikehara H, Gotoda T, Ono H, et al. Gastric perforation during endoscopic resection for gastric carcinoma and the risk of peritoneal dissemination. Br J Surg 2007;94(8):992–5.
54. Hanaoka N, Uedo N, Ishihara R, et al. Clinical features and outcomes of delayed perforation after endoscopic submucosal dissection for early gastric cancer. Endoscopy 2010;42(12):1112–5.
55. Suzuki H, Oda I, Sekiguchi M, et al. Management and associated factors of delayed perforation after gastric endoscopic submucosal dissection. World J Gastroenterol 2015;21(44):12635–43.
56. Carmack SW, Genta RM, Schuler CM, et al. The current spectrum of gastric polyps: a 1-year national study of over 120,000 patients. Am J Gastroenterol 2009;104(6):1524–32.
57. Dirschmid K, Platz-Baudin C, Stolte M. Why is the hyperplastic polyp a marker for the precancerous condition of the gastric mucosa? Virchows Arch 2006;448(1):80–4.
58. Abraham SC, Singh VK, Yardley JH, et al. Hyperplastic polyps of the stomach: associations with histologic patterns of gastritis and gastric atrophy. Am J Surg Pathol 2001;25(4):500–7.
59. Jain R, Chetty R. Gastric hyperplastic polyps: a review. Dig Dis Sci 2009;54(9):1839–46.
60. Han AR, Sung CO, Kim KM, et al. The clinicopathological features of gastric hyperplastic polyps with neoplastic transformations: a suggestion of indication for endoscopic polypectomy. Gut Liver 2009;3(4):271–5.
61. Terada T. Malignant transformation of foveolar hyperplastic polyp of the stomach: a histopathological study. Med Oncol 2011;28(4):941–4.

62. Evans JA, Chandrasekhara V, Chathadi KV, et al. The role of endoscopy in the management of premalignant and malignant conditions of the stomach. Gastrointest Endosc 2015;82(1):1–8.
63. Vogt S, Jones N, Christian D, et al. Expanded extracolonic tumor spectrum in MUTYH-associated polyposis. Gastroenterology 2009;137(6):1976–85. e1–10.
64. Worthley DL, Phillips KD, Wayte N, et al. Gastric adenocarcinoma and proximal polyposis of the stomach (GAPPS): a new autosomal dominant syndrome. Gut 2012;61(5):774–9.
65. Arnason T, Liang WY, Alfaro E, et al. Morphology and natural history of familial adenomatous polyposis-associated dysplastic fundic gland polyps. Histopathology 2014;65(3):353–62.
66. Tran-Duy A, Spaetgens B, Hoes AW, et al. Use of proton pump inhibitors and risks of fundic gland polyps and gastric cancer: systematic review and meta-analysis. Clin Gastroenterol Hepatol 2016;14(12):1706–19.e5.
67. Genta RM, Schuler CM, Robiou CI, et al. No association between gastric fundic gland polyps and gastrointestinal neoplasia in a study of over 100,000 patients. Clin Gastroenterol Hepatol 2009;7(8):849–54.
68. Attard TM, Giardiello FM, Argani P, et al. Fundic gland polyposis with high-grade dysplasia in a child with attenuated familial adenomatous polyposis and familial gastric cancer. J Pediatr Gastroenterol Nutr 2001;32(2):215–8.
69. Bertoni G, Sassatelli R, Nigrisoli E, et al. Dysplastic changes in gastric fundic gland polyps of patients with familial adenomatous polyposis. Ital J Gastroenterol Hepatol 1999;31(3):192–7.
70. Bianchi LK, Burke CA, Bennett AE, et al. Fundic gland polyp dysplasia is common in familial adenomatous polyposis. Clin Gastroenterol Hepatol 2008;6(2):180–5.
71. Zwick A, Munir M, Ryan CK, et al. Gastric adenocarcinoma and dysplasia in fundic gland polyps of a patient with attenuated adenomatous polyposis coli. Gastroenterology 1997;113(2):659–63.
72. Hofgartner WT, Thorp M, Ramus MW, et al. Gastric adenocarcinoma associated with fundic gland polyps in a patient with attenuated familial adenomatous polyposis. Am J Gastroenterol 1999;94(8):2275–81.
73. Goddard AF, Badreldin R, Pritchard DM, et al. The management of gastric polyps. Gut 2010;59(9):1270–6.
74. Ngamruengphong S, Boardman LA, Heigh RI, et al. Gastric adenomas in familial adenomatous polyposis are common, but subtle, and have a benign course. Hered Cancer Clin Pract 2014;12(1):4.
75. Tamai N, Kaise M, Nakayoshi T, et al. Clinical and endoscopic characterization of depressed gastric adenoma. Endoscopy 2006;38(4):391–4.
76. de Vries AC, van Grieken NC, Looman CW, et al. Gastric cancer risk in patients with premalignant gastric lesions: a nationwide cohort study in the Netherlands. Gastroenterology 2008;134(4):945–52.
77. Islam RS, Patel NC, Lam-Himlin D, et al. Gastric polyps: a review of clinical, endoscopic, and histopathologic features and management decisions. Gastroenterol Hepatol 2013;9(10):640–51.

Management of Non-neoplastic Gastric Lesions

Ryan K. Schmocker, MD, MS[a], Anne O. Lidor, MD, MPH[b],*

KEYWORDS

- Refractory gastric ulcer • Giant gastric ulcer • Gastric polyps
- Hyperplastic gastric polyp • Fundic gland polyp

KEY POINTS

- Refractory gastric ulcers require careful investigation into the cause of their persistence, and medical management is the mainstay for treatment of uncomplicated disease.
- Complications of persistent gastric ulcers include bleeding, perforation, and gastric outlet obstruction, with downstream management ranging from elective surgery to emergency surgery or endoscopy.
- Gastric polyps are a heterogeneous group of conditions that represent lesions which have varying risk of malignancy from rare malignant risk in fundic gland polyps to significant risk of dysplasia and malignancy in adenomas.

INTRODUCTION

Non-neoplastic gastric lesions represent a heterogeneous group of conditions, which require careful evaluation and prudent application of invasive treatments because they can mimic or degenerate into malignant lesions. This article discusses the causes, classification, and treatment of persistent gastric ulcers, giant gastric ulcers, gastric polyps, and other benign gastric lesions. Differentiation of these lesions is critical for estimating the risk of malignancy and, ultimately, offering appropriate patient counseling about management options. The relevant anatomic and pathologic considerations, diagnostic approach, and clinical outcomes of these conditions are discussed, with a particular emphasis on refractory and large gastric ulcers and gastric polyps because these can mimic or harbor gastric malignancies. An in-depth discussion of routine management of gastric peptic ulcer disease (PUD) can be found in other surgical texts.

Disclosure Statement: The authors have nothing to disclose.
[a] Department of Surgery, University of Wisconsin, 600 North Highland Avenue, MC 7375, Madison, WI 53792, USA; [b] Department of Surgery, University of Wisconsin, K4/752 CSC, 600 Highland Avenue, MC 7375, Madison, WI 53792-0001, USA
* Corresponding author.
E-mail address: lidor@surgery.wisc.edu

Surg Clin N Am 97 (2017) 387–403
http://dx.doi.org/10.1016/j.suc.2016.11.011
0039-6109/17/© 2016 Elsevier Inc. All rights reserved.

surgical.theclinics.com

REFRACTORY OR PERSISTENT GASTRIC ULCERS
Introduction

The diagnosis of refractory or persistent gastric ulceration requires endoscopic evaluation demonstrating gastric ulceration more than 5 mm in diameter that does not heal after 8 to 12 weeks of treatment with optimal proton pump inhibitor (PPI) or other antisecretory therapy.[1] These terms will be used interchangeably throughout the article. Management options include a gamut of potential therapeutic options: medical therapy, endoscopic therapies, minimally invasive surgery, and traditional surgery; therefore, refractory gastric ulcers represent a challenging clinical problem.

Pathophysiology

PUD is most commonly a result of 2 primary factors: use of nonsteroidal anti-inflammatory medications (NSAIDs) and *Helicobacter pylori* infection, with ulceration ultimately resulting from a breakdown of the body's intrinsic acid protection mechanisms. *H pylori* results in persistent inflammation of the gastric mucosa[2] by leading to increased acid section through the gastrin pathway,[2,3] as well as promoting the acid secretion response to gastrin and inhibiting the normal inhibitory response to gastric acid secretion.[3] An in-depth discussion of the pathophysiology and cause of PUD is not included here.

Persistent gastric ulcers require careful examination and history to identify factors that may be contributing to persistence of the ulceration because there are a wide range of potential explanations, including persistent *H pylori* infection or continued NSAID use, among other causes (**Box 1**). A careful history can be paramount to determining the cause of persistent gastric ulcers.

Clinical Presentation

The presentation of PUD varies greatly from asymptomatic, to dyspepsia or upper abdominal discomfort, to devastating complications such as massive upper gastrointestinal hemorrhage or hollow viscus perforation. Dyspepsia is a poorly defined phenomenon of nonspecific upper abdominal discomfort that is present in 10% to 40% of the general population,[4,5] with 5% to 15% of patients with PUD having dyspepsia.[6–8] In this vein, the most common presentation is epigastric pain, with or without associated bloating, early satiety, and nausea.[3] About 80% of patients with endoscopically diagnosed ulcers recall epigastric pain in retrospect.[9] Conversely, 70% of people with their initial presentation of peptic ulcers are asymptomatic[10] and, given the lack of symptoms, may present later or with associated complications. To this end, 43% to 87% of patients with hemorrhage from peptic ulcers present without preceding symptoms.[11–13] For patients who initially present with symptomatic PUD, persistence or recurrence of these symptoms is the primary indicator of ongoing ulceration. For those with an asymptomatic presentation, repeat endoscopy demonstrates persistent ulceration after 12 weeks of therapy, therefore meeting the definition of a persistent ulceration.

Diagnosis

Upper gastrointestinal endoscopy is the primary modality for PUD diagnosis. Recent guidelines state that upper endoscopy should be performed for all patients with dyspepsia equal to or greater than 50 years of age, or those with alarm symptoms.[14] Alarm symptoms include a family history of upper gastrointestinal malignancy, unintended weight loss, persistent nausea vomiting, iron deficiency anemia, gastrointestinal bleeding, dysphagia or odynophagia, a palpable mass, or lymphadenopathy

---

Box 1
Causes of refractory peptic ulcer disease

Persistent H pylori infection

- Poor treatment compliance

- Resistant organism

- Inadequate treatment regimen

- Unrecognized *H pylori* infection
  - False-negative testing
  - Not tested
  - Inadequate testing

Ulcers related to NSAIDs

- Continued NSAID use

- Undiscovered NSAID use

- Poor response to cotherapy with a PPI or histamine 2 receptor antagonist (H2RA)

Other mechanisms

- Impaired healing
  - Cigarette smoking

- Inadequate inhibition of acid secretion
  - Poor compliance with treatment
  - Tolerance or resistance to H2RAs
  - Resistance to PPIs
  - Rapid metabolism of PPIs

- Hypersecretory states
  - Gastrinoma
  - Antral G cell hyperfunction
  - Idiopathic hypersecretory duodenal ulcer

- Other medications
  - Glucocorticoids
  - Cytotoxic drugs
  - Other drugs such as cocaine or methamphetamines

- Uncommon causes
  - Cancer
  - Crohn disease
  - Infections other than *H pylori*
  - Eosinophilic, inflammatory, infiltrative conditions

Adapted from Vakil NB. Approach to refractory or recurrent peptic ulcer disease. UpToDate; 2015. Available at: http://www.uptodate.com/contents/approach-to-refractory-or-recurrent-peptic-ulcer-disease.

(**Box 2**).[14,15] Young patients with dyspepsia but without alarm symptoms should be evaluated by noninvasive *H pylori* testing and, if positive, appropriate medical treatment empiric treatment with acid suppression therapy or proceeding with initial endoscopy.[14] The primary reason to proceed with upper endoscopy is to rule out malignancy, because historical series put the risk of occult malignancy in gastric ulcers at 5% to 11%.[16] However, given that the rates of gastric cancer are decreasing in the United States[17] and there are certain populations for which gastric cancer is very unlikely (eg, young patient taking NSAIDs with classic appearance of NSAID ulcers), this estimation of gastric cancer incidence likely overestimates the true risk of occult malignancy even in the absence of more recent data.[15]

Box 2
Alarm symptoms in patients with dyspepsia

Alarm symptoms in patients with dyspepsia

- Age equal to or greater than 50
- Family history of upper gastrointestinal malignancy in a first-degree relative
- Unintended weight loss
- Gastrointestinal bleeding or iron deficient anemia without clear alternative cause
- Dysphagia
- Odynophagia
- Persistent nausea and vomiting
- Abnormal imaging
- Palpable mass
- Lymphadenopathy

Adapted from Shaukat A, Wang A, Acosta RD, et al. The role of endoscopy in dyspepsia. Gastrointest Endosc 2015;82:228; with permission.

Endoscopic biopsies should be performed when gastric ulcers demonstrate features concerning for malignancy. These include elevated irregular ulcer borders, mass lesion associated with the ulcer, and abnormal adjacent mucosa.[15] In general, the endoscopic appearance is an accurate predictor of malignancy.[18,19] However, some malignancies can initially appear benign so the ultimate decision for biopsy should be individualized. This is contrary to past recommendations to biopsy all gastric ulcers.[15] For certain patients who are at very low risk of malignancy (eg, young patients) or those with classic appearance of NSAID-related ulcers (shallow, flat, antral ulcer with associated erosions), biopsies may be deferred.[15] When performing biopsies, multiple samples should be taken from the base and edge of the ulcer,[20] and *H pylori* testing should be performed.[21]

Many endoscopists perform a surveillance endoscopy for patients with gastric ulcers given that some gastric cancers initially appear benign[22,23]; however, there is no major gastroenterology society guideline that recommends surveillance endoscopy. Therefore, it is recommended that the role of surveillance endoscopy should be individualized, with certain groups of patients for whom surveillance endoscopy should be strongly considered. For example, those with suspicious appearing lesions on initial endoscopy, those with persistent symptoms despite medical therapy, those with gastric ulcers of unclear cause, or those who did not undergo biopsy at the index endoscopy for reasons such as hemodynamic instability.[15] Persistence of an ulceration more than 5 mm in diameter that does not heal after 8 to 12 weeks of treatment confirms the diagnosis of a persistent gastric ulcer.[1]

Management

The ultimate goal of treatment is to elucidate the undying cause of persistent gastric ulceration and implement targeted therapy to treat the offending cause, such as those listed in **Box 1**. The first major branch point in the treatment of refractory gastric ulcers depends on whether there are complications associated with the persistent disease because patients with complicated disease proceed down a very different pathway than those with uncomplicated disease.

Uncomplicated disease

Medical management is the primary treatment modality for chronic gastric ulcers.[3] Refractory peptic ulcers (including those with complications despite treatment) require further evaluation of risk factors for persistent disease, including evaluating for false-negative *H pylori* tests, gastrinomas, and modifying lifestyle risk factors such as NSAID use, smoking, alcohol use, noncompliance with treatment,[24] as well as other more rare causes (see **Box 1**). For patients with uncomplicated persistent gastric ulcers and documented *H pylori* infection, optimal treatment includes triple therapy with a PPI, metronidazole, and clarithromycin with the addition of bismuth (quadruple therapy) in areas with high clarithromycin resistance[25]

Surveillance endoscopy should be considered on an individual basis as previously discussed. Some clinicians recommend that after 12 additional weeks of PPI therapy endoscopy should be considered to document healing, and this scar is often biopsied because some neoplastic ulcers can heal after antisecretory therapy.[26] In addition, the risk of malignancy in initially benign-appearing ulcers ranges from 0.8% to 4.3%.[27,28] Those with persistent ulceration should undergo 4-quadrant biopsies, as well as sampling of the antrum and body for *H pylori* testing.[26] For those that do not have *H pylori* on gastric biopsies, consideration should be made for subsequent testing to confirm the negative result, such as stool antigen or urease breath test, ideally off of PPI therapy for 2 weeks.

Maintenance antisecretory therapy is recommended for patients in high-risk groups, which includes patients with refractory peptic ulcers. Other indications for continued therapy include giant ulcers, *H pylori*–negative and NSAID-negative disease, failure to treat *H pylori*, greater than 2 peptic ulcer recurrences per year, continued use of NSAIDs, age greater than 50 years old, or multiple comorbidities.[29–34]

Recently, there has been concern about the long-term use of PPI therapy with studies demonstrating an increased risk of fractures[35] and cardiovascular events.[36] Given these findings, the question has been raised about the optimal approach (medical or surgical) for patients with refractory PUD. A recent Cochrane review was conducted in an attempt to answer this question.[37] Unfortunately, the available studies did not offer sufficient, high-quality evidence to make a conclusion about the comparative risks and benefits of medical versus surgical therapy for patients with uncomplicated persistent peptic ulcers. Therefore, given the lack of available evidence, it could not offer a treatment algorithm for this problem.[37] Clearly additional high quality evidence is needed to make future recommendations based on a head-to-head comparison.

In general, surgical management of uncomplicated ulcers is rarely indicated in the modern area of PPI therapy. Generally consideration of surgical therapy requires failure of twice daily PPI therapy for 24 weeks, with modification of the other factors that can contribute to persistent gastric ulcers. Surgery should be considered for those who are unable to complete medical therapy secondary to noncompliance or side-effects, recurrent ulcer despite completing treatment, and those at high risk of complications (ie, NSAID dependence).[24] Surgery offers the additional benefit of resecting potential premalignant lesions for those patients who would ultimately develop a malignancy. However, the 1% risk of mortality, as well as the complications of dumping syndrome and diarrhea, limit surgery as a primary treatment.[38] For those requiring surgery, partial gastrectomy is performed to decrease the mass of the acid producing cells[38] and vagotomy should be considered.[1]

Complicated disease

Complications of peptic ulcers (including recurrent peptic ulcers) include perforation, bleeding and gastric outlet obstruction.[39–43] These complications are associated with a high mortality, bleeding leading to a short-term mortality rate of 3%,[44] and perforation leading to a short-term mortality of 25% to 30%.[45]

In the acute phase, endoscopic and medical treatments are the mainstay of bleeding ulcer treatment,[46] with surgery as a backup for those patients who are hemodynamically unstable or for lesions that are not amenable or refractory to endoscopic therapy.[47,48] In general, for patients undergoing surgical intervention for a bleeding ulcer, partial gastrectomy should be considered because of the underlying risk of malignancy. Truncal vagotomy and pyloroplasty is another option for patients with significant comorbid conditions.[49,50] In addition, angiography and embolization for gastric ulcer bleeding is an additional nonoperative modality that can be used to treat significant hemorrhage. In fact, the American College of Radiology has issued a consensus statement with the following recommendations for upper gastrointestinal bleeding: "1. Endoscopy is the best initial diagnostic and therapeutic procedure, 2. Surgery and transcatheter arteriography and intervention (TAI) are equally effective after failed therapeutic endoscopy, but TAI should be considered particularly in patients at high risk for surgery, 3. Transcatheter arteriography and intervention is less likely to be successful in patients with impaired coagulation."[51]

Laparoscopic and open emergency surgery remains the primary treatment modality for those patients with perforated ulcers.[52] The choice of the procedure that is performed for a perforated ulcer is made at the time of the operation with special consideration given to the clinical scenario and patient comorbidities. The general approach includes partial gastrectomy because of the underlying risk of malignancy; however, for those with significant comorbidities, intraoperative instability, significant peritoneal spillage, or advanced age, less invasive procedures such as an omental patch closure should be considered.[53] For those undergoing patch closure, biopsy should be obtained to evaluate for malignancy.[53]

Management of gastric outlet obstruction is less clearly defined because there are both surgical and endoscopic modalities available. Endoscopic dilation is the primary endoscopic therapy; however, this is associated with a high risk of perforation and it does not address the underlying persistent ulcer disease contributing to a poorly emptying stomach.[39] Given these limitations, surgery is recognized as the preferred treatment approach.[39] Options for surgical therapy include a drainage procedure, in the form of a pyloroplasty or gastrojejunostomy, with possible acid-reducing procedure, such as truncal or highly selective vagotomy versus partial gastrectomy with Billroth I, Billroth II, or Roux-en-Y reconstruction plus or minus the addition of vagotomy.[39] Given the persistence of ulcer disease in this patient population, surgery usually includes a partial gastrectomy to remove the ulcer.[24] The specific operative management should also be individualized to the particular patient and clinical situation.

Summary

Refractory gastric ulcers represent a complicated clinical problem that requires careful consideration and investigation into the underlying reason for the persistent ulceration. Medical therapy remains the mainstay of therapy for uncomplicated disease, with rare indications for surgical intervention. Complicated disease management depends on the specific complication type with possible management decisions ranging from endoscopic, to elective surgery, to emergency surgery.

GIANT GASTRIC ULCER

Giant gastric ulcer is defined as an ulcer greater than 3 cm and, historically, was noted to account for 10% to 24% of all gastric ulcers.[54–56] With the routine use of PPI therapy, giant ulcers are rarely encountered today. Patients with giant gastric ulcers are generally older and often present with atypical symptoms such as anorexia and weight loss.[55] Another important consideration when a giant gastric ulcer is encountered is that these patients tend to have more complicated disease, with increased rates of urgent surgery, bleeding, and mortality.[56]

Upper endoscopy is a critical component of giant gastric ulcer diagnosis because malignancy and other rare causes of giant gastric ulcers associated with other medical problems must be ruled out.[15] Additionally, endoscopy is necessary for patients with suspected giant ulcers because barium studies may not be diagnostic, in part secondary to a large shallow base.[15] Endoscopic surveillance of these ulcers should be considered given the higher rates of complications associated with these lesions.[15]

Before availability of antisecretory therapy, medical therapy was unsuccessful, with all patients ultimately requiring operative intervention.[57] This paradigm has shifted and current medical therapies have led to greatly improved success of treatment of giant gastric ulcers nonoperatively. For example, numerous series have demonstrated the effective treatment and healing of giant gastric ulcers with histamine-2 receptor antagonist.[55,58–61] Therefore, contrary to past surgical teachings, giant gastric ulcers are no longer an absolute indication for surgical treatment.[58] Further, the presence of H pylori infection is thought to predict healing with adequate treatment and decrease the likelihood of recurrence.[62] Maintenance antisecretory should be strongly considered for patients with giant gastric ulcers.

However, indications for surgical intervention remain despite modern antisecretory therapies. The primary indication for surgery is active bleeding,[59] with 1 review suggesting that in the setting of hemodynamic instability after 4 units of packed red blood cells, failed endoscopic control, recurrent hemorrhage and shock, or continued ongoing bleeding, surgery should be pursued.[63] The second most common reason given for operative management of giant gastric ulcers is concern for malignancy. In a review of previous studies, the rate of malignancy in giant gastric ulcers was found to be 7.0% compared with an approximate risk of 2% in smaller ulcers.[62] These investigators concluded that, despite an increased risk of malignancy, giant gastric ulcers do not immediately require surgical intervention for a theoretic risk of malignancy. Instead, ulcers of all sizes should undergo multiple biopsies to evaluate for underlying malignancy.[62] Additional indications for surgical intervention reflect those previously listed, namely perforation and gastric outlet obstruction. Finally, those giant gastric ulcers that fail to heal with 8 to 12 weeks of medical therapy should be considered for surgical excision, with a similar rationale as persistent gastric ulcers. This is especially important in the elderly population given the increased risk of morbidity and mortality with emergency versus elective procedures. Finally, the type of procedure and reconstruction also echoes the considerations of a patient's anatomy and the extent of resection required; therefore, Billroth I, Billroth II, and partial gastrectomy with Roux-en-Y reconstruction can all be considered in the correct patient population.

GASTRIC POLYPS
Introduction

Gastric polyps represent a diverse set of lesions, most of which are incidental findings on upper endoscopy for a different indication. This is because most gastric polyps are asymptomatic. They are an incidental finding on approximately 6% of all upper endoscopic procedures in the United States.[64] Given the frequency that polyps are incidentally found, determining the pathologic state associated with gastric polyps is critical because certain polyps have a significant potential for malignant transformation. The common types of gastric polyps, the risk of malignancy within the various polyp types, and the resulting downstream management are discussed.

Clinical Presentation

As previously stated, most gastric polyps are asymptomatic and are incidental findings on upper endoscopy. The most common presentation for patients with symptomatic gastric polyps are bleeding (acute and chronic), as well as nonspecific complaints such as abdominal pain, weight loss, and nausea.[65]

Diagnosis

Because polyps are most commonly found as incidental findings on upper endoscopy, the initial evaluation should include evaluation of both the polyp histopathology and the associated gastric mucosa. Evaluation of small, solitary gastric polyps requires polypectomy or biopsies of the lesion for pathologic examination.[66–70] Some investigators have suggested that polyps greater than 0.5 cm should be totally removed,[67,68] with special consideration for complete polypectomy for known neoplastic polyps and those equal to or greater than 1 cm because a small foci of early gastric cancer or high-grade dysplasia can be missed with polyp biopsies.[68] Further, any polyps detected radiographically should be evaluated endoscopically with sampling for pathologic evaluation.[71] In patients with multiple polyps, the largest polyp should be completely removed with targeted biopsies of the remaining lesions.[71,72] Finally, sessile polyps may require mucosal resection for accurate diagnosis. Assessment of the remaining gastric mucosa should be performed following sampling of the gastric polyps. According to the American Society of Gastrointestinal Endoscopy Standards of Practice Committee, biopsies of the normal-appearing antrum and body mucosa should be sampled to diagnose underlying H pylori infection, as well as occult dysplasia, especially in the setting of metaplastic atrophic gastritis.[72]

The importance of clinical and pathologic correlation for determining the cause of gastric polyps cannot be overstated. It is critical that the surrounding mucosa also be sampled and sent for pathologic diagnosis because this provides an important clinical context for the pathologic examination of the polyp specimen.[73] In addition, given that a large series demonstrated that 16.1% of the time gastric polyp specimens failed to meet pathologic criteria for a defined polyp type,[64] it is common practice to attach a representative picture of the polyp in addition to the pathologic sample to assist in diagnosis.[73] For summary of features of various types of polyps please see **Table 1**.

Pathophysiology and Management of Specific Lesions

Hyperplastic polyps

Hyperplastic polyps are a type of epithelial polyp that have several synonyms, such as inflammatory polyp, regenerative polyp, and hyperplasiogenous polyp.[74] Depending on the series, hyperplastic polyps are the most commonly diagnosed polyps, accounting for 75% of all gastric polyps[64,75–78]; however, more recent data have suggested that fundic gland polyps are most common in western countries.[64] Almost all of these lesions (85%) occur in the setting of chronic gastritis[75,77,79] and likely result as an overaggressive mucosal response to the chronic inflammation associated with the underlying gastritis.[79–81] The inflammation can be a result of chemical gastritis (eg, bile reflux gastritis), H pylori gastritis, or reactive gastritis.[74] Nearly all hyperplastic polyps are less than 1 cm, with greater than 50% being less than 5 mm; however, they rarely can be greater than 10 cm.[74] They are most commonly found in the antrum; however, they can be present throughout the stomach[82] and are often multiple.

Table 1
Features of common gastric polyps

Polyp Type	Prevalence	Site	Adjacent Mucosa	Malignant Potential	Comments
Hyperplastic	18%–70%	Antrum > body	Chronic gastritis	<2%	*H pylori* often present Dysplasia in 1%–20%, greatest in polyps >2 cm and in patients >50 y
Fundic gland polyp	13%–77%	Body only	Normal	Rare	May be multiple in FAP Dysplasia in as many as 48% of FAP-associated lesions and <1% of sporadic lesions
Adenoma	0.5%–3.75% (Western Hemisphere)	Antrum > body	Normal or chronic gastritis	≥30%	Usually solitary
Inflammatory fibroid	0.1%–3%	Near Pylorus	Atrophic gastritis		Usually reactive but common genetic mutations
Juvenile	Rare	Body > antrum	Normal	Slight increase in stomach, greater elsewhere	Clinical history of polyps at other GI sites
Peutz-Jeghers	Very rare	Any site	Normal	2%–3%	Clinical history of other GI polyps, associated skin changes

Abbreviation: GI, gastrointestinal.

Data from Carmack SW, Genta RM, Graham DY, et al. Management of gastric polyps: a pathology-based guide for gastroenterologists. Nat Rev Gastroenterol Hepatol 2009;6(6):331–41; and Turner JR, Odze RD. Polyps of the stomach. In: Odze RD, Goldblum JR, eds. Surgical pathology of the GI tract, liver, biliary tract, and pancreas. 3rd edition. Philadelphia: Elsevier; 2015.

Management of hyperplastic polyps includes endoscopic sampling of the entire polyp and submission for pathologic evaluation. The overall risk of malignancy in these polyps is low (<2%); however, the rate of cancer increases with size over 2 cm.[83–85] Presence of dysplasia or intramucosal carcinoma is likely cured with complete endoscopic resection of the polyp; however, biopsies for gastric mapping should be considerd.[73] Ultimately, removal of the underlying inflammatory process, namely treatment of H pylori in those infected, leads to a significant rate of regression of the hyperplastic polyps, and repeat endoscopy after treatment should be performed to document treatment of the underlying infection and to confirm regression of the polyps.[86,87]

Fundic gland polyps

Fundic gland polyps are a very common lesion. In fact, they are commonly accepted to be the most common polyps on upper endoscopy in western countries.[64] These lesions can occur spontaneously (associated with PPI use) or in patients with familial adenomatous polyposis (FAP).[88–90] The finding of fundic gland polyps in children should prompt consideration of underlying FAP.[74] Patients with sporadic polyps are almost exclusively without H pylori infection, and polyps tend to be singular or few.[73,91] The use of PPI therapy is thought to be an important factor in the pathogenesis of these lesions[92,93]; however, this is not universally accepted.[94,95]

Sporadic fundic gland polyps are thought to have a low malignant potential (<1%).[74] In patients with small (<0.5 cm) typical fundic gland polyps, diagnosis is confirmed with biopsy of a single polyp, with the caveat that biopsies should be taken of all polyps equal to or greater than 0.5 cm.[73] PPI therapy is usually continued for small polyps but should be discontinued, if possible, for patients with greater than 1 cm polyps after complete endoscopic removal.[73] In contrast, most patients with FAP have fundic gland polyps on endoscopy (88%),[90] associated with a high risk of dysplasia (30%–50%),[89] including high-grade dysplasia (3%).[90] The risk factors for dysplasia include large size (>1 cm), antral gastritis, and severe duodenal polyposis.[90] Interestingly, PPI therapy appears to have a protective effect for familial fundic gland polyps. All polyps with dysplasia should be resected completely. Finally, there are no formal surveillance guidelines associated with patients with FAP and the utility of upper endoscopy for fundic gland polyp surveillance should be considered on an individual basis.[74]

Adenomatous polyps

Adenomatous polyps occur both spontaneously and in familial syndromes, specifically FAP. These polyps are most often located in the antrum and are usually less than 2 cm.[96] These are neoplastic lesions that are thought to fall in the classic adenoma-carcinoma sequence and are at an increased risk of malignant transformation (See Saowanee Ngamruengphong and colleagues' article, "Endoscopic Management of Early Gastric Adenocarcinoma and Pre-invasive Gastric Lesions," in this issue).

Inflammatory fibroid polyps

Inflammatory fibroid polyps (ie, Vanek tumors) are rare lesions, representing less than 1% of all gastric polyps.[73] The median size of these tumors is 1.5 cm with most less than 3 cm across.[74] They have been associated with adenomas, and a background of a hypochlorhydria and achlorhydria.[97] The vast majority (80%) occur in the antrum or pylorus,[97] and most are found incidentally. These lesions are histologically characterized by a massive eosinophilic infiltrative process[73]; however, the pathologic cause is not known.

Because most polyps are found incidentally without associated symptoms, primary management consists of excision without the need for continued surveillance because the lesions rarely recur after excision.[98] There are no reports of malignant behavior in these polyps.[74]

Juvenile polyps

Juvenile polyps are most commonly part of a genetic syndrome such as juvenile polyposis coli, which is an autosomal dominant syndrome characterized by polyps in the gastrointestinal tract.[99] Fifteen percent to 20% of patients with generalized juvenile polyposis coli have gastric polyps. These polyps are rarely encountered spontaneously. The histology of these polyps most closely resembles hyperplastic gastric polyps.[74] There is an increased risk of dysplasia and carcinoma in patients with generalized polyposis coli and there are no clear guidelines regarding management of these lesions.

Peutz-Jeghers polyps

Peutz-Jeghers syndrome is characterized by an autosomal dominant syndrome with gastrointestinal (GI) hamartomatous polyps and mucocutaneous manifestations.[100,101] These polyps can occur in any part of the GI tract but are most commonly seen in the small intestine, with 25% to 50% of patients with Peutz-Jeghers having gastric polyps.[74] These polyps tend to be small (<1 cm) and, therefore, asymptomatic. The risk of malignancy development is low (2%–3%); however, patients can present with carcinoma at young ages if it develops in these lesions.[102]

There are no consensus guidelines about surveillance and treatment of these lesions; however, it has been suggested endoscopic screening at the age of 8 years old for patients with and identified mutation. If polyps are identified, they should be removed and endoscopic surveillance should repeated every 2 years.[103]

Other polypoid lesions

There are several other pathologic diagnoses that can present with polypoid gastric lesions. These include gastrointestinal stromal tumors, carcinoid tumors, xanthomas or xanthelasma (terms are used interchangeably), and pancreatic heterotopia. In particular, xanthomas are typically small (<3 mm) and multiple, most often located in the body and fundus.[74,104,105] They develop in the setting of chronic gastritis, likely in response to tissue injury. The recognition of these lesions is important because the characteristics of gastric xanthomas (ie, intracellular glycolipids) can mimic signet cell carcinoma[106]; however, pathologic analysis can easily differentiate these lesions. In addition, gastric xanthelasma can mimic gastric carcinoids.[107] Finally, gastric xanthoma may be an early warning sign to underlying malignancy.[108]

Summary

Gastric polyps are common and represent a wide range of pathologic entities, ranging from essentially no risk of malignancy to those that have a very real risk of harboring malignancy, as well as sporadic lesions in those with a strong genetic component. Understanding the differences is critical in determining the downstream management of incidentally found polyps.

OTHER GASTRIC LESION

Lipoma

Lipomas are benign fat-containing tumors that are intramucosal and most commonly single (90%).[109] They are usually found in the antrum and are rare, representing 1% to 3% of all benign gastric tumors.[110,111] Given that they are composed of mature lipocytes, there is no malignant potential. Gastric lipomas are asymptomatic most of the time; however, GI bleeding is the most common presentation for those that are symptomatic.[112] Other presentations include abdominal pain and obstruction.[112] Diagnosis is most commonly made by classic endoscopic appearance and biopsies show normal mucosa. Those lesions that are asymptomatic and diagnosed incidentally should be managed expectantly, without need for surveillance. Local resection is the mainstay for symptomatic tumors or those that cannot be distinguished from a malignant tumor, such as liposarcoma.

SUMMARY

Non-neoplastic gastric lesions encompass a wide variety of causes and pathophysiologic entities. Given the varied underlying causes, careful history and physical examination, as well as appropriate use of adjunctive studies (eg, upper endoscopy), are required to determine the appropriate downstream management. These lesions have varying degrees of associated malignant risk; therefore, an accurate pathologic or clinical diagnosis is imperative to guide further treatment. There remain a significant number of unanswered or evolving questions related to this field that require continued scientific discovery and clinical outcome studies.

REFERENCES

1. Netchvolodoff CV. Refractory peptic lesions. Therapeutic strategies for ulcers and reflux esophagitis that resist standard regimens. Postgrad Med 1993; 93(4):143–4, 147–50, 153–4 passim.
2. Peek RM, Blasser MJ. Pathophysiology of Helicobacter pylori-induced gastritis and peptic ulcer disease. Am J Med 1997;102(2):200–7.
3. Malfertheiner P. The intriguing relationship of Helicobacter pylori infection and acid secretion in peptic ulcer disease and gastric cancer. Dig Dis 2011;29(5): 459–64.
4. El-Serag HB, Talley NJ. Systemic review: the prevalence and clinical course of functional dyspepsia. Aliment Pharmacol Ther 2004;19(6):643–54.
5. Castillo EJ, Camilleri M, Locke GR, et al. A community-based, controlled study of the epidemiology and pathophysiology of dyspepsia. Clin Gastroenterol Hepatol 2004;2(11):985–96.
6. Talley NJ, Vakil NB, Moayyedi P. American Gastroenterological Association technical review on the evaluation of dyspepsia. Gastroenterology 2005;129(5): 1756–80.
7. Vakil N, Moayyedi P, Fennerty MB, et al. Limited value of alarm features in the diagnosis of upper gastrointestinal malignancy: systematic review and meta-analysis. Gastroenterology 2006;131(2):390–401 [quiz: 659–60].
8. Wai CT, Yeoh KG, Ho KY, et al. Diagnostic yield of upper endoscopy in Asian patients presenting with dyspepsia. Gastrointest Endosc 2002;56(4):548–51.
9. Barkun A, Leontiadis G. Systematic review of the symptom burden, quality of life impairment and costs associated with peptic ulcer disease. Am J Med 2010; 123(4):358–66.e2.
10. Lu C-L, Chang S-S, Wang S-S, et al. Silent peptic ulcer disease: frequency, factors leading to "silence," and implications regarding the pathogenesis of visceral symptoms. Gastrointest Endosc 2004;60(1):34–8.
11. Gururatsakul M, Holloway RH, Talley NJ, et al. Association between clinical manifestations of complicated and uncomplicated peptic ulcer and visceral sensory dysfunction. J Gastroenterol Hepatol 2010;25(6):1162–9.

12. Matthewson K, Pugh S, Northfield TC. Which peptic ulcer patients bleed? Gut 1988;29(1):70–4.
13. Wilcox CM, Clark WS. Features associated with painless peptic ulcer bleeding. Am J Gastroenterol 1997;92(8):1289–92.
14. Shaukat A, Wang A, Acosta RD, et al. The role of endoscopy in dyspepsia. Gastrointest Endosc 2015;82(2):227–32.
15. Banerjee S, Cash BD, Dominitz JA, et al. The role of endoscopy in the management of patients with peptic ulcer disease. Gastrointest Endosc 2010;71(4): 663–8.
16. Stolte M, Seitter V, Müller H. Improvement in the quality of the endoscopic/bioptic diagnosis of gastric ulcers between 1990 and 1997-an analysis of 1,658 patients. Z Gastroenterol 2001;39(5):349–55.
17. SEER Cancer Statistics Review 1975-2006. Available at: http://seer.cancer.gov/archive/csr/1975_2006/. Accessed September 28, 2016.
18. Bustamante M, Devesa F, Borghol A, et al. Accuracy of the initial endoscopic diagnosis in the discrimination of gastric ulcers: is endoscopic follow-up study always needed? J Clin Gastroenterol 2002;35(1):25–8.
19. Maniatis AG, Eisen GM, Brazer SR. Endoscopic discrimination of gastric ulcers. J Clin Gastroenterol 1997;24(4):203–6.
20. Graham DY, Schwartz JT, Cain GD, et al. Prospective evaluation of biopsy number in the diagnosis of esophageal and gastric carcinoma. Gastroenterology 1982;82(2):228–31.
21. Marshall BJ, Warren JR. Unidentified curved bacilli in the stomach of patients with gastritis and peptic ulceration. Lancet 1984;1(8390):1311–5.
22. Eckardt VF, Giessler W, Kanzler G, et al. Does endoscopic follow-up improve the outcome of patients with benign gastric ulcers and gastric cancer? Cancer 1992;69(2):301–5.
23. Llanos O, Guzmán S, Duarte I. Accuracy of the first endoscopic procedure in the differential diagnosis of gastric lesions. Ann Surg 1982;195(2):224–6.
24. Napolitano L. Refractory peptic ulcer disease. Gastroenterol Clin North Am 2009;38(2):267–88.
25. Malfertheiner P, Megraud F, O'Morain CA, et al. Management of *Helicobacter pylori* infection—the Maastricht IV/Florence consensus report. Gut 2012;61(5): 646–64.
26. Vakil NB. Approach to refractory or recurrent peptic ulcer disease. Waltham (MA): UpToDate; 2015. Available at: https://www.uptodate.com/contents/approach-to-refractory-or-recurrent-peptic-ulcer-disease?source=search_result&search=recurrent+peptic+ulcer&selectedTitle=1%7E33#H2294659.
27. Bytzer P. Endoscopic follow-up study of gastric ulcer to detect malignancy: is it worthwhile? Scand J Gastroenterol 1991;26(11):1193–9.
28. Hopper AN, Stephens MR, Lewis WG, et al. Relative value of repeat gastric ulcer surveillance gastroscopy in diagnosing gastric cancer. Gastric Cancer 2006; 9(3):217–22.
29. Bianchi Porro G, Parente F. Long term treatment of duodenal ulcer. A review of management options. Drugs 1991;41(1):38–51.
30. Dammann HG, Walter TA. Efficacy of continuous therapy for peptic ulcer in controlled clinical trials. Aliment Pharmacol Ther 1993;7(Suppl 2):17–25.
31. Gisbert JP, Khorrami S, Carballo F, et al. Meta-analysis: *Helicobacter pylori* eradication therapy vs. antisecretory non-eradication therapy for the prevention of recurrent bleeding from peptic ulcer. Aliment Pharmacol Ther 2004;19(6): 617–29.

32. Lauritsen K, Andersen BN, Laursen LS, et al. Omeprazole 20 mg three days a week and 10 mg daily in prevention of duodenal ulcer relapse. Double-blind comparative trial. Gastroenterology 1991;100(3):663–9.

33. Penston JG. A decade of experience with long-term continuous treatment of peptic ulcers with H2-receptor antagonists. Aliment Pharmacol Ther 1993; 7(Suppl 2):27–33.

34. Penston JG, Wormsley KG. Review article: maintenance treatment with H2-receptor antagonists for peptic ulcer disease. Aliment Pharmacol Ther 1992; 6(1):3–29.

35. Yu EW, Bauer SR, Bain PA, et al. Proton pump inhibitors and risk of fractures: a meta-analysis of 11 international studies. Am J Med 2011;124(6):519–26.

36. Shah NH, LePendu P, Bauer-Mehren A, et al. Proton pump inhibitor usage and the risk of myocardial infarction in the general population. PLoS One 2015;10(6): e0124653.

37. Gurusamy KS, Pallari E. Medical versus surgical treatment for refractory or recurrent peptic ulcer. Cochrane Database Syst Rev 2016;(3):CD011523.

38. Csendes A, Burgos AM, Smok G, et al. Latest results (12-21 years) of a prospective randomized study comparing Billroth II and Roux-en-Y anastomosis after a partial gastrectomy plus vagotomy in patients with duodenal ulcers. Ann Surg 2009;249(2):189–94.

39. Barksdale AR, Schwartz RW. The evolving management of gastric outlet obstruction from peptic ulcer disease. Curr Surg 2002;59(4):404–9.

40. Hermansson M, Ekedahl A, Ranstam J, et al. Decreasing incidence of peptic ulcer complications after the introduction of the proton pump inhibitors, a study of the Swedish population from 1974-2002. BMC Gastroenterol 2009;9:25.

41. Hernández-Díaz S, Martín-Merino E, García Rodríguez LA. Risk of complications after a peptic ulcer diagnosis: effectiveness of proton pump inhibitors. Dig Dis Sci 2013;58(6):1653–62.

42. Malmi H, Kautiainen H, Virta LJ, et al. Incidence and complications of peptic ulcer disease requiring hospitalisation have markedly decreased in Finland. Aliment Pharmacol Ther 2014;39(5):496–506.

43. Zittel TT, Jehle EC, Becker HD. Surgical management of peptic ulcer disease today–indication, technique and outcome. Langenbecks Arch Surg 2000; 385(2):84–96.

44. Neumann I, Letelier LM, Rada G, et al. Comparison of different regimens of proton pump inhibitors for acute peptic ulcer bleeding. Cochrane Database Syst Rev 2013;(6):CD007999.

45. Møller MH, Vester-Andersen M, Thomsen RW. Long-term mortality following peptic ulcer perforation in the PULP trial. A nationwide follow-up study. Scand J Gastroenterol 2013;48(2):168–75.

46. Lau JYW, Barkun A, Fan D, et al. Challenges in the management of acute peptic ulcer bleeding. Lancet 2013;381(9882):2033–43.

47. Beggs AD, Dilworth MP, Powell SL, et al. A systematic review of transarterial embolization versus emergency surgery in treatment of major nonvariceal upper gastrointestinal bleeding. Clin Exp Gastroenterol 2014;7:93–104.

48. Griffiths EA, Devitt PG, Bright T, et al. Surgical management of peptic ulcer bleeding by Australian and New Zealand upper gastrointestinal surgeons. ANZ J Surg 2013;83(3):104–8.

49. Herrington JL, Sawyers JL. Gastric ulcer. Curr Probl Surg 1987;24(12):759–865.

50. Jordan PH. Surgery for peptic ulcer disease. Curr Probl Surg 1991;28(4): 265–330.

51. Millward SF. ACR appropriateness criteria on treatment of acute nonvariceal gastrointestinal tract bleeding. J Am Coll Radiol 2008;5(4):550–4.
52. Bertleff MJOE, Lange JF. Perforated peptic ulcer disease: a review of history and treatment. Dig Surg 2010;27(3):161–9.
53. Hodnett RM, Gonzalez F, Lee WC, et al. The need for definitive therapy in the management of perforated gastric ulcers. Review of 202 cases. Ann Surg 1989;209(1):36–9.
54. Meyer C, Keller D, Bur F, et al. The giant ulcer of the stomach. Notes concerning 30 cases. Sem Hop 1979;55(41–42):1917–20.
55. Raju GS, Bardhan KD, Royston C, et al. Giant gastric ulcer: its natural history and outcome in the H2RA era. Am J Gastroenterol 1999;94(12):3478–86.
56. Yii MK, Hunt PS. Bleeding giant gastric ulcer. Aust N Z J Surg 1996;66(8):540–2.
57. Cohn I, Sartin J. Giant gastric ulcers. Ann Surg 1958;147(5):749–58 [discussion: 758–9].
58. Barragry TP, Blatchford JW, Allen MO. Giant gastric ulcers. A review of 49 cases. Ann Surg 1986;203(3):255–9.
59. Chua CL, Jeyaraj PR, Low CH. Relative risks of complications in giant and non-giant gastric ulcers. Am J Surg 1992;164(2):94–7.
60. Takemoto T, Sakaki N, Tsuneoka K, et al. Clinical usefulness of ranitidine in giant gastric ulcer. J Clin Gastroenterol 1984;6(5):413–7.
61. Welch JP, Hammond JG, Nissen CW. Management of benign, giant gastric ulcers. Am Surg 1992;58(5):300–4.
62. Kennedy JS, Hanly E, Marohn MR, et al. Management of giant gastric ulcers: case report and review of the literature. Curr Surg 2004;61(2):220–3.
63. Adkins RB, DeLozier JB, Scott HW, et al. The management of gastric ulcers. A current review. Ann Surg 1985;201(6):741–51.
64. Carmack SW, Genta RM, Schuler CM, et al. The current spectrum of gastric polyps: A 1-Year National Study of over 120,000 patients. Am J Gastroenterol 2009;104(6):1524–32.
65. Goh PM, Lenzi JE. Benign tumors of the duodenum and stomach. In: Holzheimer RG, Mannick JA, editors. Surg treat evidence-based probl. Zuckschwerdt; 2001. p. 387–95.
66. Akahoshi K, Yoshinaga S, Fujimaru T, et al. Endoscopic resection with hypertonic saline-solution–epinephrine injection plus band ligation for large pedunculated or semipedunculated gastric polyp. Gastrointest Endosc 2006;63(2):312–6.
67. Ginsberg GG, Al-Kawas FH, Fleischer DE, et al. Gastric polyps: relationship of size and histology to cancer risk. Am J Gastroenterol 1996;91(4):714–7.
68. Muehldorfer SM, Stolte M, Martus P, et al, Multicenter Study Group "Gastric Polyps". Diagnostic accuracy of forceps biopsy versus polypectomy for gastric polyps: a prospective multicentre study. Gut 2002;50(4):465–70.
69. Papa A, Cammarota G, Tursi A, et al. Management of gastric polyps: the need of polypectomy also for small polyps. Am J Gastroenterol 1997;92(4):721–2.
70. Yoon WJ, Lee DH, Jung YJ, et al. Histologic characteristics of gastric polyps in Korea: emphasis on discrepancy between endoscopic forceps biopsy and endoscopic mucosal resection specimen. World J Gastroenterol 2006;12(25):4029–32.
71. Hirota WK, Zuckerman MJ, Adler DG, et al. ASGE guideline: the role of endoscopy in the surveillance of premalignant conditions of the upper GI tract. Gastrointest Endosc 2006;63(4):570–80.

72. Sharaf RN, Shergill AK, Odze RD, et al. Endoscopic mucosal tissue sampling. Gastrointest Endosc 2013;78(2):216–24.

73. Carmack SW, Genta RM, Graham DY, et al. Management of gastric polyps: a pathology-based guide for gastroenterologists. Nat Rev Gastroenterol Hepatol 2009;6(6):331–41.

74. Turner JR, Odze RD. Polyps of the stomach. In: Odze RD, Goldblum JR, editors. Surgical pathology of the GI tract, liver, biliary tract, and pancreas. 3rd edition. Philadelphia: Saunders; 2015. p. 540–78.e7.

75. Di Giulio E, Lahner E, Micheletti A, et al. Occurrence and risk factors for benign epithelial gastric polyps in atrophic body gastritis on diagnosis and follow-up. Aliment Pharmacol Ther 2005;21(5):567–74.

76. García-Alonso FJ, Martín-Mateos RM, González Martín JA, et al. Gastric polyps: analysis of endoscopic and histological features in our center. Rev Esp Enferm Dig 2011;103(8):416–20.

77. Gencosmanoglu R, Sen-Oran E, Kurtkaya-Yapicier O, et al. Gastric polypoid lesions: analysis of 150 endoscopic polypectomy specimens from 91 patients. World J Gastroenterol 2003;9(10):2236–9.

78. Morais DJ, Yamanaka A, Zeitune JMR, et al. Gastric polyps: a retrospective analysis of 26,000 digestive endoscopies. Arq Gastroenterol 2007;44(1):14–7.

79. Abraham SC, Singh VK, Yardley JH, et al. Hyperplastic polyps of the stomach: associations with histologic patterns of gastritis and gastric atrophy. Am J Surg Pathol 2001;25(4):500–7.

80. Saccá N. Hyperplastic gastric polyps and Helicobacter pylori. Scand J Gastroenterol 2003;38(8):904.

81. Gonzalez-Obeso E, Fujita H, Deshpande V, et al. Gastric hyperplastic polyps: a heterogeneous clinicopathologic group including a distinct subset best categorized as mucosal prolapse polyp. Am J Surg Pathol 2011;35(5):670–7.

82. Melton SD, Genta RM. Gastric cardiac polyps: a clinicopathologic study of 330 cases. Am J Surg Pathol 2010;34(12):1792–7.

83. Zea-Iriarte WL, Sekine I, Itsuno M, et al. Carcinoma in gastric hyperplastic polyps. A phenotypic study. Dig Dis Sci 1996;41(2):377–86.

84. Hattori T. Morphological range of hyperplastic polyps and carcinomas arising in hyperplastic polyps of the stomach. J Clin Pathol 1985;38(6):622–30.

85. Orlowska J, Jarosz D, Pachlewski J, et al. Malignant transformation of benign epithelial gastric polyps. Am J Gastroenterol 1995;90(12):2152–9.

86. Ljubičić N, Banić M, Kujundzić M, et al. The effect of eradicating Helicobacter pylori infection on the course of adenomatous and hyperplastic gastric polyps. Eur J Gastroenterol Hepatol 1999;11(7):727–30.

87. Ohkusa T, Takashimizu I, Fujiki K, et al. Disappearance of hyperplastic polyps in the stomach after eradication of Helicobacter pylori. A randomized, clinical trial. Ann Intern Med 1998;129(9):712–5.

88. Attard TM, Cuffari C, Tajouri T, et al. Multicenter experience with upper gastrointestinal polyps in pediatric patients with familial adenomatous polyposis. Am J Gastroenterol 2004;99(4):681–6.

89. Bertoni G, Sassatelli R, Nigrisoli E, et al. Dysplastic changes in gastric fundic gland polyps of patients with familial adenomatous polyposis. Ital J Gastroenterol Hepatol 1999;31(3):192–7.

90. Bianchi LK, Burke CA, Bennett AE, et al. Fundic gland polyp dysplasia is common in familial adenomatous polyposis. Clin Gastroenterol Hepatol 2008;6(2):180–5.

91. Fossmark R, Jianu CS, Martinsen TC, et al. Serum gastrin and chromogranin A levels in patients with fundic gland polyps caused by long-term proton-pump inhibition. Scand J Gastroenterol 2008;43(1):20–4.
92. Declich P, Omazzi B, Tavani E, et al. Fundic gland polyps and PPI: the Mozart effect of gastrointestinal pathology? Pol J Pathol 2006;57(4):181–2.
93. el-Zimaity HM, Jackson FW, Graham DY. Fundic gland polyps developing during omeprazole therapy. Am J Gastroenterol 1997;92(10):1858–60.
94. Raghunath AS, O'Morain C, McLoughlin RC. Review article: the long-term use of proton-pump inhibitors. Aliment Pharmacol Ther 2005;22(Suppl 1):55–63.
95. Vieth M, Stolte M. Fundic gland polyps are not induced by proton pump inhibitor therapy. Am J Clin Pathol 2001;116(5):716–20.
96. Park DY, Lauwers GY. Gastric polyps: classification and management. Arch Pathol Lab Med 2008;132(4):633–40.
97. Hasegawa T, Yang P, Kagawa N, et al. CD34 expression by inflammatory fibroid polyps of the stomach. Mod Pathol 1997;10(5):451–6.
98. Paikos D, Moschos J, Tzilves D, et al. Inflammatory fibroid polyp or Vanek's tumour. Dig Surg 2007;24(3):231–3.
99. Winkler A, Hinterleitner TA, Högenauer C, et al. Juvenile polyposis of the stomach causing recurrent upper gastrointestinal bleeding. Eur J Gastroenterol Hepatol 2007;19(1):87–90.
100. Ladd AP. Gastrointestinal tumors in children and adolescents. Semin Pediatr Surg 2006;15(1):37–47.
101. Molloy JW, Pelton JJ, Narayani RI. Peutz-Jeghers gastric polyposis. Gastrointest Endosc 2006;63(1):154.
102. Dodds WJ, Schulte WJ, Hensley GT, et al. Peutz-Jeghers syndrome and gastrointestinal malignancy. Am J Roentgenol Radium Ther Nucl Med 1972;115(2):374–7.
103. Sereno M, Aguayo C, Guillén Ponce C, et al. Gastric tumours in hereditary cancer syndromes: clinical features, molecular biology and strategies for prevention. Clin Transl Oncol 2011;13(9):599–610.
104. Isomoto H, Mizuta Y, Inoue K, et al. A close relationship between *Helicobacter pylori* infection and gastric xanthoma. Scand J Gastroenterol 1999;34(4):346–52.
105. Javdan P, Pitman ER, Schwartz IS. Gastric xanthelasma: endoscopic recognition. Gastroenterology 1974;67(5):1006–10.
106. Drude RB, Balart LA, Herrington JP, et al. Gastric xanthoma: histologic similarity to signet ring cell carcinoma. J Clin Gastroenterol 1982;4(3):217–21.
107. Luk IS, Bhuta S, Lewin KJ. Clear cell carcinoid tumor of stomach. A variant mimicking gastric xanthelasma. Arch Pathol Lab Med 1997;121(10):1100–3.
108. Sekikawa A, Fukui H, Maruo T, et al. Gastric xanthelasma may be a warning sign for the presence of early gastric cancer. J Gastroenterol Hepatol 2014;29(5):951–6.
109. Alcalde Escribano JM, Brea Hernando AJ, Molina Sánchez A, et al. Lipoma of the stomach. Presentation of a case and a review of cases reported in Spain. Rev Esp Enferm Apar Dig 1989;76(5):482–4 [in Spanish].
110. Pérez Cabañas I, Rodríguez Garrido J, De Miguel Velasco M, et al. Gastric lipoma: an infrequent cause of upper digestive hemorrhage. Rev Esp Enferm Dig 1990;78(3):163–5 [in Spanish].
111. Winants D, Arnault G. Gastric lipoma. X-ray computed tomographic diagnosis. J Radiol 1989;70(11):633–6 [in French].
112. Maderal F, Hunter F, Fuselier G, et al. Gastric lipomas–an update of clinical presentation, diagnosis, and treatment. Am J Gastroenterol 1984;79(12):964–7.

Multimodality Treatment of Gastric Lymphoma

Naruhiko Ikoma, MD[a], Brian D. Badgwell, MD, MS[a], Paul F. Mansfield, MD[b],*

KEYWORDS

- Primary gastric lymphoma • Chemotherapy • Radiation therapy
- *Helicobacter pylori* infection • Surgery

KEY POINTS

- Primary gastric lymphoma is rare.
- Appropriate use of multimodality therapy guided by tumor stage, histology subtypes, status of *Helicobacter pylori* infection, and status of t(11;18) translocation, can result in excellent outcomes in gastric lymphoma.
- Surgical resection has limited value in the treatment of gastric lymphoma.

INTRODUCTION

Non-Hodgkin lymphoma (NHL), which is more common than Hodgkin lymphoma, can be classified as nodal or extranodal. The gastrointestinal tract is the predominant site of extranodal NHL, accounting for 4% to 20% of all NHL cases and 30% to 45% of all extranodal cases.[1–4] The stomach is the most commonly affected site along the gastrointestinal tract (60%–75%) and can be a primary or secondary site.[5,6] Nevertheless, gastric NHL only accounts for 3% of gastric neoplasms and 10% of lymphomas.[7]

Primary gastric NHL has not been defined consistently. Dawson and colleagues[8] originally defined it as a case in which the tumor predominantly involves the stomach and lymphadenopathy is limited to the lymphatic drainage of the stomach, whereas the Danish Lymphoma Study Group defined it as a case in which the stomach or gastrointestinal tract represented 75% or more of the total tumor volume on clinical and radiological assessment.[1] Primary gastric lymphoma arises from the mucosa or submucosal layer, originating from lymphoid tissue in the lamina propria.

Disclosure: The authors have nothing to disclose.
[a] Department of Surgical Oncology, The University of Texas MD Anderson Cancer Center, Unit 1484, 1515 Holcombe Boulevard, Houston, TX 77030, USA; [b] Acute Care Services, The University of Texas MD Anderson Cancer Center, Unit 1485, 1515 Holcombe Boulevard, Houston, TX 77030, USA
* Corresponding author. Department of Surgical Oncology, The University of Texas MD Anderson Cancer Center, 1400 Pressler, FCT 18.6032, Houston, TX 77030.
E-mail address: pmansfie@mdanderson.org

Surg Clin N Am 97 (2017) 405–420
http://dx.doi.org/10.1016/j.suc.2016.11.012
0039-6109/17/© 2016 Elsevier Inc. All rights reserved.

surgical.theclinics.com

This article briefly summarizes diagnosis, staging, and subtypes of primary gastric NHL, and discusses multimodality treatment of primary gastric NHL by reviewing important evidences that guide current standard treatment strategy.

PRESENTATION AND DIAGNOSIS

The most common presentation of gastric lymphoma is epigastric pain (78%), followed by appetite loss (47%), unintentional weight loss (25%), bleeding (19%), and vomiting (18%).[6] B symptoms (fever and night sweats) are not common in gastric lymphoma (12%).[6] Often, no signs of disease are found on physical examination; however, palpable masses or lymphadenopathy may be found in patients with advanced disease.

The diagnosis of gastric lymphoma is based on histologic characteristics found on tissue biopsy during upper gastrointestinal endoscopy. A histologic diagnosis is crucial to guiding the treatment strategy. Endoscopic findings of gastric lymphoma include mucosal erythema, polypoid lesions (with or without ulceration), nodularity, ulceration, and mucosal thickening.[9,10] Multiple large and deep biopsies, possibly with endoscopic mucosal resection from both abnormal-appearing and normal-appearing mucosa should be obtained to improve diagnostic accuracy because the tumor can be multifocal or can infiltrate the submucosal layer under normal-appearing mucosa.[11,12]

A staging work-up is necessary to guide the treatment strategy for gastric lymphoma. Chest radiographs and computed tomography scans are the most commonly used imaging techniques for evaluating distant disease. Further evaluation with endoscopic ultrasound[13,14] and positron emission tomography may be beneficial.[15–17] Peripheral blood smear and bone marrow aspiration are fundamental to excluding metastatic disease. Patients with gastric lymphoma should be tested for *Helicobacter pylori* infection due to its importance in treatment. The t(11;18) translocation, which is detectable in one-third of gastric mucosa-associated lymphoid tissue (MALT) lymphoma cases, has demonstrated resistance to various treatments, especially *H pylori* eradication therapies.[18–20] Evaluating t(11;18) using polymerase chain reaction (PCR) or fluorescence in situ hybridization (FISH) is recommended in gastric MALT lymphoma patients.[21] Patients being considered for treatment with rituximab need to be tested for hepatitis B virus infection because rituximab can cause reactivation of the virus.

STAGING

TNM staging is ineffective for lymphoma in general and the Ann Arbor classification, or a modification by Musshoff[22] (**Table 1**), has been applied to gastrointestinal tract lymphoma.[5,6,22–25] The Lugano staging system for gastrointestinal lymphomas, which was a modification of the original Ann Arbor staging system, was introduced to incorporate measures of distant nodal involvement.[26] It has been widely used over the last 2 decades.[27] However, the lack of a uniform staging system has made some historical interstudy comparisons difficult. In brief, a stage I tumor is confined to the stomach and a stage II tumor extends outside of the primary organ but is limited to regional lymph nodes. Stages III and IV represent distant spread disease (the Lugano system has no stage III). Ruskone-Fourmestraux and colleagues[28] introduced the Paris staging system, which describes the depth of gastric wall involvement more accurately.

Disease stage is the most important prognostic factor in gastric lymphoma[6,25]; therefore, accurate staging using a combination of clinical and radiological assessment is essential to providing appropriate treatment.

Table 1 Staging systems for gastric lymphoma	
Ann Arbor Staging System with Musshoff Modification[22]	**Lugano Staging System[26]**
Stage IE: Lymphoma restricted to the gastrointestinal tract	Stage I: Lymphoma confined to the gastrointestinal tract
IE_1: Mucosa, submucosa	
IE_2: Beyond submucosa	
Stage IIE: Lymphoma infiltrating lymph nodes on the same side of the diaphragm	Stage II: Lymphoma extending into the abdomen
IIE_1: Regional lymph node involvement	II_1: Local nodal involvement
IIE_2: Distant lymph node involvement	II_2: Distant nodal involvement IIE: Penetration of serosa to involve adjacent organs or tissues
Stage III: Lymphoma involving both sides of the diaphragm	Not applicable[a]
Stage IV: Disseminated disease	Stage IV: Disseminated extranodal involvement or a gastrointestinal tract lesion with supradiaphragmatic nodal involvement

[a] The Lugano system has no stage III.
Data from Musshoff K. Clinical staging classification of non-Hodgkin's lymphomas (author's translation). Strahlentherapie 1977;153(4):218–21. [in German]; and Rohatiner A, d'Amore F, Coiffier B, et al. Report on a workshop convened to discuss the pathological and staging classifications of gastrointestinal tract lymphoma. Ann Oncol 1994;5(5):399.

The German Multicenter Study Group reported that overall survival and event-free survival durations (defined as the duration of complete or partial remission) of stage I/II patients were significantly longer than those of stage III/IV patients ($P = .0160$ and $P = .0007$, respectively), whereas tumor grade (high vs low) was not associated with survival.[6] The Hellenic Cooperative Oncology Group reported the results of a multicenter retrospective study of 128 primary gastrointestinal NHL subjects, which included gastric tumors in 68% of cases. Subjects with localized disease (stage I/II) had significantly longer survival durations than did those with advanced disease (stage III/IV) (3-year overall survival rates were 87% in stage I/II vs 60% in stage III/IV subjects; $P = .0001$).[25] Histologic subtype was not associated with survival rate.[25]

CLASSIFICATION

The histologic classification of lymphoma is a confounding matter. Many classification systems had been described by the late 1970s, with significant effort made to unify the systems afterward. In 1994, the Revised European-American Lymphoma (REAL) classification was published to classify lymphoid neoplasms.[29] According to the REAL classification, the almost all ($\geq$90%) gastric lymphomas were one of 2 histologic subtypes[30]: extranodal marginal zone B-cell lymphoma of MALT type or diffuse large B-cell lymphoma (DLBL).[6,25] In the German Multicenter Study Group's report on gastric lymphoma, low-grade MALT lymphoma accounted for 40%, high-grade lymphoma (DLBL) for 55%, and lymphoblastic or Burkitt lymphomas for a small percentage of all lymphomas (3.2%); 1.4% of cases were low-grade non-MALT type lymphoma (1.4%).[6] Because MALT and DLBL account for the almost all gastric lymphomas, this article focuses on the treatment of these 2 histologic subtypes.

TREATMENT

Although the treatment strategy for nodal NHL is well established, treatment of gastric lymphoma is not without controversy.[25] Historically, surgical excision of gastric lymphomas had been the mainstay of treatment; many studies have shown longer survival with primary resection.[31–33] Antibiotic therapy for low-grade, early-stage gastric MALT lymphoma became accepted practice after reports described tumor regression after the eradication of H pylori[34–36]; however, the benefits of surgical resection for most primary gastric lymphomas are not supported by recent studies. Multimodal therapy using surgery, chemotherapy, and radiation therapy in various combinations has been explored[37]; however, because equivalent results were reported for surgery or a combination of surgery and chemotherapy versus nonsurgical treatment such as chemotherapy and/or radiation therapy, the benefits of surgical resection were questioned.[24,37–40]

The Danish Lymphoma Study Group reported the results of a retrospective study from the population-based NHL registry, which included 175 gastric lymphoma subjects. This study revealed a shorter survival in subjects with B symptoms (relative risk, 3.3), clinical stage greater than II_1 (relative risk, 3.0), age greater than 72 years (relative risk, 2.4), and elevated lactate dehydrogenase level (relative risk, 2.0). There was no survival difference between surgically and nonsurgically treated subjects with localized disease.[1]

The German Multicenter Study group reported the results of a prospective non-randomized multicenter study that compared conservative therapy to surgery plus conservative therapy in subjects with stage IE or IIE primary gastric lymphoma.[37] Decisions regarding surgical resection were deferred to treating physicians and institutions; however, conservative treatment was stratified based on tumor grade. Low-grade tumors were treated with 30 Gy total abdominal irradiation plus a 10 Gy boost to the primary tumor if it was unresected or if residual tumor was present after resection. Stage IIE subjects underwent additional chemotherapy. Chemotherapy was given to all subjects with high-grade tumors and additional radiation therapy was given to stage IIE subjects. Of the 185 study subjects, 79 underwent surgical resection. There was no survival difference between the groups (the 5-year overall survival rates were 84% in the conservative therapy group and 82% in the surgery plus conservative therapy group).[37]

Two randomized controlled studies completed in Mexico have evaluated the benefit of surgical resection in gastric lymphoma. The first study randomly assigned 589 subjects with gastric DLBL to 1 of 4 treatment arms: chemotherapy, chemotherapy plus surgery, surgery only, and surgery plus radiation therapy. Complete response rates were similar among the groups but 10-year overall survival rates were significantly higher in the chemotherapy-only and chemotherapy plus surgery groups (10-year survival rates, 96%, 91%, 54%, and 53%, respectively; P<.001). Late toxicity was more common and severe in the surgery groups.[41] The authors concluded that chemotherapy alone should be the treatment of choice for patients with gastric DLBL.

The second study randomly assigned 241 subjects with low-grade gastric MALT lymphoma to surgery, radiation therapy, and chemotherapy. There were no differences in overall survival among the groups (10-year overall survival rates: 80% in the surgery group, 75% in the radiation therapy group, and 87% in the chemotherapy group; P = .4). H pylori eradication treatment was not used in this study. The investigators concluded that chemotherapy alone is effective and safe. Surgery or radiation therapy should be reserved for patients who are not candidates for chemotherapy.[42]

Because these studies have failed to show any benefit of surgical resection compared with conservative treatment, surgery is now only reserved for the treatment of highly selective cases of primary gastric lymphoma, such as tumors that are refractory to other therapies or that have complications, such as bleeding uncontrolled by other measures, perforation, or fistula formation (**Fig. 1**). The treatment strategy should be stratified based on the subtype, stage, *H pylori* infection status, and t(11;18) translocation. Treatment requires the coordinated efforts of multidisciplinary teams, including medical oncologists; radiation oncologists; and, rarely, surgeons.

MUCOSA-ASSOCIATED LYMPHOID TISSUE LYMPHOMA

Isaacson and Spencer[43] introduced the concept of MALT in 1983, which describes lymphoepithelial lesions with lymphoid follicles and an infiltration of plasma cells. MALT lymphoma corresponds to marginal zone cell lymphoma in the REAL classification system.[30] It typically represents low-grade tumors but one-third of high-grade gastric lymphomas contain a low-grade MALT component.[6] *H pylori* infection has been demonstrated to be strongly associated with tumorigenesis in gastric MALT lymphoma.[44–47] Wotherspoon and colleagues[44] first reported the association between *H pylori* infection and gastric lymphoma in 1991; as many as 92% of patients with primary gastric lymphoma had *H pylori* infections. The data were confirmed and supported in subsequent studies. Hussell and colleagues[34] reported that the proliferation of MALT lymphoma depends on T-cell activation by *H pylori*.

Helicobacter pylori Eradication Therapy

H pylori eradication therapy with antibiotics has been shown to be effective against gastric lymphoma; it may lead to complete remission of the tumor, as shown in several studies.[35,48–50] *H pylori* eradication regimens that combine proton pump inhibitors and clarithromycin-based triple therapy with either amoxicillin or metronidazole for 10 to 14 days are reported to be highly effective.[51] Such therapies have been reported to achieve a high success rate of *H pylori* eradication in these patients, with a high remission rate of gastric MALT lymphoma in patients with localized disease. In cases of unsuccessful eradication of *H pylori*, a second regimen should be provided, with alternative triple or quadruple therapy.[52,53]

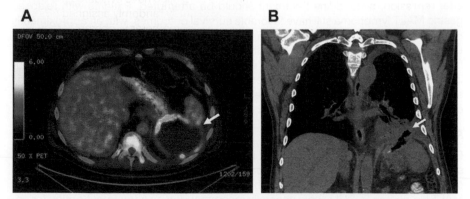

Fig. 1. A gastric DLBL in a patient who developed gastropulmonary fistula after chemotherapy. Patient underwent en bloc surgical resection of the tumor with stomach, diaphragm, lung, pancreas, and spleen for disease control. (*A*) Positron emission tomography showing 8 cm fluorodeoxyglucose (FDG)-avid tumor with central necrosis (*arrow*). (*B*) Computed tomography showing the tumor creating a gastropulmonary fistula (*arrow*).

H pylori eradication treatment is recommended for all gastric MALT lymphoma patients, regardless of stage.[27,54] *H pylori* treatment should be considered as the sole initial treatment of patients with localized *H pylori*–positive MALT lymphoma.[27] It has been reported that 50% to 80% of such patients achieve a complete remission with a long-term disease-free period in most cases.[55–59] However, there have been reports of late relapses after *H pylori* eradication treatment; thus, a long follow-up duration is recommended.[21]

Stathis and colleagues[58] reported long-term treatment outcomes in a retrospective study of 105 subjects with gastric MALT lymphoma who exclusively underwent anti-*H pylori* treatment as first-line therapy. *H pylori* was successfully eradicated after treatment with antibiotics in all 85 cases. Of all lymphoma subjects who were assessed for response (n = 102), histologic regression of the tumor was achieved in 76% and complete remission in 65%. The median time to complete remission was 15.5 months (interquartile range, 5–32 months). After a median of 6.8 years of follow-up of subjects in complete remission, disease relapse was confirmed in 22%.[58]

Tumors with t(11;18) translocation are likely to be resistant to *H pylori* eradication. Such patients should be considered candidates for alternative treatments.[57,60] Wundisch and colleagues[57] reported the results of a prospective multicenter trial of *H pylori* eradication in 120 *H pylori*–positive stage IE$_1$ gastric MALT tumor subjects. The 5-year survival rate was 90%. Ninety-six (80%) subjects achieved a complete histologic remission. The 5-year continuous complete remission rate was 71% and only 3 subjects (3%) had macroscopic disease relapse on follow-up (median follow-up, 75 months). In a subset analysis, subjects with t(11;18) translocation (n = 10) had worse outcomes; only 7% (n = 3) achieved a continuous complete remission.[57]

Failure of *H pylori* eradication treatment is not uncommon (20%–30%); however, some tumors exhibit a slow response to therapy (see previous discussion) and the median time to tumor remission after *H pylori* eradication is 15.5 months.[58] MALT tumors have an indolent nature, which allows physicians to continue watchful waiting before determining treatment responsiveness. Close follow-up is important, including periodic upper gastrointestinal endoscopy and multiple biopsies to monitor disease after *H pylori* eradication. Albeit uncommon, transformation to more aggressive lymphomas such as DLBL can occur, so the histologic type should be carefully reviewed.[61]

If *H pylori* eradication treatment fails, either because of unresponsiveness or relapse after remission, second-line treatment should be attempted. Patients with relapsed gastric MALT lymphoma still have favorable survival outcomes, with an approximately 80% to 90% 5-year survival rate. In *H pylori*–negative gastric MALT lymphoma patients, tumor regression is unlikely with *H pylori* eradication treatment. Therefore, more aggressive oncological treatment should be considered. However, *H pylori* eradication may be attempted with a higher level of caution, even with negative *H pylori* status because a response to such therapy could occur due to a false-negative test or infection by another species of *Helicobacter*.[27,53]

Radiation Therapy

Radiation therapy was commonly used in association with other treatment modalities, such as surgery or chemotherapy. More recently, multiple reports have shown that exclusive moderate-dose radiation therapy is effective against localized gastric MALT lymphoma.[62–65] It is now generally recommended as a treatment option for patients who do not experience a response to or who experience a relapse after *H pylori* treatment. It is also an appropriate initial therapy for patients with localized *H pylori*–negative gastric MALT lymphoma and those with t(11;18) translocation because they are unlikely to experience a response to *H pylori* eradication therapy. Excellent disease control after radiation therapy has been shown in several reports (response rates of close to 100%), although no large randomized control studies have compared radiation therapy and systemic treatment, such as chemotherapy, in localized gastric MALT lymphoma. Moderate-dose (24–30 Gy) radiation therapy of the involved fields, including the stomach and perigastric nodes, is generally recommended.[65–67]

A French multi-institutional study group reported the results of a prospective study of radiation therapy for gastric MALT lymphoma. The study included 53 subjects who underwent moderate-dose radiation therapy (30 Gy in 15 fractions) for localized gastric MALT lymphoma that persisted after *H pylori* eradication treatment. No acute or late toxicities were observed. A complete remission was achieved in all subjects except 1 (98%), with no relapse after a median follow-up of 4.9 years after the completion of radiation therapy. The 5-year overall survival rate was 94%.[65]

Chemotherapy and Immunotherapy

The use of chemotherapy and immunotherapy has been reported in gastric MALT lymphoma of all stages; however, there is no strong evidence to indicate the most effective chemotherapy regimen, with or without immunotherapy. Patients with localized disease who are not eligible for or who have failed to experience a response to radiation therapy should be considered for systemic treatment with chemotherapy.

The efficacy of multiple single-agent chemotherapy regimens has been reported. Hammel and colleagues[68] reported the efficacy of oral alkylating agents (daily oral cyclophosphamide or oral chlorambucil), which resulted in complete response rates of 75% (18 of 24 subjects) after a median treatment duration of 12 months. Jager and colleagues[69] reported the results of a prospective study of 25 subjects with MALT lymphoma, including 19 gastric MALT lymphoma subjects who underwent single-agent chemotherapy with cladribine. Cladribine infusion therapy resulted in a complete remission rate of 100% in gastric MALT lymphoma subjects.

Patients' translocation t(11;18) status may affect the efficacy of their chemotherapy. Levy and colleagues[19] reported a retrospective study of 53 subjects with gastric MALT lymphoma. Translocation t(11;18) was detected in 32% of subjects and it was more prevalent in *H pylori*–negative subjects (63% vs 15%; $P = .005$). All 3 t(11;18)-positive, *H pylori*–positive subjects failed to experience a response to *H pylori* eradication therapy, whereas 75% (21 of 28) of t(11;18)-negative subjects achieved a complete remission after therapy. Only 42% (5 of 12 subjects) of t(11;18)-positive subjects demonstrated remission 1 year after treatment versus 89% (8 of 9) of t(11;18)-negative subjects ($P = .07$). After long-term follow-up (median, 7 years), only 1 t(11;18)-positive subject remained in remission (8%) versus all 8 t(11;18)-negative subjects (89%; $P = .0003$).

Streubel and colleagues[20] reported that translocation t(11;18) was not predictive of response to chemotherapy with cladribine. In their retrospective analysis of 17 subjects with gastric MALT lymphoma, 8 (47%) were found to express t(11;18) translocation. Fifteen subjects (88%) experienced a response to treatment (13 complete responses) and there was no difference in treatment response between t(11;18)-positive versus t(11;18)-negative subjects. There are other factors important in predicting response to therapy, in addition to translocation status, and other treatment options for patients resistant to initial chemotherapy. The presence of perigastric lymph node involvement is reported to be a negative predictive factor of response to *H pylori* treatment and alkylating agents.[70]

Rituximab is an anti-CD20 monoclonal antibody that has been demonstrated to be effective and well-tolerated against different lymphomas, either as a single agent or in combination with other chemotherapy.[71] Similarly, rituximab is reported to be effective at treating gastric MALT lymphoma.

Martinelli and colleagues[72] reported their retrospective study of 27 subjects with gastric MALT lymphoma (any stage) who were not eligible for or experienced relapsed or refractory disease after H pylori eradication therapy. Among the 26 evaluated subjects, 77% (n = 20) achieved an objective response and 46% (n = 12) had a complete remission after rituximab treatment. Only 2 subjects (7%) received rituximab as an initial therapy; rituximab was shown to be effective as salvage therapy after the failure of other treatment modalities and t(11;18) status was not associated with treatment response to rituximab.[72]

An analysis of a surveillance epidemiology and end results (SEER)-Medicare database of gastric MALT lymphoma patients was recently reported. Among 1134 patients, 21% underwent radiation therapy and 24% underwent chemotherapy, with or without rituximab as an initial treatment (H pylori eradication data were not available in the analysis). The median overall survival duration was 6.7 years. In the subset analysis of stage IE patients who underwent radiation therapy (n = 185) or chemotherapy (n = 162), lymphoma-related death occurred more often in the chemotherapy group than in the radiation therapy group (5-year cumulative incidence, 19% vs 5%; $P<.001$). Among 321 patients who underwent chemotherapy, rituximab was associated with a lower risk of lymphoma-related death (HR = 0.53; $P = .017$). Among the 230 patients who received rituximab, there was no survival difference between patients who received rituximab alone and those who underwent combined chemoimmunotherapy.[73]

Zucca and colleagues[74] reported the results of a prospective randomized study, International Extranodal Lymphoma Study Group (IELSG)-19, that evaluated the benefits of adding rituximab to chlorambucil in the treatment of gastric MALT lymphoma subjects who did not experience a response to or were not eligible for local therapy. The complete remission rate was higher (78% vs 65%) and the 5-year event-free survival was significantly higher (68% vs 50%; $P = .002$) in the group treated with rituximab. However, there was no significant difference in the 5-year overall survival rate (89% in both groups).

In summary, H pylori eradication therapy is the recommended initial treatment in localized gastric MALT lymphoma patients with H pylori infection. The significance of t(11;18) is not well defined but it is considered a risk for treatment failure. In patients who do not experience a response to or who experience relapse after H pylori eradication and in patients without H pylori infection, radiation therapy is generally the recommended treatment option.[21,27] Systemic treatment should be considered for patients with localized gastric MALT lymphoma who fail to experience a response to or are not eligible for radiation therapy and for those with advanced gastric MALT lymphoma, although the ideal treatment regimen has not been well defined. Because of the indolent nature of MALT lymphoma, close monitoring without treatment is an option in asymptomatic or high risk patients.[21,27]

DIFFUSE LARGE B-CELL LYMPHOMA

DLBL is the most common subtype of gastric lymphoma, accounting for approximately 50% to 55% of cases.[6,24] Gastric DLBL is sometimes called high-grade gastric lymphoma. Before current multimodality therapy was established, high-grade lymphoma was recognized as a negative prognostic factor for survival. Compared with low-grade MALT lymphoma, high-grade gastric lymphoma was reported to be associated with a lower complete remission rate (68% vs 92%) and a shorter 5-year survival rate (75% vs

92%; P = .0001).[75] However, more recent studies showed no survival differences between MALT lymphoma and DLBL, likely because of improved treatment modalities.[6,25,37] As previously described, surgery is no longer a standard treatment of gastric DLBL. In general, because there is no evidence that indicates that gastric DLBL is different from other nodal or extranodal DLBL,[76] the principle of treatment of gastric DLBL follows that of general DLBL. Most patients are treated with systemic chemotherapy combined with immunotherapy, regardless of the tumor stage.[27,77]

Chemotherapy

The most commonly used chemotherapeutic regimen for DLBL of the stomach is a combination of cyclophosphamide, doxorubicin, vincristine, and prednisone (CHOP); or rituximab (R)-CHOP.

Aviles and colleagues[41] reported the results of a randomized trial comprising 589 subjects with gastric DLBL that compared CHOP, surgery plus CHOP, surgery only, and surgery plus adjuvant radiation therapy. The study revealed that chemotherapy was superior to the other treatment options (10-year survival rates of 96%, 91%, 54%, and 53%, respectively; P<.001). No survival benefit was observed with the addition of surgery. This large prospective, randomized study did not include rituximab as a treatment option and did not evaluate the benefit of adding radiation therapy to chemotherapy. However, it did show that chemotherapy is the mainstay for treatment of gastric DLBL.

Coiffier and colleagues[78] reported a multiinstitutional randomized trial of 400 subjects with nodal DLBL that compared R-CHOP and CHOP. Complete response rates (76% vs 63%; P = .005) and overall survival rates (relative risk for death, 0.64; 2-year survival rates, 70% vs 57%; P = .007) were significantly higher in the R-CHOP group than in the CHOP group. Toxicity was not significantly different between the groups.[78]

Based on its reported therapeutic benefit in nodal DLBL patients,[78–80] R-CHOP has been used increasingly as the primary treatment in patients with localized gastric DLBL. However, the addition of rituximab to CHOP chemotherapy is still controversial because no large prospective trial has proven that it is beneficial specifically in gastric DLBL.

Aviles and colleagues[81] reported the results of a phase II clinical trial to assess the benefit of adding rituximab to CHOP in subjects with CD20$^+$ localized gastric DLBL. The study included 42 subjects treated with R-CHOP who were compared with subjects from their previous study.[41] The 5-year overall survival rate was 95%, which was not significantly different from that for the historic controls. The investigators concluded that the addition of rituximab to CHOP chemotherapy does not improve outcomes in subjects with early-stage gastric DLBL.[81]

Sohn and colleagues[82] reported a retrospective study of 93 gastric DLBL subjects who received either CHOP or R-CHOP as first-line chemotherapy. The complete response rates were 94% in the CHOP group and 93% in the R-CHOP group. There was no survival difference (3-year overall survival rates, 95% vs 85%). The investigators concluded that there is no benefit to the addition of rituximab.

Leopardo and colleagues[83] reported a multi-institutional retrospective study of stage I/IV gastric DLBL subjects (n = 60) that compared chemotherapy alone to chemotherapy plus rituximab. The addition of rituximab resulted in an improved complete response rate (100% vs 76.6%; P = .041), 5-year disease-free survival rate (100% vs 73%; P = .03), and 5-year overall survival rate (100% vs 63%; P = .02).

Radiation Therapy

Several studies have reported the benefits of consolidation therapy with radiation therapy after chemotherapy in nodal DLBL.[84–86] Albeit limited, there is accumulating evidence regarding the addition of radiation therapy to chemotherapy in gastric DLBL. Martinelli and colleagues[87] reported the results of a randomized clinical trial that evaluated the role of radiation therapy in addition to chemotherapy in subjects with gastric DLBL. This study included 44 subjects. All underwent at least 4 cycles of CHOP or CHOP-like chemotherapy. The chemotherapy-only group received 2 additional cycles and the chemotherapy-radiation therapy group received a minimal dose of 30 Gy. The investigators reported a significant reduction in the incidence of local recurrence in the chemotherapy-radiation therapy group (local recurrence rate, 18% in the chemotherapy-only group vs 0% in the chemotherapy-radiation therapy group at 2 years; $P = .0381$); however, there was no difference in overall survival ($P = .774$).

Tanaka and colleagues[88] reported their multiinstitutional retrospective study, which included 58 subjects with localized gastric DLBL who were treated with 6 cycles of R-CHOP (n = 23) or 3 to 4 cycles of R-CHOP plus radiation therapy (n = 35). They reported an 88% complete response rate and a 12% partial response rate, with a 3-year overall survival rate of 93%. Subjects who underwent R-CHOP plus radiation therapy had a slightly better complete response rate (91% vs 83%) and 3-year overall survival rate (95% vs 91%) than did the R-CHOP-only group; however, these rates were not found to be statistically significant ($P = .278$) by univariate analysis.[88]

Helicobacter pylori Eradication Therapy

Several reports have found tumor remission after *H pylori* eradication therapy in gastric DLBL subjects. The remission rate is likely affected by whether the tumor contains a low-grade MALT component.

Chen and colleagues[55] reported a multi-institutional prospective study that included 24 *H pylori*–positive subjects with early-stage gastric "high-grade transformed tumors" (referred to as DLBL with features of MALT) treated with *H pylori* eradication therapy. Twenty-two (92%) subjects had successful *H pylori* eradication and 14 (65%) achieved a complete remission. Among those 14, none experienced recurrence during follow-up.

Kuo and colleagues[89] reported the results of a retrospective study that included 50 subjects with *H pylori*–positive localized gastric lymphoma who underwent *H pylori* eradication treatment (16 with "pure" or de novo DLBL [tumors without a MALT component] and 34 with "high-grade transformed MALT lymphoma" [DLBL with MALT features]). *H pylori* eradication was successful in 100% of the pure DLBL subjects and 94% of the DLBL with MALT subjects. Complete remission was achieved in 68% and 56%, respectively.[89]

In summary, gastric DLBL is generally treated similarly to general DLBL; chemotherapy is a treatment option regardless of tumor stage. The benefits of the addition of rituximab to CHOP chemotherapy have not been confirmed in gastric DLBL. The addition of radiation therapy has been considered; however, there is no strong evidence to support it, especially in the era of rituximab-containing regimens. Recent advanced technology in radiation therapy, such as intensity-modulated radiation therapy, may improve the safety and efficacy of radiation therapy.[90] *H pylori* eradication therapy may be effective for *H pylori*–positive localized gastric DLBL, especially when the tumor contains a MALT component; however, this needs to be validated in a larger prospective study.

Surgery for Treatment Complications

As previously mentioned, surgery is now reserved only for the treatment of highly selective cases of primary gastric lymphoma. The most common indication for a surgery consult in patients with gastric lymphoma at the authors' institution is "stand-by" for possible treatment complication, such as bleeding or a perforation, although it is a rare event.[6,91,92] Spectre and colleagues[93] reported their experience of treatment of 73 gastric DLBL subjects who were initially treated with chemotherapy. Chemotherapy regimens were mostly CHOP with or without rituximab, and 62% of subjects achieved complete response. During the course of treatment, 22% (16/73) of subjects experienced complications, including bleeding (11%, 8/73) and gastric outlet obstruction (11%, 8/73); however, no subjects developed perforation in this study. Of those, a total of 4 subjects (5%, 4/73; 1 subject with bleeding and 3 subjects with obstruction) required surgical resection to manage complications.[93] In the authors' experience, patients with large, bulky transmural tumors are the ones at greatest risk for perforation, given the highly responsive nature of the disease to treatment. The authors have on occasion, treated some of these patients with a 25% dose reduction for the first cycle, to minimize the neutropenia that would make surgical intervention impossible. Surgeons should be aware of that such complications can occur during gastric lymphoma treatment; however, those risks should not be overestimated.

SUMMARY

This article reviewed and summarized the available evidence regarding the treatment of gastric lymphoma, especially MALT lymphoma and DLBL. Treatment should be stratified based on histologic type, stage, *H pylori* infection, and t(11;18) translocation status. Surgery no longer plays a significant role in the treatment of most patients and should be reserved for rare situations such as refractory bleeding, perforation, or fistula formation. Multimodal treatment of gastric lymphoma, including *H pylori* eradication treatment, radiation therapy, chemotherapy, and immunotherapy, should be provided as appropriate because it can result in excellent outcomes.

REFERENCES

1. d'Amore F, Brincker H, Gronbaek K, et al. Non-Hodgkin's lymphoma of the gastrointestinal tract: a population-based analysis of incidence, geographic distribution, clinicopathologic presentation features, and prognosis. Danish Lymphoma Study Group. J Clin Oncol 1994;12(8):1673–84.

2. Hockey MS, Powell J, Crocker J, et al. Primary gastric lymphoma. Br J Surg 1987; 74(6):483–7.

3. Otter R, Gerrits WB, vd Sandt MM, et al. Primary extranodal and nodal non-Hodgkin's lymphoma. A survey of a population-based registry. Eur J Cancer Clin Oncol 1989;25(8):1203–10.

4. d'Amore F, Christensen BE, Brincker H, et al. Clinicopathological features and prognostic factors in extranodal non-Hodgkin lymphomas. Danish LYFO Study Group. Eur J Cancer 1991;27(10):1201–8.

5. Ruskone-Fourmestraux A, Aegerter P, Delmer A, et al. Primary digestive tract lymphoma: a prospective multicentric study of 91 patients. Groupe d'Etude des Lymphomes Digestifs. Gastroenterology 1993;105(6):1662–71.

6. Koch P, del Valle F, Berdel WE, et al. Primary gastrointestinal non-Hodgkin's lymphoma: I. Anatomic and histologic distribution, clinical features, and survival data of 371 patients registered in the German Multicenter Study GIT NHL 01/92. J Clin Oncol 2001;19(18):3861–73.

7. Freeman C, Berg JW, Cutler SJ. Occurrence and prognosis of extranodal lymphomas. Cancer 1972;29(1):252–60.

8. Dawson IM, Cornes JS, Morson BC. Primary malignant lymphoid tumours of the intestinal tract. Report of 37 cases with a study of factors influencing prognosis. Br J Surg 1961;49:80–9.

9. Spinelli P, Lo Gullo C, Pizzetti P. Endoscopic diagnosis of gastric lymphomas. Endoscopy 1980;12(5):211–4.

10. Fork FT, Haglund U, Hogstrom H, et al. Primary gastric lymphoma versus gastric cancer. An endoscopic and radiographic study of differential diagnostic possibilities. Endoscopy 1985;17(1):5–7.

11. Wotherspoon AC, Doglioni C, Isaacson PG. Low-grade gastric B-cell lymphoma of mucosa-associated lymphoid tissue (MALT): a multifocal disease. Histopathology 1992;20(1):29–34.

12. Suekane H, Iida M, Kuwano Y, et al. Diagnosis of primary early gastric lymphoma. Usefulness of endoscopic mucosal resection for histologic evaluation. Cancer 1993;71(4):1207–13.

13. Suekane H, Iida M, Yao T, et al. Endoscopic ultrasonography in primary gastric lymphoma: correlation with endoscopic and histologic findings. Gastrointest Endosc 1993;39(2):139–45.

14. Caletti G, Ferrari A, Brocchi E, et al. Accuracy of endoscopic ultrasonography in the diagnosis and staging of gastric cancer and lymphoma. Surgery 1993;113(1): 14–27.

15. Perry C, Herishanu Y, Metzer U, et al. Diagnostic accuracy of PET/CT in patients with extranodal marginal zone MALT lymphoma. Eur J Haematol 2007;79(3): 205–9.

16. Beal KP, Yeung HW, Yahalom J. FDG-PET scanning for detection and staging of extranodal marginal zone lymphomas of the MALT type: a report of 42 cases. Ann Oncol 2005;16(3):473–80.

17. Hoffmann M, Kletter K, Becherer A, et al. 18F-fluorodeoxyglucose positron emission tomography (18F-FDG-PET) for staging and follow-up of marginal zone B-cell lymphoma. Oncology 2003;64(4):336–40.

18. Liu H, Ruskon-Fourmestraux A, Lavergne-Slove A, et al. Resistance of t(11;18) positive gastric mucosa-associated lymphoid tissue lymphoma to Helicobacter pylori eradication therapy. Lancet 2001;357(9249):39–40.

19. Levy M, Copie-Bergman C, Gameiro C, et al. Prognostic value of translocation t(11;18) in tumoral response of low-grade gastric lymphoma of mucosa-associated lymphoid tissue type to oral chemotherapy. J Clin Oncol 2005; 23(22):5061–6.

20. Streubel B, Ye H, Du MQ, et al. Translocation t(11;18)(q21;q21) is not predictive of response to chemotherapy with 2CdA in patients with gastric MALT lymphoma. Oncology 2004;66(6):476–80.

21. Zelenetz AD, Gordon LI, Wierda WG, et al. Non-Hodgkin's lymphomas, version 4.2014. J Natl Compr Canc Netw 2014;12(9):1282–303.

22. Musshoff K. Clinical staging classification of non-Hodgkin's lymphomas (author's translation). Strahlentherapie 1977;153(4):218–21 [in German].

23. Rosenberg SA, Kaplan HS. Evidence for an orderly progression in the spread of Hodgkin's disease. Cancer Res 1966;26(6):1225–31.

24. Morton JE, Leyland MJ, Vaughan Hudson G, et al. Primary gastrointestinal non-Hodgkin's lymphoma: a review of 175 British National Lymphoma Investigation cases. Br J Cancer 1993;67(4):776–82.

25. Papaxoinis G, Papageorgiou S, Rontogianni D, et al. Primary gastrointestinal non-Hodgkin's lymphoma: a clinicopathologic study of 128 cases in Greece.

A Hellenic Cooperative Oncology Group study (HeCOG). Leuk Lymphoma 2006; 47(10):2140–6.

26. Rohatiner A, d'Amore F, Coiffier B, et al. Report on a workshop convened to discuss the pathological and staging classifications of gastrointestinal tract lymphoma. Ann Oncol 1994;5(5):397–400.

27. Zucca E, Copie-Bergman C, Ricardi U, et al. Gastric marginal zone lymphoma of MALT type: ESMO clinical practice guidelines for diagnosis, treatment and follow-up. Ann Oncol 2013;24(Suppl 6):vi144–8.

28. Ruskone-Fourmestraux A, Dragosics B, Morgner A, et al. Paris staging system for primary gastrointestinal lymphomas. Gut 2003;52(6):912–3.

29. Rosenberg SA. Classification of lymphoid neoplasms. Blood 1994;84(5): 1359–60.

30. Harris NL, Jaffe ES, Stein H, et al. A revised European-American classification of lymphoid neoplasms: a proposal from the International Lymphoma Study Group. Blood 1994;84(5):1361–92.

31. Bartlett DL, Karpeh MS Jr, Filippa DA, et al. Long-term follow-up after curative surgery for early gastric lymphoma. Ann Surg 1996;223(1):53–62.

32. Binn M, Ruskone-Fourmestraux A, Lepage E, et al. Surgical resection plus chemotherapy versus chemotherapy alone: comparison of two strategies to treat diffuse large B-cell gastric lymphoma. Ann Oncol 2003;14(12):1751–7.

33. Economopoulos T, Alexopoulos C, Stathakis N, et al. Primary gastric lymphoma–the experience of a general hospital. Br J Cancer 1985;52(3):391–7.

34. Hussell T, Isaacson PG, Crabtree JE, et al. The response of cells from low-grade B-cell gastric lymphomas of mucosa-associated lymphoid tissue to *Helicobacter pylori*. Lancet 1993;342(8871):571–4.

35. Wotherspoon AC, Doglioni C, Diss TC, et al. Regression of primary low-grade B-cell gastric lymphoma of mucosa-associated lymphoid tissue type after eradication of *Helicobacter pylori*. Lancet 1993;342(8871):575–7.

36. Isaacson PG. Gastric MALT lymphoma: from concept to cure. Ann Oncol 1999; 10(6):637–45.

37. Koch P, del Valle F, Berdel WE, et al. Primary gastrointestinal non-Hodgkin's lymphoma: II. Combined surgical and conservative or conservative management only in localized gastric lymphoma–results of the prospective German Multicenter Study GIT NHL 01/92. J Clin Oncol 2001;19(18):3874–83.

38. Cortelazzo S, Rossi A, Roggero F, et al. Stage-modified international prognostic index effectively predicts clinical outcome of localized primary gastric diffuse large B-cell lymphoma. International Extranodal Lymphoma Study Group (IELSG). Ann Oncol 1999;10(12):1433–40.

39. Mafune KI, Tanaka Y, Suda Y, et al. Outcome of patients with non-Hodgkin's lymphoma of the stomach after gastrectomy: clinicopathologic study and reclassification according to the revised European-American lymphoma classification. Gastric Cancer 2001;4(3):137–43.

40. Amer MH, el-Akkad S. Gastrointestinal lymphoma in adults: clinical features and management of 300 cases. Gastroenterology 1994;106(4):846–58.

41. Aviles A, Nambo MJ, Neri N, et al. The role of surgery in primary gastric lymphoma: results of a controlled clinical trial. Ann Surg 2004;240(1):44–50.

42. Aviles A, Nambo MJ, Neri N, et al. Mucosa-associated lymphoid tissue (MALT) lymphoma of the stomach: results of a controlled clinical trial. Med Oncol 2005; 22(1):57–62.

43. Isaacson PG, Spencer J. Malignant lymphoma of mucosa-associated lymphoid tissue. Histopathology 1987;11(5):445–62.

44. Wotherspoon AC, Ortiz-Hidalgo C, Falzon MR, et al. *Helicobacter pylori*-associated gastritis and primary B-cell gastric lymphoma. Lancet 1991;338(8776): 1175–6.

45. Cuttner J, Werther JL, McGlynn P, et al. Seroprevalence of *Helicobacter pylori* infection in patients with lymphoma. Leuk Lymphoma 2001;40(5–6):591–7.

46. Parsonnet J, Hansen S, Rodriguez L, et al. *Helicobacter pylori* infection and gastric lymphoma. N Engl J Med 1994;330(18):1267–71.

47. Eck M, Schmausser B, Haas R, et al. MALT-type lymphoma of the stomach is associated with *Helicobacter pylori* strains expressing the CagA protein. Gastroenterology 1997;112(5):1482–6.

48. Weber DM, Dimopoulos MA, Anandu DP, et al. Regression of gastric lymphoma of mucosa-associated lymphoid tissue with antibiotic therapy for *Helicobacter pylori*. Gastroenterology 1994;107(6):1835–8.

49. Carlson SJ, Yokoo H, Vanagunas A. Progression of gastritis to monoclonal B-cell lymphoma with resolution and recurrence following eradication of *Helicobacter pylori*. JAMA 1996;275(12):937–9.

50. Steinbach G, Ford R, Glober G, et al. Antibiotic treatment of gastric lymphoma of mucosa-associated lymphoid tissue. An uncontrolled trial. Ann Intern Med 1999; 131(2):88–95.

51. Fuccio L, Laterza L, Zagari RM, et al. Treatment of *Helicobacter pylori* infection. BMJ 2008;337:a1454.

52. Bertoni F, Coiffier B, Salles G, et al. MALT lymphomas: pathogenesis can drive treatment. Oncology (Williston Park) 2011;25(12):1134–42, 1147.

53. Ruskone-Fourmestraux A, Fischbach W, Aleman BM, et al. EGILS consensus report. Gastric extranodal marginal zone B-cell lymphoma of MALT. Gut 2011; 60(6):747–58.

54. Dreyling M, Thieblemont C, Gallamini A, et al. ESMO Consensus conferences: guidelines on malignant lymphoma. part 2: marginal zone lymphoma, mantle cell lymphoma, peripheral T-cell lymphoma. Ann Oncol 2013;24(4):857–77.

55. Chen LT, Lin JT, Tai JJ, et al. Long-term results of anti-*Helicobacter pylori* therapy in early-stage gastric high-grade transformed MALT lymphoma. J Natl Cancer Inst 2005;97(18):1345–53.

56. Bertoni F, Conconi A, Capella C, et al. Molecular follow-up in gastric mucosa-associated lymphoid tissue lymphomas: early analysis of the LY03 cooperative trial. Blood 2002;99(7):2541–4.

57. Wundisch T, Thiede C, Morgner A, et al. Long-term follow-up of gastric MALT lymphoma after *Helicobacter pylori* eradication. J Clin Oncol 2005;23(31):8018–24.

58. Stathis A, Chini C, Bertoni F, et al. Long-term outcome following *Helicobacter pylori* eradication in a retrospective study of 105 patients with localized gastric marginal zone B-cell lymphoma of MALT type. Ann Oncol 2009;20(6):1086–93.

59. Nakamura S, Sugiyama T, Matsumoto T, et al. Long-term clinical outcome of gastric MALT lymphoma after eradication of *Helicobacter pylori*: a multicentre cohort follow-up study of 420 patients in Japan. Gut 2012;61(4):507–13.

60. Alpen B, Neubauer A, Dierlamm J, et al. Translocation t(11;18) absent in early gastric marginal zone B-cell lymphoma of MALT type responding to eradication of *Helicobacter pylori* infection. Blood 2000;95(12):4014–5.

61. Neubauer A, Thiede C, Morgner A, et al. Cure of *Helicobacter pylori* infection and duration of remission of low-grade gastric mucosa-associated lymphoid tissue lymphoma. J Natl Cancer Inst 1997;89(18):1350–5.

62. Tomita N, Kodaira T, Tachibana H, et al. Favorable outcomes of radiotherapy for early-stage mucosa-associated lymphoid tissue lymphoma. Radiother Oncol 2009;90(2):231–5.
63. Goda JS, Gospodarowicz M, Pintilie M, et al. Long-term outcome in localized extranodal mucosa-associated lymphoid tissue lymphomas treated with radiotherapy. Cancer 2010;116(16):3815–24.
64. Vrieling C, de Jong D, Boot H, et al. Long-term results of stomach-conserving therapy in gastric MALT lymphoma. Radiother Oncol 2008;87(3):405–11.
65. Ruskone-Fourmestraux A, Matysiak-Budnik T, Fabiani B, et al. Exclusive moderate-dose radiotherapy in gastric marginal zone B-cell MALT lymphoma: results of a prospective study with a long term follow-up. Radiother Oncol 2015; 117(1):178–82.
66. Tsang RW, Gospodarowicz MK. Radiation therapy for localized low-grade non-Hodgkin's lymphomas. Hematol Oncol 2005;23(1):10–7.
67. Wirth A, Gospodarowicz M, Aleman BM, et al. Long-term outcome for gastric marginal zone lymphoma treated with radiotherapy: a retrospective, multicentre, International Extranodal Lymphoma Study Group study. Ann Oncol 2013;24(5):1344–51.
68. Hammel P, Haioun C, Chaumette MT, et al. Efficacy of single-agent chemotherapy in low-grade B-cell mucosa-associated lymphoid tissue lymphoma with prominent gastric expression. J Clin Oncol 1995;13(10):2524–9.
69. Jager G, Neumeister P, Brezinschek R, et al. Treatment of extranodal marginal zone B-cell lymphoma of mucosa-associated lymphoid tissue type with cladribine: a phase II study. J Clin Oncol 2002;20(18):3872–7.
70. Levy M, Copie-Bergman C, Traulle C, et al. Conservative treatment of primary gastric low-grade B-cell lymphoma of mucosa-associated lymphoid tissue: predictive factors of response and outcome. Am J Gastroenterol 2002;97(2):292–7.
71. Conconi A, Martinelli G, Thieblemont C, et al. Clinical activity of rituximab in extranodal marginal zone B-cell lymphoma of MALT type. Blood 2003;102(8): 2741–5.
72. Martinelli G, Laszlo D, Ferreri AJ, et al. Clinical activity of rituximab in gastric marginal zone non-Hodgkin's lymphoma resistant to or not eligible for anti-*Helicobacter pylori* therapy. J Clin Oncol 2005;23(9):1979–83.
73. Olszewski AJ, Castillo JJ. Comparative outcomes of oncologic therapy in gastric extranodal marginal zone (MALT) lymphoma: analysis of the SEER-Medicare database. Ann Oncol 2013;24(5):1352–9.
74. Zucca E, Conconi A, Laszlo D, et al. Addition of rituximab to chlorambucil produces superior event-free survival in the treatment of patients with extranodal marginal-zone B-cell lymphoma: 5-year analysis of the IELSG-19 Randomized Study. J Clin Oncol 2013;31(5):565–72.
75. Taal BG, Boot H, van Heerde P, et al. Primary non-Hodgkin lymphoma of the stomach: endoscopic pattern and prognosis in low versus high grade malignancy in relation to the MALT concept. Gut 1996;39(4):556–61.
76. Narita M, Yatabe Y, Asai J, et al. Primary gastric lymphomas: morphologic, immunohistochemical and immunogenetic analyses. Pathol Int 1996;46(9):623–9.
77. Vitolo U, Seymour JF, Martelli M, et al. Extranodal diffuse large B-cell lymphoma (DLBCL) and primary mediastinal B-cell lymphoma: ESMO Clinical Practice Guidelines for diagnosis, treatment and follow-up. Ann Oncol 2016;27(Suppl 5):v91–102.
78. Coiffier B, Lepage E, Briere J, et al. CHOP chemotherapy plus rituximab compared with CHOP alone in elderly patients with diffuse large-B-cell lymphoma. N Engl J Med 2002;346(4):235–42.

79. Feugier P, Van Hoof A, Sebban C, et al. Long-term results of the R-CHOP study in the treatment of elderly patients with diffuse large B-cell lymphoma: a study by the Groupe d'Etude des Lymphomes de l'Adulte. J Clin Oncol 2005;23(18): 4117–26.

80. Habermann TM, Weller EA, Morrison VA, et al. Rituximab-CHOP versus CHOP alone or with maintenance rituximab in older patients with diffuse large B-cell lymphoma. J Clin Oncol 2006;24(19):3121–7.

81. Aviles A, Castaneda C, Cleto S, et al. Rituximab and chemotherapy in primary gastric lymphoma. Cancer Biother Radiopharm 2009;24(1):25–8.

82. Sohn BS, Kim SM, Yoon DH, et al. The comparison between CHOP and R-CHOP in primary gastric diffuse large B cell lymphoma. Ann Hematol 2012;91(11): 1731–9.

83. Leopardo D, Di Lorenzo G, De Renzo A, et al. Efficacy of rituximab in gastric diffuse large B cell lymphoma patients. World J Gastroenterol 2010;16(20): 2526–30.

84. Phan J, Mazloom A, Medeiros LJ, et al. Benefit of consolidative radiation therapy in patients with diffuse large B-cell lymphoma treated with R-CHOP chemotherapy. J Clin Oncol 2010;28(27):4170–6.

85. Held G, Murawski N, Ziepert M, et al. Role of radiotherapy to bulky disease in elderly patients with aggressive B-cell lymphoma. J Clin Oncol 2014;32(11): 1112–8.

86. Vargo JA, Gill BS, Balasubramani GK, et al. Treatment selection and survival outcomes in early-stage diffuse large B-cell lymphoma: do we still need consolidative radiotherapy? J Clin Oncol 2015;33(32):3710–7.

87. Martinelli G, Gigli F, Calabrese L, et al. Early stage gastric diffuse large B-cell lymphomas: results of a randomized trial comparing chemotherapy alone versus chemotherapy + involved field radiotherapy. (IELSG 4). [corrected]. Leuk Lymphoma 2009;50(6):925–31.

88. Tanaka T, Shimada K, Yamamoto K, et al. Retrospective analysis of primary gastric diffuse large B cell lymphoma in the rituximab era: a multicenter study of 95 patients in Japan. Ann Hematol 2012;91(3):383–90.

89. Kuo SH, Yeh KH, Wu MS, et al. *Helicobacter pylori* eradication therapy is effective in the treatment of early-stage *H pylori*-positive gastric diffuse large B-cell lymphomas. Blood 2012;119(21):4838–44 [quiz: 5057].

90. Liu X, Fang H, Tian Y, et al. Intensity modulated radiation therapy for early-stage primary gastric diffuse large B-cell lymphoma: dosimetric analysis, clinical outcome, and quality of life. Int J Radiat Oncol Biol Phys 2016;95(2):712–20.

91. Brincker H, D'Amore F. A retrospective analysis of treatment outcome in 106 cases of localized gastric non-Hodgkin lymphomas. Danish Lymphoma Study Group, LYFO. Leuk Lymphoma 1995;18(3–4):281–8.

92. Hsu C, Chen CL, Chen LT, et al. Comparison of MALT and non-MALT primary large cell lymphoma of the stomach: does histologic evidence of MALT affect chemotherapy response? Cancer 2001;91(1):49–56.

93. Spectre G, Libster D, Grisariu S, et al. Bleeding, obstruction, and perforation in a series of patients with aggressive gastric lymphoma treated with primary chemotherapy. Ann Surg Oncol 2006;13(11):1372–8.

Role of Chemotherapy and Radiation Therapy in the Management of Gastric Adenocarcinoma

Daphna Spiegel, MD[a], Manisha Palta, MD[a],
Hope Uronis, MD, MHS[b],*

KEYWORDS

• Gastric cancer • Chemotherapy • Radiation therapy • Neoadjuvant • Adjuvant

KEY POINTS

• There is not a standard approach to the management of localized gastric adenocarcinoma, as data exist for perioperative chemotherapy, adjuvant chemotherapy, and adjuvant chemoradiation.

• Adequate staging, including cross-sectional imaging and endoscopic ultrasound, should be performed, and diagnostic laparoscopy should be considered.

• Adjuvant chemotherapy provides survival benefit in Asian studies, where D2 resection is standard, while adjuvant chemoradiotherapy is most appropriate in countries in which D2 resection is not standard.

• The role of anti-HER2 therapy in resectable gastric cancer is an area of ongoing investigation.

• Multidisciplinary evaluation is essential in the management of patients with gastric cancer.

INTRODUCTION

Gastric adenocarcinoma is the fifth most common cancer worldwide and is often diagnosed at a late stage, with nearly 50% of patients having locally advanced, unresectable or metastatic disease at the time of presentation. In 2016, an estimated 26,370 new cases of gastric cancer are projected in the United States, with an estimated 10,730 deaths.[1] Prognosis for patients diagnosed with gastric cancer is generally poor. Older population-based, surgical series demonstrated 5-year survival

Disclosure Statement: The authors have nothing to disclose.
[a] Department of Radiation Oncology, Duke University, DUMC Box 3085, Durham, NC 27710, USA; [b] Division of Medical Oncology, Duke University, DUMC Box 2823, Durham, NC 27710, USA
* Corresponding author.
E-mail address: Hope.uronis@duke.edu

Surg Clin N Am 97 (2017) 421–435
http://dx.doi.org/10.1016/j.suc.2016.11.013
0039-6109/17/© 2017 Elsevier Inc. All rights reserved.

rates for completely resected, early-stage gastric cancer (stage IA/B) at 58% to 78%; for patients with stage II or more advanced disease, 5-year survival estimates are less than 35%.[2] Efforts to improve outcomes in patients with resected as well as unresectable gastric cancer with various chemotherapy and radiation regimens are ongoing. Appropriate evaluation and management of these patients is often not straightforward and requires the input of a multidisciplinary team, including gastroenterology, medical oncology, radiation oncology, and surgery. There is no consensus as to the best approach for treatment of gastric cancer; however, the available data as well as our institutional approach to the management of gastric cancer are discussed.

INITIAL EVALUATION

Clinical staging is an essential first step in developing a treatment plan. After a diagnosis of gastric adenocarcinoma by esophagogastroduodenoscopy and biopsy, patients should undergo cross-sectional imaging to evaluate for the presence of metastatic disease. In general, contrasted computed tomography (CT) scan is recommended. Functional imaging, such as PET scan, can be considered, but may be misleading as many gastric cancers, notably diffuse tumors, are not fludeoxyglucose (FDG)-avid.[3] Once the tumor is confirmed to be localized, endoscopic ultrasound (EUS) is recommended to establish T-stage and N-stage, because as many as 15% of early-stage cancers are node-positive[4] and EUS allows appropriate classification of these patients. Finally, diagnostic laparoscopy should be considered. Although the risk of peritoneal spread increases as T-stage increases, and is highest in those with T4 disease and linitis plastica, there is still a risk in those with earlier stage tumors and its identification would change treatment recommendations.[5]

For patients with confirmed localized disease, the treatment plan is dictated by T- and N-stage. Those patients with very early disease (defined as ≤T1bN0) should undergo immediate local intervention, either endoscopic or surgical resection. Those patients with more advanced disease should be considered for combined modality therapy, either chemotherapy or chemoradiotherapy. We would advocate for multidisciplinary involvement in treatment planning.

POTENTIALLY RESECTABLE DISEASE
Neoadjuvant Treatment

Neoadjuvant/perioperative chemotherapy
Many countries primarily use neoadjuvant chemotherapy or perioperative chemotherapy for the treatment of localized gastric cancers. This approach to resectable gastric cancer serves 2 main purposes: downstaging of disease before attempted surgical resection and selection of patients for surgery based on the biology of their disease. It is not unusual for patients with gastric cancer to have micrometastatic disease at the time of diagnosis; by administering a course of neoadjuvant chemotherapy before surgical resection, patients who do not develop progressive disease can be selected to undergo resection, whereas those who do develop overt metastasis can be spared the morbidity of surgery. There are 3 major studies that examine the use of neoadjuvant or perioperative chemotherapy, including the Medical Research Council Adjuvant Gastric Infusional Chemotherapy (MAGIC) trial, the French Fédération Nationale des Centres de Lutte Contre le Cancer (FNCLCC)/Fédération Francophone de Cancérologie Digestive (FFCD) trial, and the European Organization for Research and Treatment of Cancer (EORTC) 40984 study (**Table 1**).

The MAGIC trial is the largest of the 3 studies and was performed in the United Kingdom from July 1994 and April 2002.[6] In this trial, 503 patients with stage II or

Table 1
Studies examining the role of perioperative or neoadjuvant chemotherapy

Study	Study Arms	N	Overall Survival, %	Local Recurrence, %	R0 Rate, %
MAGIC	Surgery	253	23	21	66
	ECF → Surgery → ECF	250	36[a]	14	69
FNLCC/FFCD	Surgery	111	24	26	74
	5-FU/Cisplatin → Surgery	113	38[b]	24	84
EORTC 40954	Surgery	72	69.9	—	67
	5-FU/Cisplatin → Surgery	72	73[c]	—	82

Abbreviations: ECF, epirubicin, cisplatin, 5-fluorouracil; EORTC, European Organization for Research and Treatment of Cancer; FFCD, French FNCLCC/Fédération Francophone de Cancérologie Digestive; FNCLCC, Fédération Nationale des Centres de Lutte Contre le Cancer; FU, fluorouracil; MAGIC, Medical Research Council Adjuvant Gastric Infusional Chemotherapy; NS, not significant.
  [a] P = .009 (5-year).
  [b] P = .02 (5-year).
  [c] P = NS (2-year).
Data from Refs.[6–8]

higher or locally advanced, inoperable gastric adenocarcinoma as well as distal esophageal or gastroesophageal junction (GEJ) adenocarcinomas were randomized to receive surgery alone or surgery plus perioperative chemotherapy, consisting of epirubicin, cisplatin, and infusional fluorouracil (5-FU), abbreviated collectively as ECF. The perioperative regimen consisted of 3 cycles of ECF chemotherapy before and after surgical resection. There were more patients with T1/T2 disease (51.7% vs 36.8%, P = .002) and more N0/N1 patients (84.4% vs 70.5%, P = .01) in the group that received chemotherapy. Of the 74% of patients with gastric cancer included in this study, a significant percentage of patients who received perioperative chemotherapy ultimately underwent surgery (79.3% vs 70.3%, P = .03). Rates of R0 resection were not significantly different between the 2 treatment arms, although there is little information regarding surgical technique used. With regard to overall survival, 36% of patients in the perioperative chemotherapy group versus 23% of patients in the surgery alone group were alive at 5 years (P = .009). Progression-free survival also was better in the perioperative group than the surgery alone group, with a hazard ratio (HR) for progression of 0.66 (P<.001). This trial has been criticized, as not all patients underwent EUS staging and only 42% of patients in the perioperative chemotherapy group received all therapy per protocol (with 34% of patients in this group not starting postoperative chemotherapy at all). It also should be noted that this trial was conducted before newer chemotherapy agents became available. Nevertheless, this study demonstrates a significant survival benefit with the use of perioperative chemotherapy and is considered a standard of care approach.

Another study examining the role of perioperative chemotherapy is a French randomized phase III trial from Fédération Nationale des Centers de Lutte contre le Cancer (FNCL) and the FFCD.[7] A total of 224 patients with gastric, lower esophageal, or GEJ adenocarcinomas were randomized to receive either surgery alone or perioperative infusional 5-FU and cisplatin. The study closed early because of poor accrual, but despite this limitation, patients in the perioperative chemotherapy arm had a statistically significant improvement in 5-year overall survival as compared with the surgery-alone arm (38% vs 24%, P = .02). There was a benefit in terms of R0 resection rates seen in patients who had undergone preoperative chemotherapy versus those who proceeded directly to surgery (84% vs 74%, P = .04). Similar to the MAGIC trial, only approximately 50% of patients were able to complete the intended postoperative chemotherapy. A critique of this study, with regard to its applicability to gastric cancer, is that only 25% of patients included in the trial had true gastric tumors, the remainder of patients had tumors in the lower esophagus or the GEJ.

In a study examining the role of neoadjuvant chemotherapy from the EORTC, patients with locally advanced disease within the stomach or the GEJ were randomized to receive either cisplatin, leucovorin, and infusional 5-FU followed by surgery or surgery alone.[8] Approximately 94% of patients had T3 or greater disease and approximately 50% of the primary tumors were located in the upper third/cardia region of the stomach. With only 144 of a planned 360 patients enrolled, the study closed early. Although the patients in the neoadjuvant group had higher rates of R0 resection (81.9% vs 66.7%, $P = .036$), at a median follow-up of 4.4 years, there was no significant overall survival difference (HR 0.84, 95% confidence interval [CI] 0.52–1.35; $P = .466$). Potentially contributing to the lack of a survival benefit are 4 factors: low accrual limiting the power of the study, lower-stage tumors (as compared with the MAGIC trial) that may benefit less from chemotherapy, protocol noncompliance, with only 45 patients completing all protocol-specified chemotherapy, and improved surgical techniques, with a higher D2 resection rate than in the MAGIC trial.

Given these mixed results, a meta-analysis of the aforementioned trials (MAGIC, FNCL/FFCD, and EORTC) along with other smaller trials was performed to examine the role of preoperative chemotherapy versus surgery alone.[9] This study found that preoperative chemotherapy was associated with a statistically significant improvement in terms of both overall survival (odds ratio [OR] 1.32, 95% CI 1.07–1.64) as well as progression-free survival (OR 1.82, 95% CI 1.39–2.46). As seen throughout the individual studies, there was also a statistically significant improvement in R0 resection rates with preoperative chemotherapy (OR 1.38, 95% CI 1.08–1.78). There was not a statistically significant difference in perioperative or postoperative complication rates.

The data from the randomized trials and the meta-analysis discussed previously support the use of neoadjuvant or perioperative chemotherapy. In terms of patient selection, a perioperative chemotherapy strategy is likely most appropriate for those patients with bulky tumors or bulky adenopathy, in which there is a significant risk of both micrometastatic disease as well as incomplete resection.

Neoadjuvant chemoradiation

An early randomized trial from China established a benefit for neoadjuvant radiotherapy for gastric cancers. Zhang and colleagues[10] randomized 370 patients with gastric cardia adenocarcinoma to neoadjuvant radiation therapy (40 Gy) followed by surgery versus surgery alone. Patients who were treated with neoadjuvant radiation had statistically significant improvement in overall survival, with rates at 5-year and 10-year follow-up of 30.1% and 19.75% and 20.26% and 13.3%, respectively ($P<.01$).

Given the known radiosensitizing benefits of chemotherapy, a number of small studies subsequently examined the role of neoadjuvant chemoradiation; however, there are no randomized controlled trials supporting the use of neoadjuvant chemoradiation for gastric cancers.

In a multi-institutional phase II study from M.D. Anderson Cancer Center, patients with resectable gastric carcinoma were treated with induction chemotherapy (consisting of 5-FU, leucovorin, and cisplatin) followed by chemoradiation (45 Gy plus concurrent 5-FU chemotherapy).[11] The primary endpoint of the study was pathologic complete response (pCR); secondary endpoints were R0 resection rate, survival, and safety. At a median follow-up of 50 months, survival in the 33 enrolled patients was 39%; pCR was noted in 36% of the 28 patients who ultimately underwent surgery, and the R0 resection rate in those who underwent surgery was 82%. There were no grade 4+ acute toxicities with chemoradiation. A subsequent multicenter, phase II study was conducted by the Radiation Therapy Oncology Group (RTOG); in this study, 49 patients with gastric adenocarcinoma from 21 institutions were treated with induction 5-FU, leucovorin, and cisplatin chemotherapy followed by radiation to 45 Gy with concomitant infusional 5-FU and paclitaxel.[12] The primary endpoint was pCR rate with secondary endpoints of toxicity and feasibility. Of the 43 patients who went on to surgery, 26% had a pCR; at 21.6 months of follow-up, median survival was 23.2 months. In the patients undergoing resection, 82% of patients with pCR were alive at 12 months as compared with 69% of patients with less than pCR.

Data supporting the benefit of neoadjuvant chemoradiation for other gastrointestinal sites, including esophagus, GEJ, and the gastric cardia, are more established. A landmark study, the CROSS (ChemoRadiotherapy for Oesophageal cancer followed by Surgery Study) trial, compared outcomes of neoadjuvant chemoradiation versus surgery alone and found that preoperative chemoradiotherapy improved survival (HR 0.657, 95% CI 0.495–0.871; $P = .003$).[13] Although this study primarily included patients with esophageal cancers, 24% of patients had cancers arising from within 5 cm of the GEJ, suggesting that patients with cancers within the gastric cardia may derive a survival benefit from neoadjuvant chemoradiation. A similar benefit to neoadjuvant chemoradiation was noted in the POET trial (PreOperative chemotherapy or radiochemotherapy in Esophagogastric adenocarcinoma Trial), which randomized patients to either induction chemotherapy alone or neoadjuvant chemoradiation. Although this study was limited to GEJ adenocarcinomas and results were not statistically significant (early closure due to accrual), there was certainly a clinically significant survival difference at the 3-year follow-up (27.7% vs 47.7%, HR 0.67, 95% CI 0.41–1.07; $P = .07$).[14] Whether these data can be extrapolated to all gastric cancers is unknown, but this is an area of further investigation. The TOPGEAR trial, an international study that randomizes patients to neoadjuvant chemotherapy versus chemoradiation (discussed further later in this article), is currently enrolling patients in hopes of defining the optimal neoadjuvant regimen.[15]

Adjuvant Treatment

Adjuvant chemotherapy

The use of adjuvant chemotherapy has been explored in more than 30 randomized trials, most of which have shown no benefit in overall survival as compared with surgery alone. Most of these studies have used older chemotherapy and are best viewed in aggregate in the form of a meta-analysis. One such analysis, conducted with patient-level data, is from the Global Advanced/Adjuvant Stomach Tumor Research International Collaborative (GASTRIC),[16] which looked at all randomized controlled trials comparing surgery plus adjuvant chemotherapy versus surgery alone. Seventeen trials with a total of 3838 patients were identified; median follow-up exceeded 7 years. There was a significant benefit to adjuvant chemotherapy of any type with HR for death equal to 0.82 (95% CI 0.76–0.90, $P<.001$) and an estimated median overall survival in the surgery-only group of 4.9 years (95% CI 4.4–5.5) as compared with 7.8 years in the group receiving adjuvant chemotherapy (95% CI 6.5–8.7). The absolute benefit for overall survival was estimated to be 5.8% at 5 years and 7.4% at 10 years. Interaction tests between the type of chemotherapy regimen and effect on disease-free survival and overall survival were not significant. These data support the use of adjuvant chemotherapy after complete resection of gastric adenocarcinoma, but do not necessarily identify the optimal chemotherapy regimen or if specific patients benefit more from adjuvant treatment than others.

Two recent studies using modern chemotherapy agents have shown a survival benefit with adjuvant chemotherapy; both studies were conducted in Asian countries and have been the largest to date (**Table 2**). The Japanese ACTS-GC (Adjuvant Chemotherapy Trial of S-1 for Gastric Cancer) phase III trial randomized 1059 patients with confirmed stage II (474 patients; 44.8%) or III (584 patients; 55.1%) gastric cancer to receive S-1 chemotherapy for 1 year or observation following resection.[17] All patients in the study underwent D2 lymphadenectomy. The primary endpoints were relapse-free survival and safety. At 5 years, overall survival was 71.7% versus 61.1% in the surgery plus S-1 chemotherapy arm versus surgery alone (HR 0.669, 95% CI 0.540–0.828). Relapse-free survival was also significantly improved with the addition of adjuvant chemotherapy (HR 0.653, 95% CI 0.537–0.793). Grade 3 or 4 adverse events occurred in fewer than 5% of the patients in the S-1 group. This study represents the first large clinical trial of adjuvant therapy in patients who have undergone D2 lymphadenectomy; the magnitude of benefit is comparable to that observed in both the MAGIC trial and the Intergroup 0116 (INT-0116) study (discussed later in this article), which evaluated other treatment strategies as an adjunct to surgery. Although these are exciting data, it is not clear how this result can be incorporated into therapy because S-1 is available only in Asian countries and many patients, particularly in the United States, do not undergo D2 lymphadenectomy.

The CLASSIC (Capecitabine and Oxaliplatin Adjuvant Study in Stomach Cancer) study was conducted in South Korea, China, and Taiwan. A total of 1035 patients with stage II-IIIB gastric cancer were randomized to surgery alone versus surgery followed by adjuvant capecitabine plus oxaliplatin for 6 months. All patients enrolled in the study underwent D2 gastrectomy.[18] With median follow-up of 62.4 months, patients who received adjuvant chemotherapy had a statistically significant improvement in disease-free survival as compared with the patients who underwent surgery alone (68% vs 53%, P<.0001).[19] The regimen was well tolerated with expected chemotherapy-related adverse events. Subgroup analysis confirmed survival benefit for all disease stages (II, IIIA, and IIIB). Although overall survival data from this study are not yet available, this study suggests that capecitabine and oxaliplatin is another option for adjuvant therapy after D2 gastrectomy, which is a regimen used commonly throughout the world for the treatment of gastrointestinal malignancies.

Table 2
Studies examining the role of adjuvant chemotherapy that have shown survival benefit

Study	Study Arms	N	Locoregional Recurrence, %	Overall Survival, %
ACTS-GC	Surgery alone	277	13	61
	Surgery → S1 × 1 y	282	8	72[a] (5-y)
CLASSIC	Surgery	515	44	78
	Surgery → Cape/Oxaliplatin	520	21	83[b] (3-y)

Abbreviations: ACTS-GC, Adjuvant Chemotherapy Trial of S-1 for Gastric Cancer; Cape, capecitabine; CLASSIC, Capecitabine and Oxaliplatin Adjuvant Study in Stomach Cancer.
[a] Hazard ratio = 0.67.
[b] P = .049.
Data from Sasako M, Sakuramoto S, Katai H, et al. Five-year outcomes of a randomized phase III trial comparing adjuvant chemotherapy with S-1 versus surgery alone in stage II or III gastric cancer. J Clin Oncol 2011;29(33):4387–93; and Bang YJ, Kim YW, Yang HK, et al. Adjuvant capecitabine and oxaliplatin for gastric cancer after D2 gastrectomy (CLASSIC): a phase 3 open-label, randomised controlled trial. Lancet 2012;379(9813):315–21.

Both the Japanese ACTS-GC study and the South Korean CLASSIC trial demonstrate that adjuvant chemotherapy after D2 lymphadenectomy improves outcomes. However, the data also suggest that the survival of patients in Asian countries with gastric cancer is superior to that seen in Western countries, causing many to question the generalizability of the ACTS-GC and CLASSIC studies to other patient populations. The observed differences may be potentially driven by screening (resulting in lower stage at diagnosis), tumor biology, surgeon experience, or extent of surgical resection.[20–22] Despite these factors, a meta-analysis of randomized trials from non-Asian countries comparing surgery alone versus surgery plus adjuvant chemotherapy did suggest that adjuvant chemotherapy may provide a small survival benefit even for Western populations (OR for death of 0.80 [95% CI 0.66–0.97] corresponding to a relative risk of 0.94 [95% CI 0.89–1.00]).[23] Therefore, for patients who undergo upfront surgical resection, adjuvant systemic therapy is generally considered.

Adjuvant chemoradiation
The most appropriate modality of adjuvant treatment is still debated. Although the previously discussed studies demonstrate a survival advantage for adjuvant chemotherapy alone, none of the trials compared surgery alone versus adjuvant chemoradiation or adjuvant chemotherapy versus adjuvant chemoradiation.

The INT-0116 study explored the role of adjuvant chemoradiation (**Table 3**). A total of 556 patients with GEJ/gastric adenocarcinomas ≥T3 and/or node-positive were randomized to observation (n = 277) or postoperative 5-FU and leucovorin given with concurrent radiation to 45 Gy (n = 282). Three-year disease-free survival was 48% versus 31% (P<.001) and overall survival rates were 50% versus 41% (P = .005) for the chemoradiation versus surgery alone arms, respectively.[24] These benefits persisted at the 10-year analysis with superior overall survival in the chemoradiation group (P = .0046).[25] One critique of this study is that only 65% of patients in the chemoradiation arm completed therapy as planned; 17% stopped due to toxicity, 8% declined to start, 5% developed progressive disease, and 4% stopped for other reasons. Although acute toxicity was increased in the chemoradiation arm, it is possible that this was due to lack of modern supportive care, as there was no evidence of excess treatment-related toxicity with long-term follow-up. An additional

Table 3
Adjuvant chemoradiation trials

Study	Study Arms	N	Disease-Free Survival (3-y), %	Overall Survival (3-y), %
INT 0116	Surgery alone	277	31	41
	Surgery → 5-FU/LV/RT + 5-FU	282	48[a]	50[b]
CALGB	Surgery → 5-FU/LV/RT + 5-FU	546	46	50
801010	Surgery → ECF + 5-FU/LV/RT + ECF		47[c]	52[c]

Abbreviations: CALGB, Cancer and Leukemia Group B; ECF, epirubicin, cisplatin, 5-fluorouracil; FU, fluorouracil; INT, Intergroup; LV, leucovorin; NS, not significant; RT, radiation therapy.
  [a] P<.001.
  [b] P = .005.
  [c] P = NS.
Data from Macdonald JS, Smalley SR, Benedetti J, et al. Chemoradiotherapy after surgery compared with surgery alone for adenocarcinoma of the stomach or gastroesophageal junction. N Engl J Med 2001;345(10):725–30; and Noel G, Jauffret E, Mazeron JJ. Randomized clinical trial on the combination of preoperative irradiation and surgery in the treatment of adenocarcinoma of gastric cardia (AGC)—report on 370 patients. Cancer Radiother 1999;3(4):344 [in French].

major criticism of this study is that the extent of surgical resection was not predefined. Review of nodal dissection type revealed that 299 patients (54%) underwent less than a D1 resection, 199 patients (36%) underwent a D1 resection, and 54 patients (9.6%) underwent D2 resection. This study enrolled patients at high risk of local recurrence due to bulky tumor or nodal positivity, and in the setting of less than D2 resection, it may be that chemoradiation compensated for inadequate surgery. Lack of D2 resection likely also contributed to the poor performance of the surgery-alone arm.[26] Nonetheless, publication of this study changed practice in the United States and adjuvant chemoradiation therapy remains a common approach.

Multiple chemotherapeutic regimens have been explored in the adjuvant setting with concurrent radiation. The Cancer and Leukemia Group B (CALGB) 80,101 study randomized 546 patients with resected gastric cancer to 1 of 2 chemotherapy arms (see **Table 3**). The patients on the control arm were treated according to the INT-0116 regimen with once cycle of 5-FU plus leucovorin followed by 45 Gy radiation delivered concurrently with 5-FU followed by 2 cycles of 5-FU and leucovorin chemotherapy; patients on the experimental arm were treated with 1 cycle of ECF chemotherapy followed by 45 Gy radiation with concurrent 5-FU followed by 2 cycles of reduced dose ECF. Results have been presented only in abstract form at the 2011 American Society of Clinical Oncology meeting, but overall survival, the primary endpoint of the study, was not significantly improved with the ECF-based regimen.[27]

A total of 6 trials have compared adjuvant chemotherapy and adjuvant chemoradiation; none of these trials have demonstrated a survival advantage for chemoradiation over chemotherapy alone.[28–33] The largest study, the Adjuvant Chemoradiation Therapy in Stomach Cancer (ARTIST) trial, randomized 458 patients to either chemotherapy alone (6 cycles of capecitabine and cisplatin, XP) or 2 cycles of XP chemotherapy followed by chemoradiation (45 Gy plus concurrent capecitabine) and an additional 2 cycles of XP chemotherapy (**Table 4**). In contrast to the Intergroup trial, the ARTIST study required D2 lymph node dissection. Therapy completion rates were high with 75% of patients in the chemotherapy arm completing all therapy and 82% of patients in the chemoradiotherapy arm completing all therapy; toxicity was manageable. Although there was no statistically significant disease-free survival

Table 4
Trials comparing adjuvant chemotherapy with adjuvant chemoradiation therapy

Study	Study Arms	N	Disease-Free Survival (3-y), %	Overall Survival (5-y), %
ARTIST	Surgery → Cape/Cis	458	74.2	—
	Surgery → Cape/Cis + Cape/RT + Cape/Cis		78.2[a]	—
CRITICS	ECX or EOX → Surgery → ECX or EOX	788	—	41.3
	ECX or EOX → Surgery → Cape/RT		—	40.9[b]

Abbreviations: ARTIST, Adjuvant Chemoradiation Therapy in Stomach Cancer; Cape, capecitabine; cis, cisplatin; CRITICS, ChemoRadiotherapy after Induction chemoTherapy In Cancer of the Stomach; ECX, epirubicin, cisplatin, capecitabine; EOX, epirubicin, oxaliplatin, capecitabine; RT, radiation therapy.
[a] $P = .0862$.
[b] $P = .99$.
Data from Park SH, Sohn TS, Lee J, et al. Phase III trial to compare adjuvant chemotherapy with capecitabine and cisplatin versus concurrent chemoradiotherapy in gastric cancer: final report of the adjuvant chemoradiotherapy in stomach tumors trial, including survival and subset analyses. J Clin Oncol 2015;33(28):3130–6; and Randomized phase III trial of adjuvant chemotherapy or chemoradiotherapy in resectable gastric cancer (CRITICS). Available at: https://clinicaltrials.gov/ct2/show/NCT00407186. Accessed August 19, 2016.

benefit to chemoradiation at a median of 84 months of follow-up, subgroup analysis did suggest that patients with node-positive disease had improved disease-free survival with the addition of chemoradiation (76% vs 72%, $P = .004$). Patterns of recurrence, locoregional and distant, did not differ between arms. This is the first study to address the question of adjuvant chemoradiotherapy in patients who have undergone a D2 resection. A follow-up and ongoing study, termed the ARTIST-II trial, is comparing adjuvant chemotherapy with S-1 versus S-1 and oxaliplatin chemotherapy with or without radiation therapy in patients with node-positive, resected gastric cancer.[34]

The most recent study to compare adjuvant chemotherapy with adjuvant chemoradiation is the Dutch CRITICS trial (ChemoRadiotherapy after Induction chemoTherapy In Cancer of the Stomach), which has been presented only in abstract form (see **Table 4**). This trial differs from the ARTIST study in that patients were treated preoperatively with induction chemotherapy (either epirubicin, cisplatin, and capecitabine, or epirubicin, oxaliplatin, and capecitabine) followed by surgical resection and then subsequently randomized to adjuvant chemotherapy (same as the induction regimen) or chemoradiation (45 Gy with concurrent cisplatin and capecitabine). At a median follow-up of 4.2 years, overall survival was similar across the 2 arms (40.8% and 40.9% for chemotherapy and chemoradiation, respectively).[35,36] Final publication in a peer-reviewed journal is awaited before drawing further conclusions.

LOCALLY ADVANCED UNRESECTABLE DISEASE

The optimal treatment of patients with locally advanced unresectable, but nonmetastatic gastric cancer is still being explored. Although some patients may ultimately become surgical candidates, the conversion from unresectable to resectable disease following neoadjuvant treatment is rare for these patients. Choice for initial treatment varies widely across institutions. No randomized trials have explored upfront chemotherapy alone versus chemoradiation for patients with nonmetastatic inoperable gastric cancer. A number of small, nonrandomized studies suggest that pCR rates of 5% to 15% are possible with neoadjuvant chemotherapy alone for patients with locally advanced disease.[37–40] In one of the more contemporary series, 82 patients were treated with initial ECF chemotherapy followed by reevaluation and consideration of surgical resection. All patients underwent restaging following completion of chemotherapy with CT scan, EUS, and biopsies; partial response was seen in 49% and complete response was seen in 7%. A total of 37 patients (45%) ultimately underwent resection, and 4 of those patients (5%) achieved a pCR.[37] Combined modality therapy either with or without chemotherapy (given either as induction chemotherapy or sequentially after chemoradiation) is an alternative strategy for treating patients with locally advanced unresectable disease. As discussed previously, RTOG 99 to 04 examined the effect of induction chemotherapy followed by chemoradiation in patients with initially unresectable tumors. Forty-nine patients were enrolled and 43 patients ultimately went to surgery; 26% of the patients who underwent surgery had a pCR.[12]

At our institution, patients with locally advanced, but nonmetastatic disease are generally treated with a course of induction chemotherapy alone. Following completion of chemotherapy, patients are reassessed; if disease progression is noted, then patients continue with chemotherapy alone. For those patients who do not progress on chemotherapy alone, chemoradiation with radiosensitizing 5-FU is considered with the goal of establishing local control. For patients who present with gastrointestinal bleeding, obstruction, or pain, we generally pursue upfront chemoradiation with radiosensitizing 5-FU.

METASTATIC DISEASE

Patients with advanced gastric cancer often present with uncontrolled bleeding, obstructive symptoms, or pain. Nonsurgical palliation with both radiotherapy and chemotherapy can decrease these symptoms and improve quality of life.

Local palliation with radiation therapy can be extremely effective even at low doses. A retrospective review of 115 patients treated with multiple fractionation schemes, ranging from 8 Gy in a single fraction to 40 Gy in 16 fractions, revealed that there was no difference in response rates with low radiation doses versus higher-dose regimens, defined as a biologically effective dose of ≤39 Gy or >39 Gy, respectively. Control of bleeding, obstructive symptoms, and pain was achieved in 81%, 53%, and 46% of patients, and median duration of response was 99, 97, and 233 days, respectively. Three patients developed grade 3 toxicity (nausea, vomiting, and/or anorexia).[41] Other small studies have had similar findings; a retrospective series examining short-course radiation with 30 Gy in 10 fractions for gastric bleeding revealed response rates of 73% (defined as not requiring blood transfusions for 1 or more months after radiation). No grade 3 or higher toxicity was observed in patients treated with radiation alone. Duration of response was similar at 3.3 months.[42]

ONGOING RESEARCH

The optimal multidisciplinary treatment strategy for patients with gastric cancer remains an area of active investigation (**Table 5**). For patients who are advised to undergo preoperative or perioperative chemotherapy, the MAGIC regimen is most commonly used. There is question as to whether we can improve on this regimen; the ongoing MAGIC-B trial randomized patients to epirubicin, cisplatin, and capecitabine (ECX) chemotherapy delivered with or without bevacizumab followed by surgery and then adjuvant ECX with or without maintenance bevacizumab.[43] Neoadjuvant chemoradiotherapy can also be considered, and the ongoing TOPGEAR trial is randomizing patients to either preoperative chemotherapy alone (ECF) versus 2 cycles of ECF chemotherapy followed by concurrent 5-FU–based chemoradiotherapy. Following surgery, both groups will receive adjuvant ECF.[15] Finally, the ARTIST-II trial is open in South Korea and is attempting to clarify the appropriate adjuvant treatment regimen for patients with node-positive disease; in this study, patients are being randomized to either adjuvant chemotherapy alone, with a second randomization to either S-1 versus S-1 plus oxaliplatin, versus chemoradiation.[34]

With the success of trastuzumab in the treatment of HER2-overexpressing tumors in the metastatic setting, there are several studies examining the role of targeting HER2 in the neoadjuvant setting in patients with resectable gastric cancer. A pilot study within the MAGIC-B study is enrolling 40 patients with HER2-overexpressing gastric cancer and randomizing to ECX ± lapatinib; patients are still being accrued.[43] The INNOVATION study, conducted by the EORTC, is randomizing patients to 3 neoadjuvant treatment arms (1:2:2) as follows: standard chemotherapy (cisplatin/capecitabine or cisplatin/5-FU), experimental arm 1 (cisplatin/capecitabine plus trastuzumab or cisplatin/5-FU plus trastuzumab), or experimental arm 2 (cisplatin/capecitabine plus trastuzumab plus pertuzumab or cisplatin/5-FU plus trastuzumab plus pertuzumab).[44] The ongoing RTOG 1010 is evaluating the role of trastuzumab in localized esophageal/gastroesophageal cancer. Patients with HER2-overexpressing tumors are being randomized to standard neoadjuvant chemoradiation with carboplatin/paclitaxel (CROSS regimen) or similar regimen plus trastuzumab.[45] The phase II TOXAG study is evaluating the use of trastuzumab in the adjuvant setting. Patients with resected gastric or gastroesophageal cancer with stage IB or higher disease will receive 3 cycles of

Name	Random?	Study Arms	N	Primary Outcome (s)
Table 5 Ongoing studies				
Perioperative therapy				
MAGIC-B NCT00450203	Yes	ECX → Surgery → ECX ECX-Bev → Surgery → ECX-Bev	1103	Safety Efficacy Overall survival
TOPGEAR NCT01924819	Yes	ECF → Surgery → ECF ECF + 5-FU/RT → Surgery → ECF	752	Overall survival
MAGIC-B *Her2+ pilot* NCT00450203	Yes	ECX → Surgery → ECX ECX-Lapatinib → Surgery → ECX-Lapatinib	40	Safety Efficacy Overall survival
Neoadjuvant therapy				
RTOG 1010 *Her2+* NCT01196390	Yes	Carbo/Taxol/RT → Surgery Carbo/Taxol/Trastuzumab → Surgery	591	Disease-free survival
INNOVATION *Her2+* NCT02205047	Yes (1:2:2)	FP/Cisplatin FP/Cisplatin + trastuzumab FP/Cisplatin + trastuzumab + pertuzumab	220	Near complete pathologic response rate
Adjuvant therapy				
ARTIST II NCT01761461	Yes	S1 × 8 cycles S1/oxaliplatin × 8 cycles S1/oxaliplatin × 2 cycles → S1/RT to 45 Gy → S1/oxaliplatin × 4 cycles	900	Disease-free survival
TOXAG *Her2+* NCT01748773	No	Cape/oxaliplatin/trastuzumab × 3 cycles followed by Cape/RT to 40 Gy	35	Safety

Abbreviations: ARTIST, Adjuvant Chemoradiation Therapy in Stomach Cancer; Bev, bevacizumab; Cape, capecitabine; Carbo, carboplatin; ECF, epirubicin, cisplatin, 5-fluorouracil; ECX, epirubicin, cisplatin, capecitabine; FP, fluoropyrimidine; MAGIC, Medical Research Council Adjuvant Gastric Infusional Chemotherapy; RT, radiation therapy; RTOG, Radiation Therapy Oncology Group.

capecitabine, oxaliplatin, and trastuzumab followed by chemoradiation to a total dose of 45 Gy.[46] Each of these ongoing studies addresses an important question and the results will inform practice in years to come.

DISCUSSION

Poor long-term outcomes for patients with gastric cancer have motivated research exploring numerous treatment strategies. Although curative resection is the mainstay of treatment for gastric cancer, patients who undergo surgery have high rates of both local and distant recurrence. Caring for these patients is complicated and warrants evaluation by a multidisciplinary team. All members of the multidisciplinary team, including medical oncology, radiation oncology, and surgical oncology, should evaluate the patient and determine the treatment plan. The first step is appropriate staging, including cross-sectional imaging and EUS. In patients with bulky or node-positive disease, we also consider diagnostic laparoscopy so that we can identify those patients who will not benefit from local therapy.

In the small group of patients with early-stage disease defined as ≤T1bN0 by EUS, we favor upfront surgery. Patients found to have stage II or greater disease at the time of surgical resection are generally treated with adjuvant chemoradiation in the United States, based on INT-0116; given risk of distant recurrence, we consider additional adjuvant chemotherapy (typically 5-FU/platinum-based) after chemoradiation. Treatment of T2N0 disease (stage IB) remains more controversial.

In patients with more advanced disease on EUS, multidisciplinary evaluation is imperative. In many European countries, these patients are generally treated with a course of perioperative chemotherapy. At our institution, we favor upfront chemotherapy for those patients with bulky primary tumors or node positivity on EUS. We typically pursue 2 to 4 months of 5-FU/platinum-based systemic chemotherapy before restaging. If patients can tolerate a triplet regimen, we use epirubicin, oxaliplatin, and capecitabine (EOX), a modification of ECF shown to be noninferior in the REAL-2 study.[47] In elderly or very symptomatic patients, we favor doublet chemotherapy with 5-FU and oxaliplatin on the modified FOLFOX-6 platform. If there is no evidence of metastatic disease on repeat imaging, we then consider surgical resection versus chemoradiation. Our institutional bias is toward neoadjuvant chemoradiation due to the ability to clearly identify the target volume, potentially allowing for smaller treatment fields, undisrupted vasculature, which maximizes therapeutic effect, higher rates of treatment completion compared with adjuvant delivery, and irradiation of microscopic disease extension to facilitate a margin-negative resection with tumor and nodal downstaging. For those patients who receive both induction chemotherapy and chemoradiation in the neoadjuvant setting, the decision to pursue adjuvant therapy depends on performance status in the postoperative setting as well as the pathologic stage and nodal status, although our bias is toward additional 5-FU/platinum-based chemotherapy (ie, modified FOLFOX-6). We await results of ongoing studies, as the data are certain to guide clinical practice moving forward.

REFERENCES

1. Siegel RL, Miller KD, Jemal A. Cancer statistics, 2016. CA Cancer J Clin 2016; 66(1):7–30.
2. Hundahl SA, Phillips JL, Menck HR. The National Cancer Data Base Report on poor survival of U.S. gastric carcinoma patients treated with gastrectomy: Fifth Edition American Joint Committee on Cancer staging, proximal disease, and the "different disease" hypothesis. Cancer 2000;88(4):921–32.
3. Yun M, Lim JS, Noh SH, et al. Lymph node staging of gastric cancer using (18)F-FDG PET: a comparison study with CT. J Nucl Med 2005;46(10):1582–8.
4. Roviello F, Rossi S, Marrelli D, et al. Number of lymph node metastases and its prognostic significance in early gastric cancer: a multicenter Italian study. J Surg Oncol 2006;94(4):275–80 [discussion: 274].
5. Simon M, Mal F, Perniceni T, et al. Accuracy of staging laparoscopy in detecting peritoneal dissemination in patients with gastroesophageal adenocarcinoma. Dis Esophagus 2016;29(3):236–40.
6. Cunningham D, Allum WH, Stenning SP, et al. Perioperative chemotherapy versus surgery alone for resectable gastroesophageal cancer. N Engl J Med 2006; 355(1):11–20.
7. Ychou M, Boige V, Pignon JP, et al. Perioperative chemotherapy compared with surgery alone for resectable gastroesophageal adenocarcinoma: an FNCLCC and FFCD multicenter phase III trial. J Clin Oncol 2011;29(13):1715–21.
8. Schuhmacher C, Gretschel S, Lordick F, et al. Neoadjuvant chemotherapy compared with surgery alone for locally advanced cancer of the stomach and

cardia: European Organisation for Research and Treatment of Cancer randomized trial 40954. J Clin Oncol 2010;28(35):5210–8.

9. Xiong BH, Cheng Y, Ma L, et al. An updated meta-analysis of randomized controlled trial assessing the effect of neoadjuvant chemotherapy in advanced gastric cancer. Cancer Invest 2014;32(6):272–84.

10. Zhang ZX, Gu XZ, Yin WB, et al. Randomized clinical trial on the combination of preoperative irradiation and surgery in the treatment of adenocarcinoma of gastric cardia (AGC)–report on 370 patients. Int J Radiat Oncol Biol Phys 1998;42(5):929–34.

11. Ajani JA, Mansfield PF, Janjan N, et al. Multi-institutional trial of preoperative chemoradiotherapy in patients with potentially resectable gastric carcinoma. J Clin Oncol 2004;22(14):2774–80.

12. Ajani JA, Winter K, Okawara GS, et al. Phase II trial of preoperative chemoradiation in patients with localized gastric adenocarcinoma (RTOG 9904): quality of combined modality therapy and pathologic response. J Clin Oncol 2006;24(24): 3953–8.

13. van Hagen P, Hulshof MC, van Lanschot JJ, et al. Preoperative chemoradiotherapy for esophageal or junctional cancer. N Engl J Med 2012;366(22):2074–84.

14. Stahl M, Walz MK, Stuschke M, et al. Phase III comparison of preoperative chemotherapy compared with chemoradiotherapy in patients with locally advanced adenocarcinoma of the esophagogastric junction. J Clin Oncol 2009;27(6):851–6.

15. A Randomised Phase II/III Trial of Preoperative Chemoradiotherapy Versus Preoperative Chemotherapy for Resectable Gastric Cancer. Available at: https://clinicaltrials.gov/ct2/show/NCT01924819. Accessed August 19, 2016.

16. Group G, Paoletti X, Oba K, et al. Benefit of adjuvant chemotherapy for resectable gastric cancer: a meta-analysis. JAMA 2010;303(17):1729–37.

17. Sasako M, Sakuramoto S, Katai H, et al. Five-year outcomes of a randomized phase III trial comparing adjuvant chemotherapy with S-1 versus surgery alone in stage II or III gastric cancer. J Clin Oncol 2011;29(33):4387–93.

18. Bang YJ, Kim YW, Yang HK, et al. Adjuvant capecitabine and oxaliplatin for gastric cancer after D2 gastrectomy (CLASSIC): a phase 3 open-label, randomised controlled trial. Lancet 2012;379(9813):315–21.

19. Noh SH, Park SR, Yang HK, et al. Adjuvant capecitabine plus oxaliplatin for gastric cancer after D2 gastrectomy (CLASSIC): 5-year follow-up of an open-label, randomised phase 3 trial. Lancet Oncol 2014;15(12):1389–96.

20. Gill S, Shah A, Le N, et al. Asian ethnicity-related differences in gastric cancer presentation and outcome among patients treated at a Canadian cancer center. J Clin Oncol 2003;21(11):2070–6.

21. Strong VE, Song KY, Park CH, et al. Comparison of gastric cancer survival following R0 resection in the United States and Korea using an internationally validated nomogram. Ann Surg 2010;251(4):640–6.

22. Wanebo HJ, Kennedy BJ, Chmiel J, et al. Cancer of the stomach. A patient care study by the American College of Surgeons. Ann Surg 1993;218(5):583–92.

23. Earle CC, Maroun JA. Adjuvant chemotherapy after curative resection for gastric cancer in non-Asian patients: revisiting a meta-analysis of randomised trials. Eur J Cancer 1999;35(7):1059–64.

24. Macdonald JS, Smalley SR, Benedetti J, et al. Chemoradiotherapy after surgery compared with surgery alone for adenocarcinoma of the stomach or gastroesophageal junction. N Engl J Med 2001;345(10):725–30.

25. Smalley SR, Benedetti JK, Haller DG, et al. Updated analysis of SWOG-directed intergroup study 0116: a phase III trial of adjuvant radiochemotherapy versus

observation after curative gastric cancer resection. J Clin Oncol 2012;30(19): 2327–33.

26. Noguchi Y, Yoshikawa T, Tsuburaya A, et al. Is gastric carcinoma different between Japan and the United States? Cancer 2000;89(11):2237–46.

27. Noel G, Jauffret E, Mazeron JJ. Randomized clinical trial on the combination of preoperative irradiation and surgery in the treatment of adenocarcinoma of gastric cardia (AGC)–report on 370 patients. Cancer Radiother 1999;3(4):344 [in French].

28. Bamias A, Karina M, Papakostas P, et al. A randomized phase III study of adjuvant platinum/docetaxel chemotherapy with or without radiation therapy in patients with gastric cancer. Cancer Chemother Pharmacol 2010;65(6):1009–21.

29. Kim TH, Park SR, Ryu KW, et al. Phase 3 trial of postoperative chemotherapy alone versus chemoradiation therapy in stage III-IV gastric cancer treated with R0 gastrectomy and D2 lymph node dissection. Int J Radiat Oncol Biol Phys 2012;84(5):e585–92.

30. Kwon HC, Kim MC, Kim KH, et al. Adjuvant chemoradiation versus chemotherapy in completely resected advanced gastric cancer with D2 nodal dissection. Asia Pac J Clin Oncol 2010;6(4):278–85.

31. Park SH, Sohn TS, Lee J, et al. Phase III trial to compare adjuvant chemotherapy with capecitabine and cisplatin versus concurrent chemoradiotherapy in gastric cancer: final report of the adjuvant chemoradiotherapy in stomach tumors trial, including survival and subset analyses. J Clin Oncol 2015;33(28):3130–6.

32. Yu C, Yu R, Zhu W, et al. Intensity-modulated radiotherapy combined with chemotherapy for the treatment of gastric cancer patients after standard D1/D2 surgery. J Cancer Res Clin Oncol 2012;138(2):255–9.

33. Zhu WG, Xua DF, Pu J, et al. A randomized, controlled, multicenter study comparing intensity-modulated radiotherapy plus concurrent chemotherapy with chemotherapy alone in gastric cancer patients with D2 resection. Radiother Oncol 2012;104(3):361–6.

34. Phase III randomized trial of adjuvant chemotherapy with S-1 vs S-1/oxaliplatin ± radiotherapy for completely resected gastric adenocarcinoma: the ARTIST II Trial (ARTIST-II). Available at: https://clinicaltrials.gov/ct2/show/NCT01761461. Accessed August 19, 2016.

35. Verheji M, Cats A, Jansen EPM, et al. A multicenter randomized phase III trial of neo-adjuvant chemotherapy followed by surgery and chemotherapy or by surgery and chemoradiotherapy in resectable gastric cancer: first results from the CRITICS study. J Clin Oncol 2016;34(Suppl) [Abstract 4000].

36. Randomized Phase III Trial of Adjuvant Chemotherapy or Chemoradiotherapy in Resectable Gastric Cancer (CRITICS). Available at: https://clinicaltrials.gov/ct2/show/NCT00407186. Accessed August 19, 2016.

37. Cascinu S, Scartozzi M, Labianca R, et al. High curative resection rate with weekly cisplatin, 5-fluorouracil, epidoxorubicin, 6S-leucovorin, glutathione, and filgastrim in patients with locally advanced, unresectable gastric cancer: a report from the Italian Group for the Study of Digestive Tract Cancer (GISCAD). Br J Cancer 2004;90(8):1521–5.

38. Gallardo-Rincon D, Onate-Ocana LF, Calderillo-Ruiz G. Neoadjuvant chemotherapy with P-ELF (cisplatin, etoposide, leucovorin, 5-fluorouracil) followed by radical resection in patients with initially unresectable gastric adenocarcinoma: a phase II study. Ann Surg Oncol 2000;7(1):45–50.

39. Nakajima T, Ota K, Ishihara S, et al. Combined intensive chemotherapy and radical surgery for incurable gastric cancer. Ann Surg Oncol 1997;4(3):203–8.

40. Yoshikawa T, Sasako M, Yamamoto S, et al. Phase II study of neoadjuvant chemotherapy and extended surgery for locally advanced gastric cancer. Br J Surg 2009;96(9):1015–22.
41. Tey J, Choo BA, Leong CN, et al. Clinical outcome of palliative radiotherapy for locally advanced symptomatic gastric cancer in the modern era. Medicine (Baltimore) 2014;93(22):e118.
42. Asakura H, Hashimoto T, Harada H, et al. Palliative radiotherapy for bleeding from advanced gastric cancer: is a schedule of 30 Gy in 10 fractions adequate? J Cancer Res Clin Oncol 2011;137(1):125–30.
43. A Randomised Phase II/III Trial of Peri-Operative Chemotherapy With or Without Bevacizumab in Operable Oesophagogastric Adenocarcinoma. Available at: https://clinicaltrials.gov/ct2/show/NCT00450203. Accessed August 19, 2016.
44. Neoadjuvant Study Using Trastuzumab or Trastuzumab With Pertuzumab in Gastric or Gastroesophageal Junction Adenocarcinoma (INNOVATION). Available at: https://clinicaltrials.gov/ct2/show/NCT02205047.
45. Radiation Therapy, Paclitaxel, and Carboplatin With or Without Trastuzumab in Treating Patients With Esophageal Cancer. Available at: https://clinicaltrials.gov/ct2/show/NCT01196390.
46. A Study of the Combination of Oxaliplatin, Capecitabine and Herceptin (Trastuzumab) and Chemoradiotherapy in The Adjuvant Setting in Operated Patients With HER2+ Gastric or Gastro-Esophageal Junction Cancer (TOXAG Study). Available at: https://clinicaltrials.gov/ct2/show/NCT01748773.
47. Cunningham D, Starling N, Rao S, et al. Capecitabine and oxaliplatin for advanced esophagogastric cancer. N Engl J Med 2008;358(1):36–46.

Management of Gastrointestinal Stromal Tumors

Emily Z. Keung, MD[a], Chandrajit P. Raut, MD, MSc[b,c],*

KEYWORDS

- Gastrointestinal stromal tumor • GIST • Gastric mass • Abdominal tumor
- Tyrosine kinase inhibitor • TKIs • Imatinib • Sunitinib

KEY POINTS

- Gastrointestinal stromal tumors (GISTs) are the most common mesenchymal neoplasms of the gastrointestinal tract, most commonly arising in the stomach.
- The introduction of effective molecularly targeted tyrosine kinase inhibitors (TKIs) significantly improved the prognosis of patients with GIST.
- Surgery is indicated for primary resectable GIST. Recurrence is common; patients at intermediate or high risk of recurrence should receive imatinib postoperatively.
- The standard of care for unresectable or recurrent disease is TKI therapy with first-line imatinib, second-line sunitinib, and third-line regorafenib.
- Cytoreductive surgery may be considered in recurrent GIST in carefully selected patients on TKI therapy, following a multidisciplinary approach.

INTRODUCTION

Gastrointestinal stromal tumors (GISTs) are rare neoplasms, accounting for 0.1% to 3% of all gastrointestinal malignancies.[1,2] The most common mesenchymal tumors of the gastrointestinal tract, GISTs have an annual incidence of 10 to 15 per million people and as many as 5000 to 6000 new cases in the United States each year.[2–6] GISTs can arise anywhere along the gastrointestinal tract, but develop most commonly in the stomach and small intestine as a result of activating mutations in *KIT* (*CD117*) or *PDGFRA*, genes encoding receptor protein tyrosine kinases.[3] Over

Disclosure: The authors have nothing to disclose.
[a] Department of Surgical Oncology, The University of Texas MD Anderson Cancer Center, 1400 Pressler Street, Unit 1484, Houston, TX 77030, USA; [b] Department of Surgery, Brigham and Women's Hospital, 75 Francis Street, Boston, MA 02115, USA; [c] Center for Sarcoma and Bone Oncology, Dana-Farber Cancer Institute, 450 Brookline Avenue, Boston, MA 02115, USA
* Corresponding author. Center for Sarcoma and Bone Oncology, Dana-Farber Cancer Institute, 450 Brookline Avenue, Boston, MA 02115.
E-mail address: craut@partners.org

Surg Clin N Am 97 (2017) 437–452
http://dx.doi.org/10.1016/j.suc.2016.12.001
0039-6109/17/© 2016 Elsevier Inc. All rights reserved.

surgical.theclinics.com

the past 2 decades, remarkable advances have been made in the understanding of GISTs. The identification of key signaling transduction pathways and the development of molecularly targeted therapies has dramatically changed management of GISTs and improved patient prognosis.

EPIDEMIOLOGY

The median age at diagnosis is 60 years with no gender, racial, or ethnic predilection.[2,3,7,8] Although GISTs can be secondary to germline *KIT* or *PDGFRA* mutations[9,10] or as part of familial syndromes (including von Recklinghausen neurofibromatosis [NF1]),[11] Carney triad,[12] or Carney-Stratakis syndrome[13]), most are sporadic.

CLINICAL PRESENTATION

GISTs most commonly arise in the stomach (50%–60%) and small bowel (20%–35%); less common primary sites include colon, rectum, duodenum, and esophagus.[2,3,6] Most present as a single, well-circumscribed nodule with a median size of approximately 5 cm at presentation. GISTs are generally centered on the bowel wall but may form polypoid serosal-based or mucosal-based masses. Mucosal ulceration is often associated with gastrointestinal bleeding.[3]

Two-thirds of GISTs present with symptoms related to the gastrointestinal tract, including those caused by mass effect exerted by tumor within the abdominal cavity (vague abdominal discomfort, dysphagia, early satiety, palpable mass, bowel obstruction, intestinal perforation) and bleeding (anemia, gastrointestinal bleeding).[2,4,6] The remainder are discovered incidentally, during surgery for other conditions or at autopsy.[8]

Approximately 15% to 47% of patients present with overt metastatic disease; common sites of metastasis include liver, peritoneum, and omentum.[4,6,14] Lymph node metastases are rare, usually occurring only in pediatric forms of the disease. Unlike other sarcomas, lung and bone metastases are rare and occur late in the disease course, if at all.

DIAGNOSIS
Radiographic Studies

The initial imaging study for a suspected or confirmed GIST is contrast-enhanced computed tomography (CT) of the abdomen and pelvis to characterize an abdominal mass and assess for the presence of metastasis at the initial staging work-up. Primary GISTs are typically well-circumscribed masses within the walls of hollow viscera. MRI may help characterize metastatic liver or primary perirectal disease. PET has no defined role in the evaluation of primary disease.[2,3]

Preoperative Biopsy and Endoscopy

A preoperative biopsy is not routinely necessary for a primary, resectable neoplasm suspicious for GIST if it is easily resectable and preoperative therapy is not required. Biopsy may be needed if preoperative therapy is being considered to downstage the scope of surgery (eg, from laparotomy to laparoscopy) (**Fig. 1**), for unresectable or marginally resectable tumors, or if the differential diagnosis includes entities (eg, lymphoma) that would be treated differently.[2,3] For suspected GISTs arising in the esophagus, duodenum, or rectum, where surgical management may drastically differ based on diagnosis, pretreatment diagnosis is recommended.

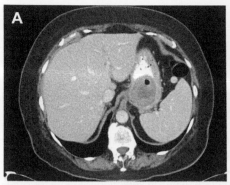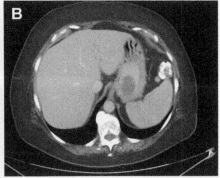

Fig. 1. GIST at gastroesophageal junction (GEJ). (*A*) A 6-cm GIST at the GEJ was treated with neoadjuvant imatinib to facilitate sparing of GEJ after a confirmatory biopsy. Intratumoral air was noted at presentation, caused by mucosal ulceration over the tumor. However, neoadjuvant imatinib was safely tolerated. (*B*) Tumor shrank sufficiently to enable a laparoscopic transgastric resection.

Endoscopically, a primary GIST may appear as a submucosal lesion with or without ulceration in the upper or lower gastrointestinal tract. Although there are reports of endoscopic treatment of small gastric GIST (<3 cm), this remains controversial because of concerns about the risk of perforation, incomplete resection, and tumor spillage.[15–18]

Obtaining adequate tumor tissue for definitive diagnosis can be challenging. GISTs are often soft and friable; preoperative biopsy may rupture a suspected GIST, increasing the risk of dissemination. Endoscopic ultrasonography (EUS)–guided fine-needle aspiration may be attempted. Although not consistently diagnostic, it is the generally favored approach for gastric and, in some cases, proximal small bowel GISTs when a diagnosis is needed. Transrectal biopsy may be feasible for presumed rectal GISTs.

CELLULAR AND MOLECULAR CLASSIFICATIONS OF GASTROINTESTINAL STROMAL TUMORS

In a landmark article, Hirota and colleagues[19] reported near-universal expression of KIT and activating gain-of-function *c-KIT* mutations in GISTs. These findings led to the use of molecularly targeted drug therapies such as imatinib mesylate (Gleevec, Novartis), which targets and inhibits the activated KIT receptor tyrosine kinase.[20–22]

More than 85% of GISTs have activating *KIT* mutations; these commonly occur in exon 11 (57%–71%), exon 9 (10%–18%), exon 13 (1%–4%), and exon 17 (1%–4%).[4,20,23,24] Of tumors lacking *KIT* mutations, ~80% have *PDGFRA* mutations and are more common in the stomach and omentum.[3] Most *PDGFRA* mutations affect exon 18, and less commonly exons 12 and 14.[3,4,24–26] A few GISTs, termed wild-type GISTs, show no detectable *KIT* or *PDGFRA* mutations and presumably have alternative pathways for pathogenesis.[27] These mutations include succinate dehydrogenase–deficient GISTs[27–30] and GISTs with *BRAF* mutations.[31]

The diagnosis of GIST is made on pathologic analysis of tumor specimens. The cellular morphology of GISTs are in 3 categories: spindle cell (70%), epithelioid (20%), or mixed (10%) types.[3,4,23] KIT, DOG1, and CD34 are key immunohistochemical markers to diagnose GIST.[3–5] Although 95% of GISTs express KIT, 5% of GISTs lack expression. DOG1, a calcium-dependent receptor-activated chloride channel protein, is a more sensitive marker for GIST than KIT, detecting 36% of KIT-negative GISTs.[4,5]

PROGNOSTIC FACTORS

The 3 established prognostic factors are tumor size, mitotic index, and tumor site of origin (Table 1).[20,32,33] Additional negative prognostic factors reported in some studies include KIT exon 9 mutations[32] and KIT exon 11 deletions involving amino acid W557 and/or K558.[24,32,34–36] Point mutations and insertions of KIT exon 11 seem to have a favorable prognosis.[32] At present, mutational analysis is not routinely recommended at initial diagnosis.[3,4] However, genotyping may become integral to the clinical management of GIST in the future, aiding in prognostication and selection of drug therapy and dosing (Fig. 2).[30] Mutational analysis may be useful in selecting patients for postoperative therapy after complete resection of primary GIST, such as to identify patients at higher risk for recurrence if considering postoperative imatinib therapy (Table 2).[3,37–39] Mutational analysis should be considered for metastatic or advanced disease; KIT exon 11 mutations are associated with higher response rates and longer progression-free survival (PFS) than KIT exon 9 mutations.[37] Exon 9 mutations are rare in gastric GISTs, thus mutational analysis should only be considered in gastric GISTs unresponsive to imatinib.[3,4]

TREATMENT OF RESECTABLE PRIMARY DISEASE
Surgery

All GISTs 2 cm or larger should be resected,[33] as should any smaller GISTs that are symptomatic (eg, gastrointestinal bleeding) or increase in size on follow-up. For patients with localized resectable GISTs, macroscopically complete (R0/R1) resection remains the standard and only potentially curative treatment.[6,40] A wedge or segmental resection of the involved stomach or bowel is generally sufficient because primary GISTs tend to displace rather than invade adjacent structures/organs beyond the site of origin. However, tumor location may determine the extent or type of operation (Fig. 3). The goal of surgery is to achieve negative microscopic margins (R0 resection), although there is no evidence to suggest that patients who have

Table 1
Risk assessment for primary gastrointestinal stromal tumors

| Mitotic Rate | Tumor Size (cm) | Patients with Progressive Disease/Risk Classification, Based on Site of Origin (%) | | | |
		Stomach	Duodenum	Jejunum/Ileum	Rectum
≤5/50 HPF	≤2	0	0	0	0
	>2, ≤5	1.9/very low	8.3/low	4.3/low	8.5/low
	>5, ≤10	3.6/low	a	24/moderate	a
	>10	12/moderate	34/high	52/high	57/high
>5/50 HPF	≤2	a	a	a	54/high
	>2, ≤5	15/moderate	50/high	73/high	52/high
	>5, ≤10	55/high	a	85/high	a
	>10	86/high	86/high	90/high	71/high

Abbreviation: HPF, high-power field.
a Insufficient data.
Adapted from Miettinen M, Lasota J. Gastrointestinal stromal tumors: pathology and prognosis at different sites. Sem Diagn Pathol 2006;23:75; with permission.

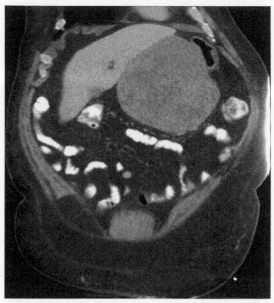

Fig. 2. Large gastric GIST. Although neoadjuvant therapy would have been ideal, this patient's GIST had a *PDGFRA* exon 18 D842V mutation that was imatinib insensitive. Therefore, the patient underwent an open partial gastrectomy.

undergone R1 resection with microscopically positive margins require reexcision.[3] McCarter and colleagues[41] reviewed outcomes among 819 patients who underwent primary GIST resection from the American College of Surgeons Oncology Group (ACOSOG) Z9000 and Z9001 clinical trials and found no difference in recurrence-free survival (RFS) for patients undergoing R1 versus R0 resection, with or without adjuvant imatinib. However, tumor rupture or tumor capsule violation during resection is associated with an increased risk of recurrence.[2] Because GISTs do not typically spread to lymph nodes in adults, lymphadenectomy is not warranted.

Management of GISTs less than 2 cm is still debated. Given the more aggressive behavior of GISTs of the small bowel and colon, tumors of any size in these locations should be resected. However, small gastric GISTs are common. Subcentimeter gastric GISTs were found in 22.5% of autopsies in adults more than 50 years old in Germany[42] and microscopic gastric GISTs were found in 35% of patients undergoing gastrectomy for gastric cancer in Japan.[43] Few seem to become clinically relevant, thus management of these small tumors is uncertain. National Comprehensive Cancer Network (NCCN) guidelines recommend surgical resection for gastric GISTs less than 2 cm with high-risk features on EUS (irregular border, cystic spaces, ulceration, echogenic foci, heterogeneity) followed by surveillance with abdominal/pelvic CT with contrast every 3 to 6 months for 3 to 5 years, then annually.[3]

In the preimatinib era, RFS at 1, 2, and 5 years among 127 patients at the Memorial Sloan Kettering Cancer Center with completely resected primary GIST was 83%, 75%, and 63%.[32] Recurrence was associated with increased mitotic rate (>5/50 high-power field [HPF]), tumor size (>10 cm), and tumor location (small bowel, hazard ratio [HR], 3.3 relative to gastric). These findings are consistent with those of pooled population-based cohorts reported by Joensuu and colleagues[44] in 2012. In addition, tumor rupture was reported to be associated with poor patient outcomes.

Table 2
KIT and PDGFRA genotype and response to imatinib in published clinical trials

Gene	Exon	US-Finnish B222 Phase II Trial (n = 127)[36]				EORTC-62005 Phase III Trial (n = 377)[35]				SWOGS0033/CALGB150105 Phase III Trial (N = 428)[37]			
		Objective Response (%)[a]	Stable Disease (%)	Progressive Disease (%)	Not Assessable (%)	Objective Response (%)[a]	Stable Disease (%)	Progressive Disease (%)	Not Assessable (%)	Objective Response (%)[a]	Stable Disease (%)	Progressive Disease (%)	Not Assessable (%)
KIT	9	47.8	26.1	17.4	8.7	34.5	46.6	17.2	1.7	37.5	37.5	9.4	15.6
	11	83.5	8.2	4.7	3.5	67.8	25.4	3.2	3.6	63.6	18.7	6.4	11.3
	13	100	0	0	0	66.7	33.3	0	0	40	20	20	20
	17	50	0	50	0	66.7	33.4	0	0	25	50	25	0
PDGRFA	12	66.7	0	33.3	0	30	30	40	0	100	0	0	0
	18	0	0	66.7	33.3					25	50	25	0
WT-GIST	—	0	33.3	55.6	11.1	23.1	50	19.2	7.7	37.3	28.4	17.9	16.4

Abbreviations: CALGB, Cancer and Leukemia Group B; EORTC, European Organisation for Research And Treatment of Cancer; GIST, gastrointestinal stromal tumor; NR, not reported; SWOG, Southwest Oncology Group; WT, wild type (no *KIT* or *PDGFRA* mutation).

[a] Complete or partial response by RECIST (Response Evaluation Criteria for Solid Tumors) criteria.

Adapted from Demetri GD, von Mehren M, Antonescu CR, et al. NCCN Task Force report: update on the management of patients with gastrointestinal stromal tumors. J Natl Compr Canc Netw 2010;8(Suppl 2):S1–7; with permission.

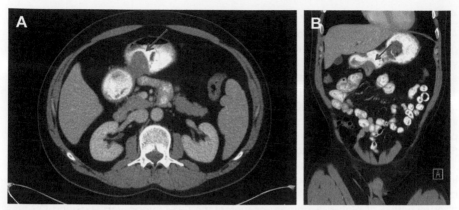

Fig. 3. (*A, B*) Prepyloric gastric GIST (*red arrows*). Gastric GIST was suspected based on radiographic and endoscopic findings in this patient presenting with symptomatic anemia from an upper gastrointestinal bleeding episode. No preoperative biopsy was performed, because neoadjuvant therapy would not have altered management. Laparoscopic wedge resection would have narrowed the pyloric channel. Therefore, laparoscopic distal gastrectomy with Billroth II gastrojejunostomy was performed. Tumor measured 5 cm with a low mitotic count. Adjuvant imatinib was not recommended.

The role of laparoscopic resection of gastric GISTs continues to expand, although data on laparoscopic resection of GISTs at other anatomic sites are limited. Two early studies showed the safety and feasibility of this approach.[45,46] Otani and colleagues[46] reported a series of 35 gastric GISTs (2–5 cm) resected laparoscopically with no local or distant recurrences seen for tumors less than 4 cm during a median follow-up of 53 months. Novitsky and colleagues[45] performed 50 laparoscopic or laparoscopic-assisted gastric GIST resections (1–8.5 cm), all with negative microscopic margins. At mean follow-up of 3 years, 92% of patients were disease free. Recent larger studies show no oncologic difference between laparoscopic versus open resection of gastric GISTs and report shorter hospital stays and low morbidity associated with laparoscopic resection.[47–51]

Neoadjuvant Therapy for Primary Disease

Neoadjuvant therapy may be considered for patients with large or unresectable tumors or poorly positioned small GISTs that are considered marginally resectable on technical grounds.[3,4,52–55] In select cases, neoadjuvant imatinib may also facilitate laparoscopic resection of GISTs that otherwise would require open resection (see **Fig. 1**).

The Radiation Therapy Oncology Group (RTOG) 0132 was the first prospective non-randomized phase II trial to evaluate the efficacy of neoadjuvant imatinib in patients with potentially resectable disease. Patients with advanced primary GIST (n = 30) and potentially operable metastatic/recurrent disease (n = 22) received imatinib 600 mg/d for 8 to 12 weeks.[52] Postoperatively imatinib was continued for 2 years. Neoadjuvant imatinib was well tolerated and the delay in time to surgery did not seem to have any adverse effects. RFS at 2 years was 82.6% and compared favorably with historical single-institutional surgical series for patients with intermediate-risk/high-risk GIST. However, it is unclear whether the RFS benefit seen among patients in RTOG 0132 was attributable to the 2 years of postoperative imatinib therapy or to the neoadjuvant imatinib.

Adjuvant Therapy for Primary Disease

Among patients with localized resectable GISTs at high risk of recurrence after surgery, multiple studies have shown improved RFS and overall survival (OS) with adjuvant imatinib.[28,56–58] The ACOSOG Z9000 multicenter, single-arm, phase 2 trial showed that 1 year of adjuvant imatinib prolonged RFS after complete resection in 106 patients with primary GIST at high risk of recurrence based on clinicopathologic factors.[58] The ACOSOG Z9001 phase 3 double-blind randomized trial showed increased RFS among patients treated with 1 year of adjuvant imatinib following complete resection of GISTs 3 cm or larger compared with patients who received placebo (97% 1-year RFS vs 83% placebo).[28]

More recently, several trials have evaluated the impact of duration of postoperative imatinib on RFS.[56,59,60] The Scandinavian/German SSG XVIII/AIO trial was a randomized, open-label trial of 1 year versus 3 years of postoperative imatinib at 400 mg daily after resection of high-risk primary or metastatic GIST. Improved RFS and OS was observed with 3 years of adjuvant imatinib treatment compared with 1 year among patients with primary resectable GIST with high-risk features (at least 1 of the following: tumor diameter >10 cm, mitotic count >10/50 HPFs, tumor diameter >5 cm and mitotic count >5/50 HPFs, or tumor rupture before or at surgery).[56]

In 2013, the European Organisation for Research and Treatment of Cancer (EORTC) 62024 phase III trial reported outcomes of patients with localized, surgically resected, high-risk/intermediate-risk GIST randomized to receive 2 years of postoperative imatinib versus no further therapy. The primary end point was originally OS but was modified in 2009 to imatinib-free survival (time to death or starting a tyrosine kinase inhibitor [TKI] other than imatinib).[59] Median follow-up was 4.7 years. Three-year and 5-year RFS were 87% and 69% in patients treated with imatinib following surgery compared with 66% and 63% in patients who underwent surgery alone.

Observation is the current standard of care for patients with primary GIST of low recurrence risk after complete macroscopic resection. Patients with primary GIST at intermediate or high risk of recurrence should be treated with imatinib for 3 years postoperatively. Those who received preoperative neoadjuvant imatinib should continue imatinib postoperatively for a cumulative 3-year course. The rationale for continuing all patients who receive neoadjuvant imatinib on adjuvant imatinib is that once a patient has been treated with neoadjuvant therapy, mitotic count is no longer reliable and patient risk for recurrence can no longer be assessed accurately. Therefore, the recommendation is to continue adjuvant imatinib to complete a total of 3 years of therapy (cumulative preoperative and postoperative course) under the assumption that risk of recurrence may have been intermediate or high at presentation. Dosing for imatinib is usually 400 mg/d, although patients with *KIT* exon 9 mutations may benefit from a dose of 800 mg/d, although this has not been confirmed prospectively. Patients who progress on the lower dose of imatinib may respond to dose escalation to 800 mg/ daily.[1,61]

TREATMENT OF ADVANCED/UNRESECTABLE PRIMARY, RECURRENT, OR METASTATIC DISEASE
Targeted Therapy

Although surgery is the treatment of choice and is effective for patients with resectable disease, recurrence is common and occurs in up to 50% of patients. However, conventional intravenous chemotherapy for advanced GIST is highly ineffective, with median survival of 10 to 20 months and 5-year survival less than 10%.[62] Since the introduction of imatinib in 2002, multiple studies have shown the efficacy of tyrosine kinase inhibition in GIST with manageable toxicities. In a landmark multicenter phase II study of 147 patients with advanced unresectable or metastatic GIST, imatinib (400 or 600 mg daily) showed impressive objective partial response (PR) rates of 53.7% and achieved stable disease (SD) in 27.9%. Overall median time to disease progression was 24 months and median OS was 57 months.[63]

The starting dose for imatinib is generally 400 mg once daily. Although initial therapy with a higher dose of imatinib confers a small PFS advantage, this is primarily in patients with KIT exon 9 mutations[64] and is associated with greater toxicity. Imatinib should be continued indefinitely, with multiple studies showing that patients with GIST on imatinib who stop imatinib therapy after 1 and 3 years had significantly higher rates of disease progression compared with those who continued on therapy.[65,66]

However, imatinib is not curative. Both primary and secondary drug resistance are well described and studied. Fourteen percent of GISTs have primary resistance to imatinib and progress within 6 months of initiating imatinib therapy. These tumors either lack mutations in KIT or PDGFRA or have a specific imatinib-resistant PDGFRA exon 18 D842V mutation. Secondary resistance occurs in patients who initially respond to imatinib and develops as a result of clonal evolution with accumulation of additional secondary mutations that render them resistant to the drug (most commonly in KIT exons 13, 14, 17, and 18).[67] Among patients who have an initial PR or SD with imatinib therapy, the median time to progression on first-line imatinib is 2 to 2.5 years.[61] In these patients who develop disease progression, dose escalation to imatinib 400 mg twice daily is effective.[68,69]

In patients who develop resistance and disease progression on imatinib at standard (400 mg daily) and higher (600 or 800 mg daily) dosing, sunitinib is started as second-line therapy. Sunitinib is a second-generation, multitargeted TKI that has shown significant improvement in time to progression compared with placebo in a phase III, double-blinded study of patients with advanced GISTs that had progressed on or were intolerant of imatinib.[70] The primary end point was time to tumor progression with secondary end points that included PFS and OS. Patients treated with sunitinib showed increased time to tumor progression compared with placebo (27.3 vs 6.4 weeks; HR, 0.33 [95% confidence interval, 0.23–0.47; P<.0001]). Initially dosed at 50 mg daily in a 4-weeks-on-2-weeks-off cycle, George and colleagues[71] showed that continuous daily dosing at 37.5 mg is as effective but better tolerated.

Regorafenib is third-line treatment of GIST based on phase III data showing improved PFS and disease control rate (disease control rate [DCR]; defined as rate of durable SD lasting >12 weeks plus complete response or PR) compared with placebo in patients with advanced GIST after imatinib and sunitinib failure (median PFS, 4.8 vs 0.9 months; DCR, 52.6% vs 9.1%).[72]

Patients failing existing lines of systemic treatment should be considered for protocol-based therapies.

Surgery

The current indications for considering cytoreductive surgery in recurrent or metastatic GIST include[3]:

1. For SD (disease that is stable or responsive to TKI therapy) when complete gross resection is possible
2. For limited disease progression (isolated clones progressing on TKI therapy after initial response, indicating secondary drug resistance)
3. For oncologic emergencies, including hemorrhage, perforation, obstruction, or abscess

Surgery alone

In the preimatinib era, surgical resection of metastatic GIST was associated with improved survival if R0/R1 resection could be achieved. Gold and Dematteo[7] reported a single-institution experience of 119 patients with metastatic GIST before the introduction of imatinib. Median OS was 19 months, with 41% and 25% 2-year and 5-year OS. Eighty-one patients (68%) underwent resection of metastatic GIST and 50 patients (42%) received conventional chemotherapy. Surgery was associated with improved median OS (27 vs 8 months) and longer 2-year OS (53%), with the best outcomes observed among patients in whom R0 resection had been achieved at some point in their disease course (median OS, 61 months; 2-year and 5-year OS, 84% and 52%).

Surgery after treatment with imatinib

With the introduction of imatinib and the marked improvement in patient outcomes associated with its use in metastatic GIST, multiple groups have examined the question of whether patients with metastatic GIST on imatinib would benefit further from surgery. Although 2 clinical trials to address this question were started (NCT00956072 in Europe, ChiCTR-TRC-00000244 in China), both failed to recruit fast enough to meet target accrual. However, multiple retrospective studies have consistently reported that patients whose disease responds to imatinib treatment benefit more from cytoreductive surgery than those with disease progression on imatinib.[73–85] Cytoreduction before initiation of imatinib offers no benefit.[86]

Maximal response to imatinib is typically achieved within 2 to 6 months after treatment initiation, with a median time to recurrence/progression on imatinib of less than 2 years. Although the benefit of surgery in selected patients with metastatic GIST after treatment with imatinib has not been proved in a randomized clinical trial, surgery should be considered in patients whose disease is rendered resectable on medical therapy.[1,3] The authors and others recommend considering cytoreductive surgery of residual metastatic disease no earlier than 6 months after TKI initiation (to confirm whether patients have PR or SD) and preferably no later than 2 years after TKI initiation.[77,80,83,87] The best candidates for surgery among patients with metastatic GIST are those with tumors that are stable or responsive to TKI therapy, fewer metastatic foci, and the possibility of a macroscopically complete resection. Imatinib can be given to patients up until 24 hours before surgery and restarted as early as possible postoperatively once the patient is tolerating a regular diet (because imatinib should be given with food).[3]

Surgery after treatment with sunitinib

The impact of surgery in patients with imatinib-resistant GIST on sunitinib is unclear. Raut and colleagues[84] showed that cytoreductive surgery on sunitinib in heavily pretreated patients is feasible (R0/R1 resection achieved in 25 of 50 patients), although incomplete resections were frequent and complication rates were high. Sunitinib is stopped 5 to 7 days before surgery and restarted 2 weeks postoperatively.[3] As always, patient selection is important.

SURVEILLANCE

The NCCN consensus panel recommends that patients who have had resection of a primary GIST undergo a history, physical examination, and abdomen/pelvis CT scans with intravenous contrast every 3 to 6 months during the first 3 to 5 years and then annually thereafter.[2,3]

SUMMARY

Remarkable advances have been made in the management of GIST over the preceding 2 decades. Surgery remains the only potentially curative treatment of GIST when complete resection (R0/R1) can be achieved. Although TKI therapy has dramatically improved patient prognosis, development of drug resistance is common and new drugs are needed. The optimal management of GIST requires multidisciplinary management involving medical oncology, surgical oncology, and radiologic and pathology expertise at both initial evaluation and follow-up.

REFERENCES

1. Keung EZ, Fairweather M, Raut CP. The role of surgery in metastatic gastrointestinal stromal tumors. Curr Treat Options Oncol 2016;17(2):8.
2. Raut CP. Gastrointestinal stromal tumors. In: Zinner MJ, Ashley SW, editors. Maingot's abdominal operations. 12th edition. New York: McGraw-Hill; 2013. p. 493–505.
3. Demetri GD, von Mehren M, Antonescu CR, et al. NCCN Task Force report: update on the management of patients with gastrointestinal stromal tumors. J Natl Compr Cancer Netw 2010;8(Suppl 2):S1–41.
4. Ho MY, Blanke CD. Gastrointestinal stromal tumors: disease and treatment update. Gastroenterology 2011;140(5):1372–6.e2.
5. Maki RG, Blay J-Y, Demetri GD, et al. Key issues in the clinical management of gastrointestinal stromal tumors: an expert discussion. Oncologist 2015;20: 823–30.
6. Quek R, George S. Gastrointestinal stromal tumor: a clinical overview. Hematol Oncol Clin North Am 2009;23(1):69–78.
7. Gold JS, Dematteo RP. Combined surgical and molecular therapy: the gastrointestinal stromal tumor model. Ann Surg 2006;244(2):176–84.
8. Nilsson B, Bumming P, Meis-Kindblom JM, et al. Gastrointestinal stromal tumors: The incidence, prevalence, clinical course, and prognostication in the preimatinib mesylate era – A population-based study in western Sweden. Cancer 2005; 103(4):821–9.
9. Beghini A, Tibiletti MG, Roversi G, et al. Germline mutation in the juxtamembrane domain of the kit gene in a family with gastrointestinal stromal tumors and urticaria pigmentosa. Cancer 2001;92(3):657–62.
10. Li FP, Fletcher JA, Heinrich MC, et al. Familial gastrointestinal stromal tumor syndrome: phenotypic and molecular features in a kindred. J Clin Oncol 2005;23(12): 2735–43.
11. Miettinen M, Fetsch JF, Sobin LH, et al. Gastrointestinal stromal tumors in patients a clinicopathologic and molecular genetic study of 45 cases. Am J Surg Pathol 2006;30(1):90–6.
12. Carney JA. Gastric stromal sarcoma, pulmonary chondroma, and extra-adrenal paraganglioma (Carney triad): natural history, adrenocortical component, and possible familial occurrence. Mayo Clin Proc 1999;74(6):543–52.
13. McWhinney SR. Familial gastrointestinal stromal tumors and germ-line mutations. N Engl J Med 2007;357(10):1054–6.
14. DeMatteo RP, Lewis JJ, Leung D, et al. Two hundred gastrointestinal stromal tumors: recurrence patterns and prognostic factors for survival. Ann Surg 2000; 231(1):51–8.
15. Joo MK, Park J-J, Kim H, et al. Endoscopic versus surgical resection of GI stromal tumors in the upper GI tract. Gastrointest Endosc 2016;83(2):318–26.

16. Park J-J. Long-term outcomes after endoscopic treatment of gastric gastrointestinal stromal tumor. Clin Endosc 2016;49:232–4.
17. Scherubl H, Faiss S, Knoefel W-T, et al. Management of early asymptomatic gastrointestinal stromal tumors of the stomach. World J Gastrointest Endosc 2014;6(7):266–71.
18. Yegin E, Duman D. Small EUS-suspected gastrointestinal stromal tumors of the stomach: an overview for the current state of management. Endosc Ultrasound 2016;5(2):69–77.
19. Hirota S, Isozaki K, Moriyama Y, et al. Gain-of-function mutations of c-kit in human gastrointestinal stromal tumors. Science 1998;279(5350):577–80.
20. Heinrich MC, Blanke CD, Druker BJ, et al. Inhibition of KIT tyrosine kinase activity: a novel molecular approach to the treatment of KIT-positive malignancies. J Clin Oncol 2002;20(6):1692–703.
21. Heinrich MC, Griffith DJ, Druker BJ, et al. Inhibition of c-kit receptor tyrosine kinase activity by STI 571, a selective tyrosine kinase inhibitor. Blood 2000;96(3):925–32.
22. Tuveson DA, Willis NA, Jacks T, et al. STI571 inactivation of the gastrointestinal stromal tumor c-KIT oncoprotein: biological and clinical implications. Oncogene 2001;20(36):5054–8.
23. Corless CL, Fletcher JA, Heinrich MC. Biology of gastrointestinal stromal tumors. J Clin Oncol 2004;22(18):3813–25.
24. Lasota J, Miettinen M. Clinical significance of oncogenic KIT and PDGFRA mutations in gastrointestinal stromal tumours. Histopathology 2008;53(3):245–66.
25. Heinrich MC, Corless CL, Duensing A, et al. PDGFRA activating mutations in gastrointestinal stromal tumors. Science 2003;299(5607):708–11.
26. Hirota S, Ohashi A, Nishida T, et al. Gain-of-function mutations of platelet-derived growth factor receptor alpha gene in gastrointestinal stromal tumors. Gastroenterology 2003;125(3):660–7.
27. Boikos SA, Pappo AS, Killian JK, et al. Molecular subtypes of KIT/PDGFRA wild-type gastrointestinal stromal tumors. JAMA Oncol 2016;2(7):922–8.
28. Corless CL, Ballman KV, Antonescu CR, et al. Pathologic and molecular features correlate with long-term outcome after adjuvant therapy of resected primary GI stromal tumor: the ACOSOG Z9001 trial. J Clin Oncol 2014;32(15):1563–70.
29. Gleeson FC, Kipp BR, Kerr SE, et al. Kinase genotype analysis of gastric gastrointestinal stromal sequencing. Clin Gastroenterol Hepatol 2015;13(1):202–6.
30. Pogorzelski M, Falkenhorst J, Bauer S. Molecular subtypes of gastrointestinal stromal tumor requiring specific treatments. Curr Opin Oncol 2016;28:331–7.
31. Agaram NP, Wong GC, Guo T, et al. Novel V600E BRAF mutations in imatinib-naive and imatinib-resistant gastrointestinal stromal tumors. Genes Chromosomes Cancer 2008;47:853–9.
32. DeMatteo RP, Gold JS, Saran L, et al. Tumor mitotic rate, size, and location independently predict recurrence after resection of primary gastrointestinal stromal tumor (GIST). Cancer 2008;112(3):608–15.
33. Miettinen M, Lasota J. Gastrointestinal stromal tumors: pathology and prognosis at different sites. Semin Diagn Pathol 2006;23(2):70–83.
34. Capelli L, Petracci E, Quagliuolo V, et al. Gastric GISTs: analysis of c-Kit, PDGFRA and BRAF mutations in relation to prognosis and clinical pathological characteristics of patients – A GIRCG study. Eur J Surg Oncol 2016;42(8):1206–14.
35. Martin J, Poveda A, Llombart-Bosch A, et al. Deletions affecting codons 557-558 of the c-KIT gene indicate a poor prognosis in patients with completely resected

gastrointestinal stromal tumors: a study by the Spanish Group for Sarcoma Research (GEIS). J Clin Oncol 2005;23(25):6190–8.

36. Wozniak A, Rutkowski P, Schöffski P, et al. Tumor genotype is an independent prognostic factor in primary gastrointestinal stromal tumors of gastric origin: a European multicenter analysis based on ConticaGIST. Clin Cancer Res 2014;20(23): 6105–16.

37. Heinrich BMC, Corless CL, Demetri GD, et al. Kinase mutations and imatinib response in patients with metastatic gastrointestinal stromal tumor. J Clin Oncol 2003;21(23):4342–9.

38. Heinrich MC, Owzar K, Corless CL, et al. Correlation of kinase genotype and clinical outcome in the North American intergroup phase III trial of imatinib mesylate for treatment of advanced gastrointestinal stromal tumor: CALGB 150105 Study by Cancer and Leukemia Group B and Southwest Oncology Group. J Clin Oncol 2008;26(33):5360–7.

39. Debiec-Rychter M, Sciot R, Le A, et al. KIT mutations and dose selection for imatinib in patients with advanced gastrointestinal stromal tumours. Eur J Cancer 2006;2:1093–103.

40. Gronchi A, Raut CP. The combination of surgery and imatinib in GIST: a reality for localized tumors at high risk, an open issue for metastatic ones. Ann Surg Oncol 2012;19(4):1370.

41. McCarter MD, Antonescu CR, Ballman KV, et al. Microscopically positive margins for primary gastrointestinal stromal tumors: analysis of risk factors and tumor recurrence. J Am Coll Surg 2012;215(1):53–9.

42. Agaimy A, Wunsch PH, Hofstaedter F, et al. Minute gastric sclerosing stromal tumors (GIST tumorlets) are common in adults and frequently show c-KIT mutations. Am J Surg Pathol 2007;31(1):113–20.

43. Kawanowa K, Sakuma Y, Sakurai S. High incidence of microscopic gastrointestinal stromal tumors in the stomach B. Hum Pathol 2006;37:1527–35.

44. Joensuu H, Vehtari A, Riihimäki J, et al. Risk of recurrence of gastrointestinal stromal tumour after surgery: an analysis of pooled population-based cohorts. Lancet Oncol 2012;13(3):265–74.

45. Novitsky YW, Kercher KW, Sing RF, et al. Long-term outcomes of laparoscopic resection of gastric gastrointestinal stromal tumors. Ann Surg 2006;243(6):14–8.

46. Otani Y, Furukawa T, Yoshida M, et al. Operative indications for relatively small (2-5 cm) gastrointestinal stromal tumor of the stomach based on analysis of 60 operated cases. Surgery 2006;139:484–92.

47. Bellorin O, Kundel A, Ni M, et al. Surgical management of gastrointestinal stromal tumors of the stomach. JSLS 2014;18(1):46–9.

48. Goh BKP, Goh Y, Eng AKH, et al. Outcome after laparoscopic versus open wedge resection for suspected gastric gastrointestinal stromal tumors: a matched-pair case-control study. Eur J Surg Oncol 2015;41(7):905–10.

49. Lin J, Huang C, Wang J, et al. Laparoscopic versus open gastric resection for larger than 5 cm primary gastric gastrointestinal stromal tumors (GIST): a size-matched comparison. Surg Endosc 2014;28:2577–83.

50. Piessen G, Lefevre JH, Cabau M, et al. Laparoscopic versus open surgery for gastric gastrointestinal stromal tumors: what is the impact on postoperative outcome and oncologic results? Ann Surg 2015;262(5):831–40.

51. Vogelaere KD, Hoorens A, Haentjens P, et al. Laparoscopic versus open resection of gastrointestinal stromal tumors of the stomach. Surg Endosc 2013;117: 1546–54.

52. Eisenberg BL, Harris J, Blanke CD, et al. Phase II trial of neoadjuvant/adjuvant imatinib mesylate (IM) for advanced primary and metastatic/recurrent operable gastrointestinal stromal tumor (GIST): Early results of RTOG 0132/ACRIN 6665. J Surg Oncol 2009;99(1):42–7.

53. Hohenberger P, Langer C, Wendtner CMHA, et al. Neoadjuvant treatment of locally advanced GIST: results of APOLLON, a prospective, open label phase II study in KIT- or PDGFRA-positive tumors. J Clin Oncol 2012;30(Suppl) [abstract: 10031].

54. McAuliffe JC, Hunt KK, Lazar AJF, et al. A randomized, phase II study of preoperative plus postoperative imatinib in GIST: evidence of rapid radiographic response and temporal induction of tumor cell apoptosis. Ann Surg Oncol 2009;16(4):910–9.

55. Wang D, Zhang Q, Blanke CD, et al. Phase II trial of neoadjuvant/adjuvant imatinib mesylate for advanced primary and metastatic/recurrent operable gastrointestinal stromal tumors: long-term follow-up results of Radiation Therapy Oncology Group 0132. Ann Surg Oncol 2012;19(4):1074–80.

56. Joensuu H. One vs three years of adjuvant imatinib for operable gastrointestinal stromal tumor a randomized trial. JAMA 2012;307(12):1265–72.

57. Joensuu H. Risk factors for gastrointestinal stromal tumor recurrence in patients treated with adjuvant imatinib. Cancer 2014;120:2325–33.

58. Dematteo RP. Long-term results of adjuvant imatinib mesylate in localized, high-risk, primary gastrointestinal stromal tumor. Ann Surg 2013;258:422–9.

59. Casali PG. Imatinib failure-free survival (IFS) in patients with localized gastrointestinal stromal tumors (GIST) treated with adjuvant imatinib (IM): the EORTC/AGITG/FSG/GEIS/ISG randomized controlled phase III trial. J Clin Oncol 2013;31(Suppl):abstr 10500.

60. Raut CP, Espat NJ, Maki RG, et al. Adjuvant imatinib (IM) for patients (pts) with primary gastrointestinal stromal tumor (GIST) at significant risk of recurrence: PERSIST-5 planned 3-year interim analysis. J Clin Oncol 2015;(Suppl) [abstract: 10537].

61. Vadakara J, von Mehren M. Gastrointestinal stromal tumors. management of metastatic disease and emerging therapies. Hematol Oncol Clin North Am 2013; 27(5):905–20.

62. Dematteo RP, Heinrich MC, El-Rifai WM, et al. Clinical management of gastrointestinal stromal tumors: before and after STI-571. Hum Pathol 2002;33(5):466–77.

63. Demetri GD, von Mehren M, Blanke CD, et al. Efficacy and Safety of Imatinib Mesylate in advanced gastrointestinal stromal tumors. N Engl J Med 2002;347(7): 472–80.

64. Gastrointestinal Stromal Tumor Meta-Analysis Group (MetaGIST). Comparison of two doses of imatinib for the treatment of unresectable or metastatic gastrointestinal stromal tumors: a meta-analysis of 1,640 patients. J Clin Oncol 2010;28(7): 1247–53.

65. Blay JY, Le Cesne A, Ray-Coquard I, et al. Prospective multicentric randomized phase III study of imatinib in patients with advanced gastrointestinal stromal tumors comparing interruption versus continuation of treatment beyond 1 year: the French Sarcoma Group. J Clin Oncol 2007;25(9):1107–13.

66. Le Cesne A, Ray-Coquard I, Bui BN, et al. Discontinuation of imatinib in patients with advanced gastrointestinal stromal tumours after 3 years of treatment: an open-label multicentre randomised phase 3 trial. Lancet Oncol 2010;11(10): 942–9.

67. Haller F, Detken S, Schulten H Jr, et al. Surgical management after neoadjuvant imatinib therapy in gastrointestinal stromal tumours (GISTs) with respect to imatinib resistance caused by secondary KIT mutations. Ann Surg Oncol 2007;14(2): 526–32.
68. Blanke CD, Rankin C, Demetri GD, et al. Phase III randomized, intergroup trial assessing imatinib mesylate at two dose levels in patients with unresectable or metastatic gastrointestinal stromal tumors expressing the kit receptor tyrosine kinase: S0033. J Clin Oncol 2008;26(4):626–32.
69. Zalcberg JR, Verweij J, Casali PG, et al. Outcome of patients with advanced gastro-intestinal stromal tumours crossing over to a daily imatinib dose of 800 mg after progression on 400 mg. Eur J Cancer 2005;41(12):1751–7.
70. Demetri GD, van Oosterom AT, Garrett CR, et al. Efficacy and safety of sunitinib in patients with advanced gastrointestinal stromal tumour after failure of imatinib: a randomised controlled trial. Lancet 2006;368(9544):1329–38.
71. George S, Blay JY, Casali PG, et al. Clinical evaluation of continuous daily dosing of sunitinib malate in patients with advanced gastrointestinal stromal tumour after imatinib failure. Eur J Cancer 2009;45(11):1959–68.
72. Demetri GD, Reichardt P, Kang YK, et al. Efficacy and safety of regorafenib for advanced gastrointestinal stromal tumours after failure of imatinib and sunitinib (GRID): an international, multicentre, randomised, placebo-controlled, phase 3 trial. Lancet 2013;381(9863):295–302.
73. Andtbacka RHI, Ng CS, Scaife CL, et al. Surgical resection of gastrointestinal stromal tumors after treatment with imatinib. Ann Surg Oncol 2007;14(1):14–24.
74. Bischof DA, Kim Y, Blazer DG, et al. Surgical management of advanced gastrointestinal stromal tumors: an international multi-institutional analysis of 158 patients. J Am Coll Surg 2014;219(3):439–49.
75. DeMatteo RP, Maki RG, Singer S, et al. Results of tyrosine kinase inhibitor therapy followed by surgical resection for metastatic gastrointestinal stromal tumor. Ann Surg 2007;245(3):347–52.
76. Gronchi A, Fiore M, Miselli F, et al. Surgery of residual disease following molecular-targeted therapy with imatinib mesylate in advanced/metastatic GIST. Ann Surg 2007;245(3):341–6.
77. Mussi C, Ronellenfitsch U, Jakob J, et al. Post-imatinib surgery in advanced/metastatic GIST: Is it worthwhile in all patients? Ann Oncol 2010;21(2):403–8.
78. Rutkowski P, Nowecki Z, Nyckowski P, et al. Surgical treatment of patients with initially inoperable and/or metastatic gastrointestinal stromal tumors (GIST) during therapy with imatinib mesylate. J Surg Oncol 2006;93(4):304–11.
79. Scaife CL, Hunt KK, Patel SR, et al. Is there a role for surgery in patients with "unresectable" cKIT+ gastrointestinal stromal tumors treated with imatinib mesylate? Am J Surg 2003;186(6):665–9.
80. Sym SJ, Ryu M-H, Lee J-L, et al. Surgical intervention following imatinib treatment in patients with advanced gastrointestinal stromal tumors (GISTs). J Surg Oncol 2008;98(1):27–33.
81. Tielen R, Verhoef C, van Coevorden F, et al. Surgery after treatment with imatinib and/or sunitinib in patients with metastasized gastrointestinal stromal tumors: is it worthwhile? World J Surg Oncol 2012;10:111.
82. Zaydfudim V, Okuno SH, Que FG, et al. Role of operative therapy in treatment of metastatic gastrointestinal stromal tumors. J Surg Res 2012;177(2):248–54.
83. Bonvalot S, Eldweny H, Pechoux CL, et al. Impact of surgery on advanced gastrointestinal stromal tumors (GIST) in the imatinib era. Ann Surg Oncol 2006;13(12):1596–603.

84. Raut CP, Posner M, Desai J, et al. Surgical management of advanced gastrointestinal stromal tumors after treatment with targeted systemic therapy using kinase inhibitors. J Clin Oncol 2006;24(15):2325–31.

85. Rubio-Casadevall J, Martinez-Trufero J, Garcia-Albeniz X, et al. Role of surgery in patients with recurrent, metastatic, or unresectable locally advanced gastrointestinal stromal tumors sensitive to imatinib: a retrospective analysis of the Spanish Group for Research on Sarcoma (GEIS). Ann Surg Oncol 2015;22(9):2948–57.

86. An HJ, Ryu M-H, Ryoo B-Y, et al. The effects of surgical cytoreduction prior to imatinib therapy on the prognosis of patients with advanced GIST. Ann Surg Oncol 2013;20(13):4212–8.

87. Barnes G, Bulusu VR, Hardwick RH, et al. A review of the surgical management of metastatic gastrointestinal stromal tumours (GISTs) on imatinib mesylate. Int J Surg 2005;3(3):206–12.

East Versus West

Differences in Surgical Management in Asia Compared with Europe and North America

Tomio Ueno, MD, PhD[a],*, Michihisa Iida, MD, PhD[b],
Shigefumi Yoshino, MD, PhD[b], Shigeru Takeda, MD, PhD[b],
Hisako Kubota, MD, PhD[a], Masaharu Higashida, MD, PhD[a],
Yasuo Oka, MD, PhD[a], Atushi Tsuruta, MD, PhD[a],
Hideo Matsumoto, MD, PhD[a], Hiroaki Nagano, MD, PhD[b]

KEYWORDS

- Gastric cancer • D2 lymph node dissection • Adjuvant therapy
- Surgical management

KEY POINTS

- Gastrectomy with a modified D2 lymphadenectomy (sparing the distal pancreas and spleen) has increasingly gained acceptance as a preferable standard surgical approach among surgeons in the East and the West.
- Despite growing consensus significant differences still exist in surgical techniques in clinical trials and clinical practices secondary to variations in epidemiology, clinicopathologic features, and surgical outcomes among geographic regions.
- D2 lymphadenectomy is the standard in Japan, with exceptions.
- S-1 is the most standard adjuvant chemotherapy used in Japan after curative resection.

INTRODUCTION

Gastric cancer is an aggressive disease that remains the fifth most common type of cancer.[1] It is the second most common cancer in Asia, with more than half of the world's gastric cancer cases arising in Eastern Asia. In Western countries, most patients with gastric cancer have advanced-stage, unresectable disease at presentation,

Disclosure Statement: Dr T. Ueno has no relevant financial or nonfinancial relationships to disclose.

[a] Department of Digestive Surgery, Kawasaki Medical School, 577 Matsushima, Kurashiki, Okayama 701-0192, Japan; [b] Department of Gastroentelogical, Breast and Endocrine Surgery, Yamaguchi University Graduate School of Medicine, 1-1-1 Minami-kogushi, Yamaguchi 755-8505, Japan
* Corresponding author. Department of Digestive Surgery, Kawasaki Medical School, 577 Matsushima, Kurashiki, Okayama 701-0192, Japan.
E-mail address: tommy@med.kawasaki-m.ac.jp

which contrasts with Eastern countries, such as Japan and South Korea, where an established national screening program permits frequent diagnosis of early stage disease.[1] In addition, most of Asia's cases are predominantly located in the distal part of the stomach,[2] whereas in the West there is an increasing frequency of these tumors in the proximal portion of the stomach.

Although clinicopathologic presentations of gastric cancer are known to vary widely between Eastern and Western countries, including histology, tumor location, and stage at presentation, it remains unclear whether these factors account for differences in survival. Survival outcomes differ considerably between Eastern and Western populations, with better overall survival reported in Eastern series.[3] Many authors have sought explanations for this finding based on the following: stage migration, differences in tumor biology, or differences in treatment.[4]

Surgical treatment differs in that extended lymph node dissection is routinely practiced in Asian countries,[5,6] resulting in greater lymph node retrieval. Whether this leads to stage migration or to a direct therapeutic effect has yet to be resolved. Furthermore, adjuvant therapy differs between the two regions.

In this article comparisons are made between the Japanese Gastric Cancer Treatment Guidelines 2014 (version 4; J-guidelines)[7] and the National Comprehensive Cancer Network (NCCN) Clinical Practice Guidelines in Oncology (NCCN Guidelines) Gastric Cancer Version 2.2016, to elucidate differences in surgical treatment and adjuvant therapy.

HISTORY OF THE JAPANESE CLASSIFICATION OF GASTRIC CARCINOMA AND THE JAPANESE GASTRIC CANCER TREATMENT GUIDELINES

In 2010, the Japanese Gastric Cancer Association (JGCA) published new versions of the Japanese Classification of Gastric Carcinoma (J-classification) and the J-guidelines.[7,8] The primary aim of the revision was to integrate a different understanding concerning the terms D1 and D2 between Japan and Western countries, and to provide an updated guide to the diagnosis and treatment of gastric cancer for clinicians and researchers worldwide. English editions are available on the Web site for free. The following descriptions were cited from a paper by Sano and Aiko,[9] who detailed the history of the J-classification and the J-guidelines.

The first edition of the J-classification was published in 1962 to standardize the surgical and pathologic documentation of gastric cancer. At that time, the Union for International Cancer Control (UICC) and the American Joint Committee on Cancer had not yet established a staging system for gastric cancer. Since then, the JGCA has made periodic revisions and expanded the J-classification into an original comprehensive guide covering all aspects of the diagnostic and therapeutic procedures for the disease, ranging from the handling of resected specimens for pathologic investigation to the extent of lymphadenectomy. Documentation using these guidelines has become standard in Japan to record all cases of gastric cancer in hospital databases in accordance with the J-classification. The first English edition of the J-classification published in 1981 is still referred to as a reference (number 95) in the section involving lymph node dissection, even in the latest NCCN guidelines.[10]

In 2001, the JGCA launched the first edition of the J-guidelines apart from the J-classification. The primary aim of the J-guidelines was to provide general and specialized clinicians with knowledge concerning standard treatments, based on evidence where available, and consensus; the purpose was to offer a patient with gastric cancer standard treatments anywhere in Japan. Because novel treatment modalities and novel handling of clinical issues are constantly being proposed in Japan, the

J-guidelines proposed two independent lists of stage-specific treatments: a standard list and an investigational list. This concept has been gradually and widely accepted in the clinical setting and has changed the general practice in Japan.

MAJOR POINTS REVISED IN THE LATEST JAPANESE CLASSIFICATION OF GASTRIC CARCINOMA

Major revisions of the J-classification and J-guidelines occurred in 2010. For the description of tumor status in the J-classification (T/N/M categories, stage grouping, and so forth), definitions identical to those in the UICC/TNM seventh edition were adopted so that the Japanese experience could be expressed using the international terminology (**Tables 1** and **2**). The modification of the N-category was the most significant change not only in this revision but also in the whole history of the J-classification.

Traditionally, the lymph node stations in the gastric drainage area have been classified into three groups (or four in some editions) depending on the anatomic position of the station in relation to the location of the primary tumor (**Fig. 1**). The JGCA grouped the regional and distant draining lymph nodes into 16 stations: stations one to six are perigastric lymph nodes, whereas the remaining 10 lymph nodes are located along the major vessels, posterior to the pancreas, and along the aorta. D1 lymphadenectomy involved limited dissection of only the perigastric lymph nodes. D2 lymphadenectomy involved extended dissection that encompassed the removal of nodes

Table 1
Differences in T category in Japanese classification of gastric cancer between second and third English edition

	Second English Edition	Third English Edition
TX	Unknown	Depth of tumor unknown
T0	Not described	No evidence of primary tumor
Tis	Not described	No description
T1	Tumor invasion of mucosa and/or muscularis mucosa (M) or submucosa (SM)	Tumor confined to the mucosa (M) or submucosa (SM)
T1a	Not described	Tumor confined to the mucosa (M)
T1b	Not described	Tumor confined to the submucosa (SM)
T2	Tumor invasion of muscularis propria (MP) or subserosa (SS)	Tumor invades the muscularis propria (MP)
T3	Tumor penetration of serosa (SE)	Tumor invades the subserosa (SS)
T4	Tumor invasion of adjacent structures (SI)	Tumor invasion is contiguous to or exposed beyond the serosa (SE) or tumor invades adjacent structures (SI)
T4a	Not described	Tumor invasion is contiguous to the serosa or penetrates the serosa and is exposed to the peritoneal cavity (SE)
T4b	Not described	Tumor invades adjacent structures (SI)

Adapted from Japanese Gastric Cancer Association (JGCA). Japanese classification of gastric carcinoma: 3rd English edition. Gastric Cancer 2011;14:101–12; and Japanese Gastric Cancer Association (JGCA). Japanese classification of gastric carcinoma: 2nd English edition. Gastric Cancer 1998;1:10–24.

Table 2
Differences in N category in Japanese classification of gastric cancer between second and third English edition

	Second English Edition	Third English Edition
NX	Unknown	Regional lymph node cannot be assessed
N0	No evidence of lymph node metastasis	No regional lymph node metastasis
N1	Metastasis to group 1 lymph nodes, but no metastasis to group 2 or 3 lymph nodes	Metastasis in 1–2 regional lymph nodes
N2	Metastasis to group 2 lymph nodes, but no metastasis to group 3 lymph nodes	Metastasis in 3–6 regional lymph nodes
N3	Metastasis to group 3 lymph nodes	Metastasis in 7 or more regional lymph nodes
N3a	Not described	Metastasis in 7–15 regional lymph nodes
N3b	Not described	Metastasis in 16 or more regional lymph nodes

Adapted from Japanese Gastric Cancer Association (JGCA). Japanese classification of gastric carcinoma: 3rd English edition. Gastric Cancer 2011;14:101–12; and Japanese Gastric Cancer Association (JGCA). Japanese classification of gastric carcinoma: 2nd English edition. Gastric Cancer 1998;1:10–24.

located along the left gastric artery, common hepatic artery, celiac axis, splenic artery, splenic hilum, and the perigastric nodes (stations 1–12). These numbers were also used to express the grade of nodal metastasis (N1–3) and the extent of lymphadenectomy (D1–3); for example, cancer with metastasis to the second group node was

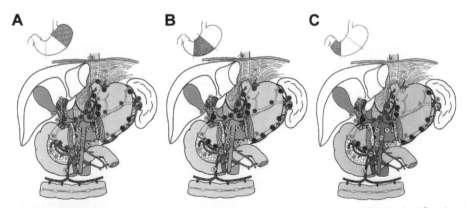

Fig. 1. Lymph node groupings in the previous J-classification. In the previous J-classification, grouping of lymph nodes of the stomach was classified by the location of the primary tumor. The location of the main tumor was in the upper third of the stomach (*A*), in the middle third of the stomach (*B*), and in the lower third of the stomach (*C*). Red nodes denote the first group; blue nodes the second group; yellow nodes the third group; and white nodes the fourth group. (*From* Japanese Gastric Cancer Association (JGCA). Japanese gastric cancer treatment guidelines 2014 (ver. 4). Gastric Cancer 2017;20(1):1–19.)

designated as N2 regardless of the number of metastatic lymph nodes, and complete dissection of up to the second group nodes was defined as D2. This terminology was often used in studies in which Japanese researchers participated. This rule has been consistent throughout the history of the J-classification, until the latest revision, although details regarding classification of the nodal groups has been modified in each edition.

In the latest version of the J-classification, this nodal grouping has been completely abandoned, and the N-number solely signifies the number of metastatic lymph nodes as determined in the UICC/TNM seventh edition. The extent of lymphadenectomy had to be newly defined independently from the N-category in the new J-guidelines (see **Table 2**). The same stage grouping as that in the UICC/TNM seventh edition has also been adopted in the new J-classification (**Table 3**). It should be noted that survival analyses involving a large number of Japanese and Korean patients contributed to the determination of this UICC/TNM stage grouping.

ANATOMIC DEFINITION OF LYMPH NODES AND REGIONAL GASTRIC LYMPH NODES IN THE LATEST JAPANESE CLASSIFICATION OF GASTRIC CARCINOMA

The lymph nodes of the stomach are defined and given station numbers, as shown in **Fig. 2** and **Table 4**. Note that the figure numbers presented in the original paper regarding the J-classification (third English edition) were incorrect. Lymph node stations 1 to 12 and 14v (a part of the no. 6 station) are defined as regional gastric lymph nodes; metastasis to any other nodes is classified as M1.

RECORDING OF LYMPH NODE METASTASIS IN ACCORDANCE WITH THE LATEST JAPANESE CLASSIFICATION OF GASTRIC CARCINOMA

For surgical resection specimens, the total number of lymph nodes and the number of involved lymph nodes at each nodal station are recorded (see **Table 2**). When a tumor nodule without histologic evidence of lymph node structure is found in the lymphatic drainage area of the primary tumor, it is recorded as extranodal metastasis and counted as a metastatic lymph node in the N determination. The same N determination as that in the UICC/TNM seventh edition has also been adopted in the new J-classification.

Table 3
Differences on staging in Japanese classification of gastric cancer between the second and the third English edition

	Second English Edition					Third English Edition			
	N0	N1	N2	N3		N0	N1	N2	N3
T1	IA	IB	II	IV	T1a (M), T1b (SM)	IA	IB	IIA	IIB
T2	IB	II	IIIA	IV	T2 (MP)	IB	IIA	IIB	IIIA
T3	II	IIIA	IIIB	IV	T3 (SS)	IIA	IIB	IIA	IIIB
T4	IIIA	IIIB	IV	IV	T4a (SE)	IIB	IIA	IIB	IIIC
					T4b (SI)	IIB	IIB	IIIC	IIIC
H1, P1, CY1, M1	IV				M1 (any T, any N)	IV			

Adapted from Japanese Gastric Cancer Association (JGCA). Japanese classification of gastric carcinoma: 3rd English edition. Gastric Cancer 2011;14:101–12; and Japanese Gastric Cancer Association (JGCA). Japanese classification of gastric carcinoma: 2nd English edition. Gastric Cancer 1998;1:10–24.

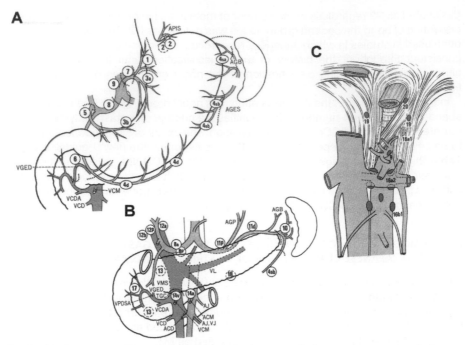

Fig. 2. (*A–C*) Location of lymph node stations in the stomach. (*From* Japanese Gastric Cancer Association (JGCA). Japanese classification of gastric carcinoma: 3rd English edition. Gastric Cancer 2011;14:101–12.)

MAJOR POINTS REVISED IN THE LATEST JAPANESE GASTRIC CANCER TREATMENT GUIDELINES

The terms D1/D2/D3 were originally defined in the J-classification and have been widely used worldwide to describe the extent of lymphadenectomy. Most randomized controlled trials (RCTs) involving gastric cancer surgery, including the Dutch,[11,12] Medical Research Council,[13] and Taipei D1/D2 trials,[14] were conducted using the classical definitions from the J-classification.

However, outside of these clinical studies, the terms D1/D2/D3 have not always been used with accuracy in the strict sense. It is generally and mistakenly believed outside of Japan, where the first group of nodes are equal to the perigastric nodes and the second group of nodes are those located along the celiac artery and its branches, and that the dissections of these nodes are designated as D1 and D2, respectively. The original definitions of N1-3 and D1-3 are far more complicated: the location of the primary tumor is determined (see **Fig. 1**), and accordingly each lymph node station is given a group number (1, 2, 3, or M) based on the primary tumor's location. For example, the left paracardial lymph nodes (station 2) are classified as group 1 nodes for a tumor located in the upper third of the stomach (see **Fig. 1**A), but as group 3 nodes for a middle or middle/lower tumor (see **Fig. 1**B), and as group M nodes (distant metastasis) for a tumor confined to the lower third of the stomach (see **Fig. 1**C).

Because this complicated definition of the nodal groups was established based on the results of detailed efficacy analysis of each lymph node station,[15] surgeons would have the best chance to cure patients if they strictly obeyed the rule for D2.

Table 4	
Definition of lymph node stations in the stomach	
1	Right paracardial LNs, including those along the first branch of the ascending limb of the left gastric artery
2	Left paracardial LNs including those along the esophagocardiac branch of the left subphrenic artery
3a	Lesser curvature LNs along the branches of the left gastric artery
3b	Lesser curvature LNs along the second branch and distal part of the right gastric artery
4sa	Left greater curvature LNs along the short gastric arteries (perigastric area)
4sb	Left greater curvature LNs along the left gastroepiploic artery (perigastic area)
4d	Right greater curvature LNs along the second branch and distal part of the right gastroepiploic artery
5	Suprapyloric LNs along the first branch and proximal part of the right gastric artery
6	Infrapyloric LNs along the first branch and proximal part of the right gastroepiploic artery down to the confluence of the right gastroepiploic vein and the anterior superior pancreatoduodenal vein
7	LNs along the trunk of left gastric artery between its root and the origin of its ascending branch
8a	Anterosuperior LNs along the common hepatic artery
8p	Posterior LNs along the common hepatic artery
9	Celiac artery LNs
10	Splenic hilar LNs including those adjacent to the splenic artery distal to the pancreatic tail, and those on the roots of the short gastric arteries and those along the left gastroepiploic artery proximal to its first gastric branch
11p	Proximal splenic artery LNs from its origin to halfway between its origin and the pancreatic tail end
11d	Distal splenic artery LNs from halfway between its origin and the pancreatic tail end to the end of the pancreatic tail
12a	Hepatoduodenal ligament LNs along the proper hepatic artery, in the caudal half between the confluence of the right and left hepatic ducts and the upper border of the pancreas
12b	Hepatoduodenal ligament LNs along the bile duct, in the caudal half between the confluence of the right and left hepatic ducts and the upper border of the pancreas
12p	Hepatoduodenal ligament LNs along the portal vein in the caudal half between the confluence of the right and left hepatic ducts and the upper border of the pancreas
13	LNs on the posterior surface of the pancreatic head cranial to the duodenal papilla
14v	LNs along the superior mesenteric vein
15	LNs along the middle colic vessels
16a1	Para-aortic LNs in the diaphragmatic aortic hiatus
16a2	Para-aortic LNs between the upper margin of the origin of the celiac artery and the lower border of the left renal vein
16b1	Para-aortic LNs between the lower border of the left renal vein and the upper border of the origin of the inferior mesenteric artery
16b2	Para-aortic LNs between the upper border of the origin of the inferior mesenteric artery and aortic bifurcation

Abbreviation: LN, lymph node.

However, the grouping in Japan was too complicated to be accurately applied worldwide; the tumor location may not have been correctly categorized by surgeons/pathologists as the JGCA had intended. In the latest J-guidelines, the definition of lymphadenectomy has been remarkably simplified; the lymph node stations to be dissected in D1, D1+, and D2 are defined for total and distal gastrectomy regardless of the tumor location. **Fig. 3** shows the extent of lymphadenectomy during each procedure. D3 is no longer defined in the latest J-guidelines, because the rationale for the recommendation of this extended surgery was not supported by the negative results in the RCT reported by Sasako and colleagues.[16]

Apart from the two major types of gastrectomy (total or distal), pylorus-preserving gastrectomy and proximal gastrectomy are proposed as options for early gastric cancers, for each of which D1 and D1+ (but not D2) have been defined (see **Fig. 3**; **Table 5**). It should be noted that the lymph nodes along the left gastric artery (No. 7), which used to be classified as N2 for tumors in any location, is now included in

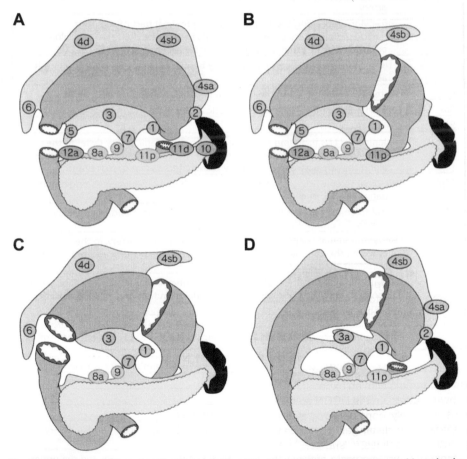

Fig. 3. The extent of lymphadenectomy in the latest J-guidelines. The extent of lymphadenectomy in the latest J-guidelines after total gastrectomy (*A*), distal partial gastrectomy (*B*), pylorus-preserving gastrectomy (*C*), and proximal gastrectomy (*D*). Complete dissection of the nodes shown in blue denotes D1 dissection, the nodes in orange D1+ dissection, and the nodes in red D2 dissection. (*From* Japanese Gastric Cancer Association (JGCA). Japanese gastric cancer treatment guidelines 2014 (ver. 4). Gastric Cancer 2017;20(1):1–19.)

Table 5
The extent of lymphadenectomy during each surgical procedure

	Total Gastrectomy			Distal Gastrectomy			Pylorus-Preserving Gastrectomy		Proximal Gastrectomy	
	D1	D1+	D2	D1	D1+	D2	D1	D1+	D1	D1+
1	■	■	■	■	■	■	■	■	■	■
2	■	■	■				▨	▨	■	■
3a	■	■	■	■	■	■	■	■	■	■
3b	■	■	■	■	■	■	■	■		
4sa	■	■	■						■	■
4sb	■	■	■	■	■	■	■	■	■	■
4d	■	■	■	■	■	■	■	■		
5	■	■	■	■	■	■	■	■		
6	■	■	■	■	■	■	■	■		
7	■	■	■	■	■	■	■	■	■	■
8a		▨	▨		▨	▨		▨		▨
8p										
9		▨	▨		▨	▨		▨		▨
10		▨	■							
11p		▨	■			■				▨
11d		▨	■							
12a		▨	■			■				
12b										
12p										

the D1 for any type of gastrectomy. The JGCA expects that these simplified definitions of lymphadenectomy will help specialized surgeons worldwide to standardize gastrectomy and to obtain the best surgical results.

GASTRIC RESECTION: JAPAN VERSUS THE WEST

In the J-guidelines, a proximal margin of at least 3 cm is recommended for T2 or deeper tumors with an expansive growth pattern, and 5 cm for those with an infiltrative growth pattern. In the NCCN guidelines, complete resection with 4 cm or greater margins is widely considered a standard goal. Subtotal gastrectomy is the preferred approach for distal gastric cancers. According to the ESMO-ESSO-ESTRO clinical practice guidelines,[17] subtotal gastrectomy is recommended to obtain a proximal margin of 5 cm; a margin of 8 cm for diffuse type cancers is also recommended.

TERMINOLOGY OF LYMPH NODE DISSECTION: JAPAN VERSUS THE WEST

The latest NCCN guidelines and ESMO-ESSO-ESTRO clinical practice guidelines do not include the revision of the latest J-guidelines published in 2014. They indicate that the perigastric lymph node stations along the lesser curvature (stations 1, 3, and 5) and greater curvature (stations 2, 4, and 6) of the stomach are grouped together as N1, and that the nodes along the left gastric artery (station 7), common hepatic artery (station 8), celiac artery (station 9), and splenic artery (stations 10 and 11) are grouped together as N2. The NCCN guidelines indicate that D1 involves gastrectomy and the removal of the involved proximal or distal part of the stomach or the entire stomach, including the greater and lesser omental lymph nodes (which would be the right and left cardiac lymph nodes along lesser and greater curvature, and suprapyloric nodes along the right gastric artery and infrapyloric area). They also indicated that D2 involves D1 plus the removal of all of the nodes along the left gastric artery. In relation to the terminology for D1 and D2, the ESMO-ESSO-ESTRO clinical practice guidelines, and the NCCN guidelines, also indicate that D1 involves the removal of perigastric lymph nodes and D2 involves the removal of perigastric lymph nodes plus those located along the left gastric, common hepatic, and splenic arteries and celiac axis. The lymph nodes along the left gastric artery (station 7), which used to be classified as N2 for tumors in any location in the previous J-classification, are now included in the D1 for any type of gastrectomy in the latest J-guidelines. The definition of the regional lymph node station in the NCCN guidelines may be reconsidered based on the current revision of the J-guidelines.

LYMPH NODE DISSECTION: JAPAN VERSUS THE WEST

Although the extent of lymphadenectomy is controversial and has been a greatly debated topic throughout the last few decades, most Japanese and Korean surgeons would agree that an extended lymphadenectomy (D2) leads to improved outcomes and survival.[2,5,6] Furthermore, in the latest J-guidelines, the JGCA recommends that nonearly potentially curable gastric cancers should be treated using D2 lymphadenectomy. D1 or D1+ should be considered as an option for T1 tumors. D1+ can be substituted for D2 in a poor-risk patient or under circumstances where D2 cannot be safely performed. Although it is not a prerequisite, the examination of 16 or more regional lymph nodes is recommended for the determination of N status.

Western proponents for a limited D1 resection or less-extensive lymph node dissection have been driven by two large RCTs carried out in the 1990s from the Netherlands (Dutch D1D2 trial) and the United Kingdom (Medical Research Council ST01trial) that failed to demonstrate a significant survival benefit for D2 over D1 lymph node dissection.[11,13,18] However, long-term follow-up data from the Netherlands have confirmed a survival benefit for D2 lymph node dissection.[12] The 15-year overall survival rates were 21% and 29%, for the D1 and D2 group, respectively. D2 lymph node dissection was also associated with lower rates of local (12% vs 22%) and regional recurrence (13% vs 19%). More importantly, the gastric cancer–related death rate was significantly lower in the D2 group relative to the D1 group (37% vs 48%). Dependent on the latest NCCN guidelines, recent reports from Western countries also suggest that D2 lymph node dissection is associated with a lower level of postoperative complications and a trend toward improved overall survival, when performed in high-volume centers that have sufficient experience with the operation and postoperative management. In the NCCN guidelines for patients with localized resectable cancer, at present, gastrectomy with D1 or a modified D2 lymph node dissection is recommended, with the goal of examining at least 15 lymph nodes. The current UICC/American Joint Committee on Cancer TNM classification recommendations (seventh edition) also include excision of a minimum of 15 lymph nodes to allow reliable staging.

One study demonstrated a median age difference of 10 years between Korea and the US cohorts.[3] Western populations also had a higher body mass index.[3,19] Increased obesity has been associated with a significant increase in perioperative complications, even in gastric cancer. Postoperative mortality at 30 days was 0.2%, which is the same in Japan, but runs higher in US studies at around 2%. In this study 97% of patients with gastric cancer in Korea and 78% in the United States received D2 or D3 lymph node dissection.[3] Therefore, the NCCN guidelines emphasize that D2 lymph node dissection is a recommended but not required procedure, and that D2 lymph node dissection should be performed by experienced surgeons in high-volume centers. In the East, D2 lymphadenectomy is indicated for potentially curable T2-T4 tumors and T1 tumors with suspicion of nodal involvement.

RESECTION OF OTHER ORGANS: JAPAN VERSUS THE WEST

The role of splenectomy for complete resection of lymph node stations 10 and 11 has long been a controversial issue. Recently, the final results of an RCT (JCOG 0110) that compared splenectomy and spleen preservation in total gastrectomy have been reported with survival analysis.[20] This is the largest RCT studying splenectomy in gastric cancer. It included 505 patients (splenectomy, 254; spleen preservation, 251) and demonstrated significant noninferiority of splenic preservation for the first time. In total gastrectomy for proximal gastric cancer that does not invade the greater curvature, prophylactic splenectomy should be avoided; this is true not only for surgical safety but also for survival benefit. The NCCN guidelines also recommend that a routine or prophylactic splenectomy should be avoided if possible, based on the findings of a Korean study by Yu and colleagues[21] in Korea. The NCCN guidelines recommend splenectomy only when the spleen or hilum is involved.

ADJUVANT THERAPY: JAPAN VERSUS THE WEST

Adjuvant chemotherapy is the main strategy adopted for curatively resected gastric cancer in the East, where relatively high curative resection rates are achieved and local tumor control is adequate using standard D2 lymphadenectomy. Various regimens have been tested in numerous clinical trials in Japan without producing solid evidence in support of adjuvant chemotherapy. Recently, two large randomized phase III trials have been performed in East Asia. One is the ACTS-GC trial (Adjuvant Chemotherapy trial of S-1 for Gastric Cancer); the other is the CLASSIC (Capecitabine and Oxaliplatin Adjuvant Study in Stomach Cancer) trial. The objective of the Japanese ACTS-GC trial was to examine the efficacy of adjuvant S-1 (tegafur, gimeracil, and oteracil) in stage II and III gastric cancer where 1034 patients were randomized to 12 months of oral S-1 or surgery alone.[22,23] The surgical quality control was excellent with all centers performing 100 cases annually; all but one patient underwent a D2 or D3 lymphadenectomy. The results of the trial regarding chemotherapy and surgery demonstrated an improvement in 5-year overall survival of 71.1% versus 61.1%. This finding secured the place of postoperative chemotherapy with S-1 as a standard of care (recommendation category 1). Subsequently, the feasibility of several combinations of anticancer drugs in combination with S-1 has been explored in the postoperative setting,[24,25] with some of the combinations currently under evaluation in phase III trials.

Additional evidence in support of postoperative chemotherapy was provided in 2012 by the CLASSIC trial conducted in South Korea, China, and Taiwan.[26] In this trial, 1035 patients with stage II or III gastric cancer were randomized to XELOX (a combination of capecitabine and oxaliplatin) or surgery alone; significant prolongation of recurrence-free survival was shown in the XELOX arm. Following the results of the J-CLASSIC and SOX-adjuvant trials,[27,28] capecitabine or S-1 plus oxaliplatin have been approved as an adjuvant regimen in Japan. Indications for these studies were as follows. The patients eligible for the ACTS-GC trial were those with a tumor of pathologic stage II, IIIA, or IIIB, excluding those classified as stage II because of pTI/pN2-N3 status as defined by the previous J-classification (second English edition), who had undergone R0 gastrectomy with greater than or equal to D2 1ymphadenectomy. The eligibility for postoperative adjuvant chemotherapy remains the same in the current version of the treatment guidelines.

However, in the latest J-classification (third English edition) whose staging scheme is the same as the seventh edition of the UICC/TNM classification, stage IIA includes pT3(SS)/N0 status. This had been classified as stage IB in the 13th edition and therefore was ineligible for the ACTS-GC. Thus, the eligibility criteria remain unchanged by excluding this population and the pT1/pN2-pN3population from stage II/III. Additionally, the information stated regarding "chemotherapy as a general practice" applies also to chemotherapy in the adjuvant setting, except that the response to treatment cannot be evaluated using imaging modalities until disease recurrence.

S-1 should be initiated within 6 weeks following surgery, after sufficient recovery from surgical intervention. A 6-week cycle consisting of 4 weeks of daily oral administration of S-1 at a dose of 80 mg/m^2 followed by 2 weeks of rest is repeated during the 12 months after surgery (eight cycles). Because postoperative patients are generally more vulnerable to hematologic and nonhematologic adverse events, appropriate dose reduction and schedule modification should be considered, including a switch to a schedule of 2 weeks of administration followed by I week of rest.

Approaches in the West have been driven by two RCTs that demonstrated a benefit regarding adjuvant therapy: the US Intergroup study (INT 0116) and the MAGIC (UK Medical Research Council Adjuvant Gastric Cancer Infusional Chemotherapy) study. In the INT 0116 trial, patients were randomized to radiotherapy at a total dose of 45 Gy and 5-FU/leucovorin or surgery alone; the study demonstrated improved local control and a significant survival benefit with a 3-year overall survival rate of 50% versus 41%.[29] In the MAGIC trial, patients were randomized to epirubicin, cisplatin, and 5-FU for three cycles preoperatively and three cycles postoperatively; the results of the trial demonstrated an improved overall and progression-free survival in the perioperative chemotherapy group, with 5-year survivals of 36% and 23%, respectively.[30] However, Eastern investigators have made several criticisms regarding these trials.[2,4] In the INT 0116 trial only 10% of patients had a D2 lymphadenectomy. Similarly, in the MAGIC trial, only 41% of patients had a D2 lymphadenectomy and in 40% of the patients the lymphadenectomy status was unknown. Japanese surgeons would argue that perioperative chemotherapy or adjuvant chemoradiotherapy compensates for inadequate surgery. Lending support to this is that patient survival in the surgery-alone arm is much lower in both Western trials than that seen in Japanese trials or series. Japanese surgeons would argue that the use of these modalities is unproven in patients who underwent a D2 lymphadenectomy.[2]

SUMMARY

In recent decades, there has been considerable worldwide progress in the treatment of gastric cancer. Gastrectomy with a modified D2 lymphadenectomy (sparing the distal pancreas and spleen) is now accepted as a preferable standard of surgical option in the East and the West. However, differences in surgical techniques still exist in clinical trials and practices from region to region according to variations in epidemiology, clinicopathologic features, and surgical outcomes among geographic regions. In addition, Western physicians would focus on adjuvant chemotherapy using S-1.

REFERENCES

1. Ryun Park S. Management of gastric cancer: East vs West. Curr Probl Cancer 2015;39:315–41.
2. Sasako M, Inoue M, Lin JT, et al. Gastric Cancer Working Group report. Jpn J Clin Oncol 2010;40(Suppl 1):i28–37.
3. Strong VE, Song KY, Park CH, et al. Comparison of gastric cancer survival following R0 resection in the United States and Korea using an internationally validated nomogram. Ann Surg 2010;251:640–6.
4. Bickenbach K, Strong VE. Comparisons of gastric cancer treatments: East vs. West. J Gastric Cancer 2012;12:55–62.
5. Sasako M, Saka M, Fukagawa T, et al. Surgical treatment of advanced gastric cancer: Japanese perspective. Dig Surg 2007;24:101–7.
6. Yoon SS, Yang HK. Lymphadenectomy for gastric adenocarcinoma: should West meet East? Oncologist 2009;14:871–82.
7. Japanese Gastric Cancer Association (JGCA). Japanese gastric cancer treatment guidelines 2014 (ver. 4). Gastric Cancer 2017;20:1–19.
8. Japanese Gastric Cancer Association (JGCA). Japanese classification of gastric carcinoma: 3rd English edition. Gastric Cancer 2011;14:101–12.
9. Sano T, Aiko T. New Japanese classifications and treatment guidelines for gastric cancer: revision concepts and major revised points. Gastric Cancer 2011;14: 97–100.
10. Kajitani T. The general rules for the gastric cancer study in surgery and pathology. Part I. Clinical classification. Jpn J Surg 1981;11:127–39.
11. Bonenkamp JJ, Songun I, Hermans J, et al. Randomised comparison of morbidity after D1 and D2 dissection for gastric cancer in 996 Dutch patients. Lancet 1995; 345:745–8.
12. Songun I, Putter H, Kranenbarg EM, et al. Surgical treatment of gastric cancer: 15-year follow-up results of the randomised nationwide Dutch D1D2 trial. Lancet Oncol 2010;11:439–49.
13. Cuschieri A, Weeden S, Fielding J, et al. Patient survival after D1 and D2 resections for gastric cancer: long-term results of the MRC randomized surgical trial. Surgical Co-operative Group. Br J Cancer 1999;79:1522–30.
14. Wu CW, Hsiung CA, Lo SS, et al. Nodal dissection for patients with gastric cancer: a randomised controlled trial. Lancet Oncol 2006;7:309–15.
15. Sasako M, McCulloch P, Kinoshita T, et al. New method to evaluate the therapeutic value of lymph node dissection for gastric cancer. Br J Surg 1995;82:346–51.
16. Sasako M, Sano T, Yamamoto S, et al. D2 lymphadenectomy alone or with para-aortic nodal dissection for gastric cancer. N Engl J Med 2008;359:453–62.
17. Waddell T, Verheij M, Allum W, et al. Gastric cancer: ESMO-ESSO-ESTRO Clinical Practice Guidelines for diagnosis, treatment and follow-up. Ann Oncol 2013; 24(Suppl 6):vi57–63.
18. Hartgrink HH, van de Velde CJ, Putter H, et al. Extended lymph node dissection for gastric cancer: who may benefit? Final results of the randomized Dutch gastric cancer group trial. J Clin Oncol 2004;22:2069–77.
19. Noguchi Y, Yoshikawa T, Tsuburaya A, et al. Is gastric carcinoma different between Japan and the United States? Cancer 2000;89:2237–46.

20. Sano T, Sasako M, Mizusawa J, et al. Randomized controlled trial to evaluate splenectomy in total gastrectomy for proximal gastric carcinoma. Ann Surg 2016. http://dx.doi.org/10.1097/SLA.0000000000001814.
21. Yu W, Choi GS, Chung HY. Randomized clinical trial of splenectomy versus splenic preservation in patients with proximal gastric cancer. Br J Surg 2006; 93:559–63.
22. Sakuramoto S, Sasako M, Yamaguchi T, et al. Adjuvant chemotherapy for gastric cancer with S-1, an oral fluoropyrimidine. N Engl J Med 2007;357:1810–20.
23. Sasako M, Sakuramoto S, Katai H, et al. Five-year outcomes of a randomized phase III trial comparing adjuvant chemotherapy with S-1 versus surgery alone in stage II or III gastric cancer. J Clin Oncol 2011;29:4387–93.
24. Takahari D, Hamaguchi T, Yoshimura K, et al. Feasibility study of adjuvant chemotherapy with S-1 plus cisplatin for gastric cancer. Cancer Chemother Pharmacol 2010;67:1423–8.
25. Kodera Y, Ishiyama A, Yoshikawa T, et al. A feasibility study of postoperative chemotherapy with S-1 and cisplatin (CDDP) for gastric carcinoma (CCOG0703). Gastric Cancer 2010;13:197–203.
26. Noh SH, Park SR, Yang HK, et al. Adjuvant capecitabine plus oxaliplatin for gastric cancer after D2 gastrectomy (CLASSIC): 5-year follow-up of an open-label, randomised phase 3 trial. Lancet Oncol 2014;15:1389–96.
27. Fuse N, Bando H, Chin K, et al. Adjuvant capecitabine plus oxaliplatin after D2 gastrectomy in Japanese patients with gastric cancer: a phase II study. Gastric Cancer 2016. [Epub ahead of print].
28. Shitara K, Chin K, Yoshikawa T, et al. Phase II study of adjuvant chemotherapy of S-1 plus oxaliplatin for patients with stage III gastric cancer after D2 gastrectomy. Gastric Cancer 2017;20(1):175–81.
29. Macdonald JS, Smalley SR, Benedetti J, et al. Chemoradiotherapy after surgery compared with surgery alone for adenocarcinoma of the stomach or gastro-esophageal junction. N Engl J Med 2001;345(10):725–30.
30. Cunningham D, Allum WH, Stenning SP, et al. Perioperative chemotherapy versus surgery alone for resectable gastroesophageal cancer. N Engl J Med 2006; 355(1):11–20.

The Evaluation and Management of Suspicious Gastric Lesions Following Bariatric Surgery

Guillermo Gomez, MD

KEYWORDS

- Gastric lesions • Barrett metaplasia • Gastroesophageal reflux disease
- Bariatric surgery

KEY POINTS

- Obesity has reached epidemic proportions worldwide and is associated with a higher mortality from several diseases, including adenocarcinoma of the esophagus and of the gastric cardia.
- Increased body mass index is associated with an increased incidence of gastroesophageal reflux disease (GERD), Barrett metaplasia (BE), and adenocarcinoma of the cardia.
- Bariatric surgery remains the most effective treatment of morbid obesity and has the potential to improve weight-related GERD.
- Currently, there are no separate practice guidelines for the diagnosis and management of BE disease in the obese; similarly, bariatric surgery may have the potential to reduce the incidence of obesity-related adenocarcinoma of the foregut.
- Consideration should be given to the bariatric technique in the presence of pathologic GERD, BE, or intestinal metaplasia, especially when other risk factors for adenocarcinoma of the esophagus or stomach are present.

INTRODUCTION

Obesity has reached epidemic proportions worldwide and is associated with a higher mortality from several diseases, including cancer.[1] The prevalence of obesity (body mass index [BMI] $\geq$30 kg/m^2) in the United States exceeds 30% in most age groups.[2] A recent pooled analysis reported a 6% prevalence for class III obesity (BMI $\geq$40 kg/m^2) in the United States.[3] Among these patients, heart disease, diabetes, and cancer contributed the greatest to increased mortality. This increased mortality was associated with an elevation in BMI in a dose-dependent manner, translating into a net loss of life between 6.7 to 13.7 years as BMI increased from 40 kg/m^2 to 59 kg/m^2.

General Surgery, The University of Texas Medical Branch, Galveston, TX, USA
E-mail address: ggomez@utmb.edu

Surg Clin N Am 97 (2017) 467–474
http://dx.doi.org/10.1016/j.suc.2016.12.003
0039-6109/17/© 2016 Elsevier Inc. All rights reserved.

surgical.theclinics.com

Above a BMI of 50 kg/m^2, the loss of life expectancy exceeded that observed from to-bacco smoking. Furthermore, a special report predicted a potential decline in life ex-pectancy due to obesity in the twenty-first century.[4]

Bariatric surgery has evolved into the most effective treatment modality for adequate and durable weight loss when compared with traditional noninvasive ther-apy (including diet, exercise, behavior modification, and pharmacotherapy).[5] Bariatric surgery effectively ameliorates obesity-related comorbidities with low morbidity and very low mortality.[6] Studies have also shown that bariatric surgery is associated with improved overall and cause-specific mortality for cancer.[7–10] Given that the num-ber of patients presenting at risk for foregut neoplasia in the setting of obesity is ex-pected to increase, it is important for the general surgeon to understand the relationship between obesity and foregut neoplasia and to be cognizant to ensure early diagnosis of lesions.

OBESITY, BARIATRIC SURGERY, AND ESOPHAGEAL NEOPLASIA

Increased BMI is strongly associated with the development of esophageal adenocar-cinoma (EAC) in both men and women.[11] In contrast, the incidence of squamous cell carcinoma does not increase with obesity.[11]

The pathway to the development of EAC is well recognized, starting with pathologic gastroesophageal reflux disease (GERD), causing chronic esophagitis, resulting in Barrett metaplasia (BE), which eventually progresses into dysplasia and carcinoma. Increased BMI, particularly from central obesity, is associated with an increased inci-dence of GERD and BE.[12,13] Furthermore, being overweight was found to be an inde-pendent predictor for progression from BE to EAC.[14–16] As bariatric surgery is the treatment of choice for antireflux surgery in the morbidly obese, special attention should be given to investigate the effect of bariatric procedures on GERD and BE.

The cause of increased GERD incidence in obesity is multifactorial.[17] Among impor-tant etiologic factors mentioned include increased intra-abdominal pressure (direct correlation with BMI and waist circumference), increased prevalence of defective lower esophageal sphincter, increased frequency of transient lower sphincter relaxa-tion (direct correlation with BMI and waist circumference), altered esophageal motility, higher prevalence of hiatal hernia, and delayed gastric emptying (eg, gastroparesis). Overall, all bariatric procedures have the potential to improve GERD symptoms, an ef-fect that is related to the amount of weight loss.[18] However, Roux-en-Y gastric bypass (RNYGB) has shown a superior therapeutic effect for GERD resolution when compared with restrictive operations, including gastric band and sleeve gastrec-tomy.[18,19] Importantly, RNYGB has shown the ability to induce regression of BE in the obese in terms of decreased length of BE, improvement in the degree of dysplasia, and reconstitution of cardiac mucosa.[20–22] In this regard, RNYGB reproduced the re-sults given by antireflux surgery encompassing acid suppression along with aversion of biliopancreatic duodenal refluxate from the esophagus.[23] A recent literature review by an expert panel concluded that RNYGB is the best treatment option for morbid obesity complicated with Barrett esophagus.[24,25]

The diagnosis and management of BE should follow current practice guidelines rec-ommended by professional societies.[26,27] Endoscopic screening for BE in unselected (ie, without risk factors for BE) patients with GERD symptoms is not supported at the present time. Obesity, however, represents a major risk factor for BE. In the presence of other risk factors such as chronic (>5 years) GERD symptoms, age greater than 50 years, history of smoking, and family history of BE or EAC, endoscopic screening for BE is indicated. If the finding of BE will alter surgical decision making, BE screening is indicated. Equally important, as many centers perform routine preoperative upper endoscopic examination for reasons other than BE screening, this can also be an incidental finding that must be addressed.[28]

BE can develop several years after bariatric procedures. BE has been reported after gastric band[29] and sleeve gastrectomy.[30] The real incidence of BE after bariatric surgery is not known, and it may be procedure specific. Currently, there are no separate practice guidelines available for BE after bariatric surgery.

When BE is diagnosed, the patient should be treated according to current practice guidelines at a minimum.[26,27] For BE without dysplasia, endoscopic surveillance should be performed at 3- to 5-year intervals. Yearly surveillance for nondysplastic BE is not supported. For BE with indefinite dysplasia, a repeat endoscopy should take place after 3 to 6 months of acid suppressive therapy. Options for BE with low-grade dysplasia include endoscopic therapy or surveillance every 12 months. BE with confirmed high-grade dysplasia should receive endoscopic therapy. Most importantly, BE with dysplasia should be referred to specialized centers. In addition, in bariatric patients with BE, a consideration should be given to a bariatric technique capable of preventing progression to EAC (namely RNYGB as either primary or revisional bariatric technique). However, BE formation and progression to EAC have also been reported to occur late (14 and 21 years) after RNYGB.[31]

EAC has developed at different intervals (a few months to several years) after various bariatric procedures, including gastric bypass, gastric band, jejunoileal bypass, vertical banded gastroplasty, and sleeve gastrectomy.[31–35] The real incidence of EAC after bariatric surgery is not known. Once EAC is diagnosed, patients are treated according to the cancer type and stage.

At this point, data regarding the association between bariatric surgery, BE, and EAC are still immature due to the retrospective nature, relatively small sample size, and short follow-up for most of the studies. Therefore, clinical discretion using current understanding of pathogenic factors is necessary to individualize screening and surveillance of BE and EAC after bariatric surgery.

OBESITY, BARIATRIC SURGERY, AND GASTRIC NEOPLASIA

There is heterogeneity in the epidemiology of gastric cancer. The overall incidence and mortality from gastric cancer have declined over the past 30 years.[36] However, the incidence of cancer of the gastric cardia has been increasing on par with the obesity epidemic, reminiscent of the increased incidence of BE and EAC. Recent cohort and meta-analysis studies[37,38] revealed an increased risk of gastric cardia cancer with increasing BMI (relative risk 1.4 in BMI 25–30, and 2.06 in BMI > 30). Higher socioeconomic status is also associated with gastric cardia cancers (as it is with EAC). However, no increased risk for noncardia gastric cancer has been found with obesity nor with *Helicobacter pylori*. In contrast, *H pylori* infection is the main etiologic factor for noncardia gastric cancer. Tobacco smoking shows a significant association with cardia as well as noncardia gastric cancer. Obesity and tobacco smoking may synergize in the risk for gastric cancer,[6] and therefore, comprehensive interventions in gastric cancer are to address both environmental risk factors, that is obesity and tobacco smoking. In the absence of established algorithms for gastric neoplasia and obesity, current epidemiology should help to tailor the screening and surveillance of specific populations at risk.

Bariatric surgeons have attempted to determine the impact of bariatric surgery on gastric cancer. Interestingly, preliminary observations suggest that some bariatric operations may exert a protective effect. An analysis of the Utah Cancer Registry showed that gastric bypass resulted in a significant 46% reduction in mortality from obesity-related cancers (including EAC) after a mean follow-up of 12.5 years.[39] Another descriptive study using all reported cases of gastric neoplasia following gastric bypass surgery found an incidence of gastric cancer that was significantly lower than expected when compared with a population of obese individuals without gastric bypass.[40] Furthermore, in an experimental model of chemically induced gastric cancer in rats, gastric bypass resulted in a 4-fold reduction in the development of gastric cancer.[41] It is reassuring to find that bariatric surgery has not been threatened by increased gastric cancer formation. To the contrary, understanding of risks factors and pathophysiology for esophagogastric cancer can be used in planning for bariatric surgery.

GASTRIC NEOPLASIA AFTER BARIATRIC SURGERY

Neoplasia of the esophagus and stomach has been reported following nearly all types of bariatric operations (eg, gastric banding, vertical banded gastroplasty, sleeve gastrectomy, gastric bypass), and at different intervals following bariatric surgery. Although most of reported tumors are adenocarcinomas, other entities have been described such as carcinoid, lymphoma, and gastrointestinal stromal tumors.[42] Neoplasia can develop in the esophagus or esophagogastric junction,[32,43] gastric pouch,[44] or gastric remnant.[45,46] The diagnostic workup is triggered by symptoms and is conducted by established endoscopic, imaging, and surgical techniques. The first challenge for early diagnosis is the recognition of new symptoms, because bariatric surgery and eating behaviors can cause the same complaints as foregut neoplasia. A higher index of suspicion is recommended particularly for patients at risk for esophageal or gastric cancer. For example, geographic areas endemic for cancer, the presence of BE or intestinal metaplasia, tobacco smoking, or a personal or family history for gastrointestinal malignancy should all signal the need for heightened awareness. Postoperative surveillance can be facilitated by thoughtful preoperative planning. For example, expert centers would recommended avoiding sleeve gastrectomy in favor of gastric bypass in BE disease.[24] In cases of known gastric intestinal metaplasia, gastric mucosa at risk should not be left unattended from endoscopic surveillance, and resection of the gastric remnant is recommended if gastric bypass is to be performed given the difficulty in accessing this later due to anatomic constraints.[47,48]

EXAMINATION OF GASTRIC REMNANT AFTER ROUX-EN-Y GASTRIC BYPASS

Evaluation for neoplastic processes after bariatric surgery is indicated for symptoms, such as abdominal pain, nausea, vomiting, exaggerated weight loss, hematochezia, melena, iron deficiency anemia, particularly when symptoms develop years after an uneventful index operation and when symptoms do not improve following diet and behavior modification. The indication for evaluation for cancer grows stronger in the presence of risk factors such as tobacco smoking and patients who live in endemic areas for cancer.

The presence of the Roux-en-Y configuration presents a barrier for endoscopic assessment of the remnant stomach, and different approaches have been described. The workup depends largely upon the local expertise and resources available.

Endoscopic examination is paramount and usually represents the first step in the workup because there is need for direct mucosal examination and tissue diagnosis. Endoscopic examination can be accomplished by retrograde duodenogastroscopy following the biliopancreatic limb.[49] Using conventional endoscopic techniques (push enteroscopy), retrograde duodenogastroscopy fails in over one-third of the patients. Technical advances in endoscopy have provided new avenues for retrograde duodenogastroscopy. One technique is the double balloon enteroscopy.[50,51] Another technical advancement is due to the shape-locking technology (overtube guide through which a standard endoscope is advanced).[52] Unfortunately, despite these endoscopic advances, a significant number of patients (10%–20%) cannot complete retrograde endoscopy due to difficult anatomy (eg, narrow anastomosis). Furthermore, capability for advanced enteroscopy may not be readily available.

A hybrid approach using both laparoscopy and endoscopy can be used to reach the gastric remnant. Laparoscopic-assisted transgastric endoscopy uses conventional laparoscopic techniques to localize the gastric remnant. A small gastrostomy is made in the gastric remnant and then a trocar is placed directly into the remnant, through which a conventional flexible endoscope can be used.[53] Subsequently, the gastrotomy is either closed or converted to a tube gastrostomy according to clinical needs. Laparoscopy is also used for tissue sampling and clinical staging as pertinent.

Image-guided percutaneous gastrostomy tube placement is another approach to access the excluded stomach remnant for endoscopic examination. Using ultrasound, fluoroscopy, or computed tomography (CT) guidance, a gastrostomy catheter is placed; later, the gastrostomy channel is dilated to accommodate a small-diameter flexible endoscope.[54]

Virtual gastroduodenoscopy using 3-dimensional CT has been investigated as a new technique for minimally or noninvasive examination of the gastric remnant. In one version of the technique, air or saline is injected via CT-guided percutaneous puncture to obtain distension of the gastric remnant.[55] Another version of virtual CT gastroduodenoscopy uses retrograde reflux of gas produced by swallowed effervescent granules to obtain gastric distension.[56,57] These imaging modalities do not allow for tissue sampling, and their role in diagnosis of premalignant lesions or early gastric cancer has not been established.

SUMMARY

Obesity has reached epidemic proportions worldwide and is associated with a higher mortality from several diseases, including adenocarcinoma of the esophagus and of the gastric cardia. Increased BMI is associated with an increased incidence of GERD, BE, and adenocarcinoma of the cardia. Bariatric surgery remains the most effective treatment of morbid obesity and has the potential to improve weight-related GERD. Currently, there are no separate practice guidelines for the diagnosis and management of BE disease in the obese. Similarly, bariatric surgery may have the potential to reduce the incidence of obesity-related adenocarcinoma of the foregut. However, consideration should be given to the bariatric technique in the presence of pathologic GERD, BE, or intestinal metaplasia, especially when other risk factors for adenocarcinoma of the esophagus or stomach are present. A high index of suspicion is paramount for early detection of foregut neoplasia after bariatric surgery.

REFERENCES

1. Whitlock G, Lewington S, Sherliker P, et al. Body-mass index and cause-specific mortality in 900 000 adults: collaborative analyses of 57 prospective studies. Lancet 2009;373:1083–96.

2. Flegal KM, Carroll MD, Ogden CL, et al. Prevalence and trends in obesity among US adults, 1999-2008. JAMA 2010;303:235–41.

3. Kitahara CM, Flint AJ, Berrington de Gonzalez A, et al. Association between class III obesity (BMI of 40-59 kg/m2) and mortality: a pooled analysis of 20 prospective studies. PLoS Med 2014;11:e1001673.

4. Olshansky SJ, Passaro DJ, Hershow RC, et al. A potential decline in life expectancy in the United States in the 21st century. N Engl J Med 2005;352:1138–45.

5. Wolfe BM, Morton JM. Weighing in on bariatric surgery: procedure use, readmission rates, and mortality. JAMA 2005;294:1960–3.

6. Chang SH, Stoll CR, Song J, et al. The effectiveness and risks of bariatric surgery: an updated systematic review and meta-analysis, 2003-2012. JAMA Surg 2014; 149:275–87.

7. Sjostrom L, Narbro K, Sjostrom CD, et al. Effects of bariatric surgery on mortality in Swedish obese subjects. N Engl J Med 2007;357:741–52.

8. Adams TD, Gress RE, Smith SC, et al. Long-term mortality after gastric bypass surgery. N Engl J Med 2007;357:753–61.

9. Casagrande DS, Rosa DD, Umpierre D, et al. Incidence of cancer following bariatric surgery: systematic review and meta-analysis. Obes Surg 2014;24: 1499–509.

10. Funk LM, Jolles S, Fischer LE, et al. Patient and referring practitioner characteristics associated with the likelihood of undergoing bariatric surgery: a systematic review. JAMA Surg 2015;150:999–1005.

11. Renehan AG, Tyson M, Egger M, et al. Body-mass index and incidence of cancer: a systematic review and meta-analysis of prospective observational studies. Lancet 2008;371:569–78.

12. Kendall BJ, Macdonald GA, Hayward NK, et al. The risk of Barrett's esophagus associated with abdominal obesity in males and females. Int J Cancer 2013; 132:2192–9.

13. Navab F, Nathanson BH, Desilets DJ. The impact of lifestyle on Barrett's esophagus: a precursor to esophageal adenocarcinoma. Cancer Epidemiol 2015;39: 885–91.

14. Krishnamoorthi R, Borah B, Heien H, et al. Rates and predictors of progression to esophageal carcinoma in a large population-based Barrett's esophagus cohort. Gastrointest Endosc 2016;84:40–6.e7.

15. Oberg S, Wenner J, Johansson J, et al. Barrett esophagus: risk factors for progression to dysplasia and adenocarcinoma. Ann Surg 2005;242:49–54.

16. Csendes A, Burdiles P, Braghetto I, et al. Dysplasia and adenocarcinoma after classic antireflux surgery in patients with Barrett's esophagus: the need for long-term subjective and objective follow-up. Ann Surg 2002;235:178–85.

17. Nadaleto BF, Herbella FA, Patti MG. Gastroesophageal reflux disease in the obese: pathophysiology and treatment. Surgery 2016;159:475–86.

18. Pallati PK, Shaligram A, Shostrom VK, et al. Improvement in gastroesophageal reflux disease symptoms after various bariatric procedures: review of the Bariatric Outcomes Longitudinal Database. Surg Obes Relat Dis 2014;10:502–7.

19. Li J, Lai D, Wu D. Laparoscopic Roux-en-Y gastric bypass versus laparoscopic sleeve gastrectomy to treat morbid obesity-related comorbidities: a systematic review and meta-analysis. Obes Surg 2016;26:429–42.

20. Houghton SG, Romero Y, Sarr MG. Effect of Roux-en-Y gastric bypass in obese patients with Barrett's esophagus: attempts to eliminate duodenogastric reflux. Surg Obes Relat Dis 2008;4:1–4.

21. Csendes A, Burgos AM, Smok G, et al. Effect of gastric bypass on Barrett's esophagus and intestinal metaplasia of the cardia in patients with morbid obesity. J Gastrointest Surg 2006;10:259–64.

22. Cobey F, Oelschlager B. Complete regression of Barrett's esophagus after Roux-en-Y gastric bypass. Obes Surg 2005;15:710–2.
23. Csendes A, Bragheto I, Burdiles P, et al. Regression of intestinal metaplasia to cardiac or fundic mucosa in patients with Barrett's esophagus submitted to vagotomy, partial gastrectomy and duodenal diversion. A prospective study of 78 patients with more than 5 years of follow up. Surgery 2006;139:46–53.
24. Braghetto I, Csendes A. Patients having bariatric surgery: surgical options in morbidly obese patients with Barrett's esophagus. Obes Surg 2016;26:1622–6.
25. Gagner M. Is sleeve gastrectomy always an absolute contraindication in patients with Barrett's? Obes Surg 2016;26:715–7.
26. Shaheen NJ, Falk GW, Iyer PG, et al, American College of Gastroenterology. ACG clinical guideline: diagnosis and management of Barrett's esophagus. Am J Gastroenterol 2016;111:30–50.
27. Fitzgerald RC, di Pietro M, Ragunath K, et al. British Society of Gastroenterology guidelines on the diagnosis and management of Barrett's oesophagus. Gut 2014; 63:7–42.
28. Munoz R, Ibanez L, Salinas J, et al. Importance of routine preoperative upper GI endoscopy: why all patients should be evaluated? Obes Surg 2009;19:427–31.
29. Braghetto I, Csendes A. Prevalence of Barrett's esophagus in bariatric patients undergoing sleeve gastrectomy. Obes Surg 2016;26:710–4.
30. Varela JE. Barrett's esophagus: a late complication of laparoscopic adjustable gastric banding. Obes Surg 2010;20:244–6.
31. Allen JW, Leeman MF, Richardson JD. Esophageal carcinoma following bariatric procedures. JSLS 2004;8:372–5.
32. Melstrom LG, Bentrem DJ, Salvino MJ, et al. Adenocarcinoma of the gastro-esophageal junction after bariatric surgery. Am J Surg 2008;196:135–8.
33. Korswagen LA, Schrama JG, Bruins Slot W, et al. Adenocarcinoma of the lower esophagus after placement of a gastric band. Obes Surg 2009;19:389–92.
34. Stauffer JA, Mathew J, Odell JA. Esophageal adenocarcinoma after laparoscopic gastric band placement for obesity. Dis Esophagus 2011;24:E8–10.
35. Scheepers AF, Schoon EJ, Nienhuijs SW. Esophageal carcinoma after sleeve gastrectomy. Surg Obes Relat Dis 2011;7:e11–2.
36. de Martel C, Forman D, Plummer M. Gastric cancer: epidemiology and risk factors. Gastroenterol Clin North Am 2013;42:219–40.
37. Yang P, Zhou Y, Chen B, et al. Overweight, obesity and gastric cancer risk: results from a meta-analysis of cohort studies. Eur J Cancer 2009;45:2867–73.
38. Cho Y, Lee DH, Oh HS, et al. Higher prevalence of obesity in gastric cardia adenocarcinoma compared to gastric non-cardia adenocarcinoma. Dig Dis Sci 2012;57:2687–92.
39. Adams TD, Stroup AM, Gress RE, et al. Cancer incidence and mortality after gastric bypass surgery. Obesity (Silver Spring) 2009;17:796–802.
40. Menendez P, Padilla D, Villarejo P, et al. Does bariatric surgery decrease gastric cancer risk? Hepatogastroenterology 2012;59:409–12.
41. Inoue H, Rubino F, Shimada Y, et al. Risk of gastric cancer after Roux-en-Y gastric bypass. Arch Surg 2007;142:947–53.
42. Raghavendra RS, Kini D. Benign, premalignant, and malignant lesions encountered in bariatric surgery. JSLS 2012;16:360–72.
43. Trincado MT, del Olmo JC, Garcia Castano J, et al. Gastric pouch carcinoma after gastric bypass for morbid obesity. Obes Surg 2005;15:1215–7.
44. Babor R, Booth M. Adenocarcinoma of the gastric pouch 26 years after loop gastric bypass. Obes Surg 2006;16:935–8.

45. Escalona A, Guzman S, Ibanez L, et al. Gastric cancer after Roux-en-Y gastric bypass. Obes Surg 2005;15:423–7.
46. Magge D, Holtzman MP. Gastric adenocarcinoma in patients with Roux-en-Y gastric bypass: a case series. Surg Obes Relat Dis 2015;11:e35–8.
47. Voellinger DC, Inabnet WB. Laparoscopic Roux-en-Y gastric bypass with remnant gastrectomy for focal intestinal metaplasia of the gastric antrum. Obes Surg 2002;12:695–8.
48. Csendes A, Burdiles P, Papapietro K, et al. Results of gastric bypass plus resection of the distal excluded gastric segment in patients with morbid obesity. J Gastrointest Surg 2005;9:121–31.
49. Flickinger EG, Sinar DR, Pories WJ, et al. The bypassed stomach. Am J Surg 1985;149:151–6.
50. Sakai P, Kuga R, Safatle-Ribeiro AV, et al. Is it feasible to reach the bypassed stomach after Roux-en-Y gastric bypass for morbid obesity? The use of the double-balloon enteroscope. Endoscopy 2005;37:566–9.
51. Ross AS, Semrad C, Alverdy J, et al. Use of double-balloon enteroscopy to perform PEG in the excluded stomach after Roux-en-Y gastric bypass. Gastrointest Endosc 2006;64:797–800.
52. Pai RD, Carr-Locke DL, Thompson CC. Endoscopic evaluation of the defunctionalized stomach by using ShapeLock technology (with video). Gastrointest Endosc 2007;66:578–81.
53. Gill KR, McKinney JM, Stark ME, et al. Investigation of the excluded stomach after Roux-en-Y gastric bypass: the role of percutaneous endoscopy. World J Gastroenterol 2008;14:1946–8.
54. Roberts KE, Panait L, Duffy AJ, et al. Laparoscopic-assisted transgastric endoscopy: current indications and future implications. JSLS 2008;12:30–6.
55. Sundbom M, Nyman R, Hedenstrom H, et al. Investigation of the excluded stomach after Roux-en-Y gastric bypass. Obes Surg 2001;11:25–7.
56. Silecchia G, Catalano C, Gentileschi P, et al. Virtual gastroduodenoscopy: a new look at the bypassed stomach and duodenum after laparoscopic Roux-en-Y gastric bypass for morbid obesity. Obes Surg 2002;12:39–48.
57. Alva S, Eisenberg D, Duffy A, et al. A new modality to evaluate the gastric remnant after Roux-en-Y gastric bypass. Surg Obes Relat Dis 2008;4:46–9.

Index

Note: Page numbers of article titles are in **boldface** type.

Surg Clin N Am 97 (2017) 475–485
http://dx.doi.org/10.1016/S0039-6109(17)30024-5
0039-6109/17

surgical.theclinics.com

Moving?

Make sure your subscription moves with you!

To notify us of your new address, find your **Clinics Account Number** (located on your mailing label above your name), and contact customer service at:

Email: journalscustomerservice-usa@elsevier.com

800-654-2452 (subscribers in the U.S. & Canada)
314-447-8871 (subscribers outside of the U.S. & Canada)

Fax number: 314-447-8029

**Elsevier Health Sciences Division
Subscription Customer Service
3251 Riverport Lane
Maryland Heights, MO 63043**

*To ensure uninterrupted delivery of your subscription, please notify us at least 4 weeks in advance of move.

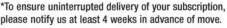

Printed and bound by CPI Group (UK) Ltd, Croydon, CR0 4YY

07/10/2024

01040502-0008